Optimizing Exercise and Physical Activity in Older People

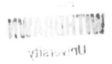

For Butterworth Heinemann:

Senior Commissioning Editor: Heidi Allen
Associate Editor: Robert Edwards
Project Manager: Samantha Ross
Designer: George Ajayi
Illustration Manager: Bruce Hogarth

Optimizing Exercise and Physical Activity in Older People

Edited by

Meg E Morris

PhD, MAppSc, BAppSc, GradDip(Gerontol), MAPA, FACP

Adrian M M Schoo

PhysioD, MH1thSc, GradDipMT/Acup/Manag/Ed, DipPT

BUTTERWORTH
HEINEMANN

EDINBURGH LONDON NEW YORK OXFORD PHILADELPHIA ST LOUIS SYDNEY TORONTO 2004

BUTTERWORTH-HEINEMANN
An imprint of Elsevier Science Limited

First published 2004

ISBN 0 7506 5479 1

British Library Cataloguing in Publication Data
A catalogue record for this book is available from the British Library

Library of Congress Cataloging in Publication Data
A catalog record for this book is available from the Library of Congress

Notice
Medical knowledge is constantly changing. Standard safety precautions must be followed, but as new research and clinical experience broaden our knowledge, changes in treatment and drug therapy may become necessary or appropriate. Readers are advised to check the most current product information provided by the manufacturer of each drug to be administered to verify the recommended dose, the method and duration of administration, and contraindications. It is the responsibility of the practitioner, relying on experience and knowledge of the patient, to determine dosages and the best treatment for each individual patient. Neither the Publisher nor the editors assume any liability for any injury and/or damage to persons or property arising from this publication.

The Publisher

ELSEVIER
SCIENCE

your source for books,
journals and multimedia
in the health sciences

www.elsevierhealth.com

The
publisher's
policy is to use
**paper manufactured
from sustainable forests**

Printed in China

Contents

Contributors   vii

Introduction   ix

1 Health benefits of physical activity for older adults – epidemiological approaches to the evidence   1

Adrian Bauman

2 Grandmothers on the move: benefits, barriers and best practice interventions for physical activity in older women   26

Wendy J Brown and Christina Lee

3 Assisting health professionals to promote physical activity and exercise in older people   38

Colette Browning, David Menzies and Shane Thomas

4 Physical activity and health in an ageing workforce   63

John Carlson and Geraldine Naughton

5 Biomechanical and neuromuscular considerations in the maintenance of an active lifestyle   76

Bruce Elliott, David Lloyd and Tim Ackland

6 Reducing the risk of osteoporosis: the role of exercise and diet   99

Shona L Bass, Caryl Nowson and Robin M Daly

7 Strength training for older people   125

Karen J Dodd, Nicholas F Taylor and Scott Bradley

8 Declining muscle function in older people – repairing the deficits with exercise   158

Dennis R Taaffe

9 Therapeutic exercise guidelines for the rehabilitation of older people following fracture 187

Nicholas F Taylor and Tania Pizzari

10 Physical activity and exercise in people with osteoarthritis 213

Adrian M M Schoo and Meg E Morris

11 Common foot problems that can impair performance of regular physical activity and exercise in older people: prevention and treatment 229

Hylton B Menz

12 Physical activity and falls prevention 247

Keith Hill and Kate Murray

13 Effects of dual task interference on postural control, movement and physical activity in healthy older people and those with movement disorders 267

Sandra G Brauer and Meg E Morris

14 Precautions and contraindications for exercise in elderly people with cardiorespiratory or musculoskeletal conditions 288

Helen McBurney and Jill Cook

15 Exercise training for older people with type 2 diabetes 303

Scott Bradley

Appendix: WHO classifications for overweight and obesity 328

Index 329

Contributors

Tim Ackland PhD, MPE, BPE(Hons)
Associate Professor, School of Human Movement and Exercise Science, University of Western Australia, Crawley, Perth, Australia

Shona L Bass PhD, MSc, BAppSc
Senior Research Fellow, Centre for Physical Activity and Nutrition, Deakin University, Victoria, Australia

Adrian Bauman PhD, FAFPHM
Professor, School of Public Health, University of New South Wales, Sydney, Australia

Scott Bradley PhD, BSc(Hons), BAppSc(Physio), GradDipExercSportsSci
Lecturer, School of Physiotherapy, La Trobe University, Victoria, Australia

Sandra G Brauer PhD, BPhty(Hons)
Conjoint Lecturer, Department of Physiotherapy, Princess Alexandra Hospital and University of Queensland, St Lucia, Australia

Wendy J Brown PhD, MSc, BSc(Hons)
Professor, School of Human Movement Studies, University of Queensland, St Lucia, Australia

Colette Browning PhD, MSc, BSc(Hons)
Associate Professor, School of Public Health, La Trobe University, Victoria, Australia

John Carlson PhD, MSc, BSc
Professor, Centre for Rehabilitation, Exercise and Sport Science, Victoria University, Melbourne, Australia

Jill Cook PhD, PostGradDipManipTher, BAppSc(Phty)
School of Physiotherapy, La Trobe University, Victoria, Australia

Robin M Daly PhD, BAppSc
Research Fellow, Centre for Physical Activity and Nutrition, Burwood, Victoria, Australia

Karen J Dodd PhD, BAppSc(Physio)
Senior Lecturer, School of Physiotherapy, La Trobe University, Victoria, Australia

Bruce Elliott PhD, MEd, BEd
Professor, School of Human Movement and Exercise Science, University of Western Australia, Crawley, WA, Australia

Keith Hill PhD, BAppSc(Physio), GradDip(Physio)
Senior Research Fellow, National Ageing Research Institute, Melbourne, Victoria, Australia

Christina Lee PhD, BA
Director, Research Centre for Gender and Health, University of Newcastle, Newcastle, Australia

David Lloyd PhD, BSc(MechEng)
Senior Lecturer – Biomechanics Group, School of Human Movement and Exercise Science, University of Western Australia, Crawley, Australia

Helen McBurney PhD
School of Physiotherapy, La Trobe University, Victoria, Australia

Hylton B Menz PhD, BAppSc(Pod)Hons
Falls and Balance Research Group, Prince of Wales Medical Research Institute, Australia

David Menzies GradDipEx, RehabBEd, PhysEd
School of Public Health, La Trobe University, Victoria, Australia

Meg E Morris PhD, MAppSc, BAppSc, GradDip(Gerontol), MAPA, FACP
Professor and Head of School of Physiotherapy, La Trobe University, Victoria, Australia

Kate Murray MSc(Neurology), BAppSc(Physio)
Research Officer, Division of Public Health, National Ageing Research Institute, Melbourne, Victoria, Australia

Geraldine Naughton PhD, MAppSc, BAppSc(Dist), BEd
Associate Professor, Children's Hospital Institute of Sports Medicine, The Children's Hospital, Westmead, Australia

Caryl Nowson PhD, BSc, DipNutrDiet, DipEd, DipEval
Associate Professor, Centre for Physical Activity and Nutrition, Deakin University, Burwood, Victoria, Australia

Tania Pizzari PhD, BPhysio(Hons)
School of Physiotherapy, La Trobe University, Victoria, Australia

Adrian M M Schoo PhysioD, MH1thSc, GradDipMT/Acup/Manag/Ed, DipPT
Clinical Education, Research and Practice, ProActive Health, Bendigo, Victoria, Australia

Dennis R Taaffe PhD, MSc, BSc, DipTeach
School of Human Movement Studies, University of Queensland, St Lucia, Australia

Nicholas F Taylor PhD, BSc, BAppSc(Physio)
School of Physiotherapy, La Trobe University, Victoria, Australia

Shane Thomas PhD, BA, DipPubPol, MAPS
Professor and Director of Research, Australian Institute for Primary Care, La Trobe University, Victoria, Australia

Introduction

Physical activity, exercise and health: the growing needs of an ageing population

One of the biggest challenges that faces healthcare professionals and policy makers in the 21st century is how to enable older people to adopt lifestyle choices that promote physical activity and regular exercise, in order to enhance health, well-being and participation in society. Older people themselves are also becoming increasingly aware that regular physical activity can improve health outcomes, although uncertainty exists regarding which activities are most beneficial for people who are healthy, frail or disabled. Healthcare professionals and policy makers need access to up-to-date information on the evidence for the outcomes of different population-based health promotion strategies, therapeutic exercise programmes and physical activities, to guide them in designing and implementing the most effective interventions.

It is now well established that health-related problems increase with both age and inactivity (Mathers et al 1999, US Department of Health and Human Services 1996, World Health Organization 1996). With the rapid population-ageing that is currently occurring throughout industrialized nations, the number of elders seeking information, advice, support or treatment in order to regain, maintain or improve their physical abilities will rapidly increase. Compared with young adults, people over the age of 65 years have a high incidence of chronic conditions such as osteoarthritis, diabetes, depression, stroke and Parkinson's disease (WHO 1996). More than 85% of individuals aged 65–100 years have at least one chronic condition and the number continues to increase with advancing age (Hoffman et al 1996, Rice et al 1996). Evidence is accumulating that the onset, rate of progression and severity of many diseases in older people can be prevented, minimized or delayed with the provision of effective health promotion programmes, therapeutic exercises or physical activities (Australian Institute of Health and Welfare 1996, Harvey 1991, Nutbeam et al 1993).

Older people not only have higher levels of disability than the population as a whole: they are heavy users of healthcare services (Hoffman et al 1996, Hopman-Rock et al 1997). Healthcare costs in the aged-care sector are therefore expected to increase dramatically over the next 50 years. A key question is whether programmes are best aimed at individuals, environments or communities (Baum 1998). Methods of influencing behaviour include the use of government legislative and regulatory policies to promote higher levels of physical activity, tax incentives for activities such as riding a bicycle to work, and encouragement to walk regularly and take the stairs instead of elevators (King 1994), and involvement in community-based or home exercise programmes.

The type of exercise or physical activity that is most beneficial varies according to the person's health status, age, gender and values. Although aerobic exercises can enable some older individuals to achieve health benefits (Fisher and Pendergast 1994, Ries et al 1996, 1997, Sashika et al 1996), vigorous physical activity is not always necessary to acquire or maintain optimal health and well-being (US Department of Health and Human Services 1996). Weight-bearing activities, progressive resistance exercises and regular sustained performance of routine daily activities such as walking, stair-climbing, gardening and home duties can improve health, regardless of age (Andersen et al 1999, Blair et al 1995, Dunn et al 1999, Rantanen et al 1997). Several short exercise sessions throughout the day can have a cumulative effect (Paffenberg et al 1994), although at least 30 minutes of moderate-intensity physical activity on all days (minimum of 5 days per week) has been recommended (Commonwealth Department of Health and Aged Care 1999, US Department of Health and Human Services 1996).

Inactivity is a key obstacle to the health of older people (Bassett and Howley 1998). Inactivity can be associated with deconditioning, weight gain (Bar-Or et al 1998), osteoarthritis in later life (Cicuttini et al 1996, Felson and Chaisson 1997, Felson et al 1997), depression (Gabriel et al 1997, Hopman-Rock et al 1997) and cardiovascular disease (Philbin et al 1996, Ries et al 1997). Prolonged periods of inactivity and a sedentary lifestyle can also predispose some older individuals to osteopenia and sarcopenia, which in turn can contribute to disability (Åstrand 1992, Bassett and Howley 1998). There are several reasons for reduced physical activity in older people. These include misconceptions about the ability to exercise in the presence of disability, lack of time and lack of confidence (Smith et al 1999). A seasonal reduction in physical activity has also been reported, particularly in winter (Bank et al 1997, Uitenbroek 1993). Cars and other forms of motorized transport now compete with walking or riding a bicycle as a means of transport. Sedentary leisure activities such as watching television and computer use have recently increased in older people (McGinnis 1995). Other factors related to inactivity include the presence of multiple disabling conditions, very advanced age and lack of knowledge on the benefits and need to exercise.

The negative effects of inactivity can be reduced or sometimes even reversed by the adoption of exercise, even after long periods of inactivity (Convertino et al 1997). Clinical studies and epidemiological research have suggested that physical activity can sometimes counteract the development and progression of chronic conditions such as obesity, cardiovascular disease, hypertension, type 2 diabetes, colon cancer, depression, muscle and joint disorders and osteoporosis (Lopez and Murray 1996, Victorian Department of Human Services 2000). The risk of falls in older people might also be reduced by regular physical activity and exercise (Shumway Cook et al 1997, Wolf et al 1996, Wolfson et al

1996). As shown by Dodd et al (Chapter 7 in this volume), progressive resistance strength training is a particularly effective method for reducing muscle weakness, as well as for increasing mobility and well-being.

One of the challenges with the introduction and maintenance of physical activity and exercise in older people is optimizing adherence. Motivating individuals and developing an infrastructure that supports lifelong participation in physical activity are key factors that influence exercise adherence over the long-term (Smith et al 1999). Potential obstacles to exercise adherence in very old people can include reduced comprehension and processing of complex information, reading difficulties and memory loss (Smith et al 1998, Whiting and Smith 1997). Some older people require specific methods of exercise instruction due to poor vision or hearing loss (Keller et al 1999), literacy problems (Weiss et al 1995) or difficulty accessing and using audiovisual technology (Steinberg et al 1998). Exercises need to be specific to individual needs and performed correctly, consistently and with an appropriate intensity to achieve beneficial outcomes. Instructions should therefore be specific, clear and accessible to optimize exercise outcomes, whether they be provided verbally (Friedrich et al 1996), by illustrated handouts (Delp and Jones 1996, Jackson 1994, Schneiders et al 1997), audiotapes (Terpstra et al 1992), videotapes (Brubaker et al 1998, Jette et al 1998, 1999) or interactive computer/web-based systems (Minor et al 1998).

The aim of this book is to provide healthcare professionals, policy makers, administrators and older people with evidenced-based information on how to optimize physical activities, therapeutic exercises and movement rehabilitation strategies for older people. In Chapter 1, the epidemiological data are presented on the health benefits of physical activity for older people. Chapter 2 extends this theme by examining the benefits, barriers and best practice interventions for physical activity in older women. Chapter 3 uses data from research on the psychology of ageing to assist health professionals to promote physical activity and exercise in older people. In the fourth chapter the benefits of promoting physical activity and exercise in older workers are presented. Chapters 5–11 explore in detail the effects of different exercise and physical activity programmes for people with conditions such as arthritis, osteoporosis, muscle weakness and disorders of the feet. The ways in which falls can be reduced by physical activity are investigated in Chapter 12. This is followed by a summary of the effects of dual task interference during physical activities in healthy older people and those with neurological disabilities. Chapter 14 summarizes the risks, precautions and procedures to increase safety during exercises and physical activities in older people. The final chapter looks at exercise training for older people with type 2 diabetes. Together this information provides readers with a comprehensive account of how to promote health and reduce impairments, activity limitations and participation restrictions in older people through effective physical activity, exercise and movement rehabilitation programmes.

References

Andersen R E, Wadden T A, et al 1999 Effects of lifestyle activity vs structured aerobic exercise in obese women: a randomized trial. JAMA 281(4):335–340

Åstrand P O 1992 Physical activity and fitness. American Journal of Clinical Nutrition 55(Suppl):1231–1236

Australian Institute of Health and Welfare 1996 Australia's Health 1996. Canberra, Australian Government Publishing Service

Bank R A, Bayliss M T, et al 1997 Prevalence of leisure-time physical activity among persons with arthritis and other rheumatic conditions – United States, 1990–1991. Morbidity and Mortality Weekly Report 46(18):389–393

Bar-Or O, Foreyt J, et al 1998 Physical activity, genetic, and nutritional considerations in childhood weight management. Medicine and Science in Sports and Exercise 30(1):2–10

Bassett D R, Jr, Howley E T 1998 American College of Sports Medicine Position Stand. Exercise and physical activity for older adults. Medicine and Science in Sports and Exercise 30(6):992–1008

Baum F 1998 The new public health: an Australian perspective. Oxford University Press, Melbourne

Blair S N, Kohl H W, et al 1995 Changes in physical fitness and all-cause mortality: A prospective study of healthy and unhealthy men. JAMA 273:1093–1098

Brubaker J, Davis M, et al 1998 A comparison of videotape and written instruction for learning therapeutic exercises [Abstract]. Journal of Sport and Exercise Psychology 20(Suppl. 104)

Cicuttini F M, Baker J R, et al 1996 The association of obesity with osteoarthritis of the hand and knee in women: a twin study. Journal of Rheumatology 23(7):1221–1226

Commonwealth Department of Health and Aged Care 1999 National physical activity guidelines for Australians. CDHAC, Canberra

Convertino V A, Bloomfield S A, et al 1997 An overview of the issues: physiological effects of bed rest and restricted physical activity. Medicine and Science in Sports and Exercise 29(2):187–190

Delp C, Jones J 1996 Communicating information to patients: the use of cartoon illustrations to improve comprehension of instructions. Academic Emergency Medicine 3(3):264–270

Dunn A L, Marcus B H, et al 1999 Comparison of lifestyle and structured interventions to increase physical activity and cardiorespiratory fitness: a randomized trial. JAMA 281(4):327–334

Felson D T, Chaisson C E 1997 Understanding the relationship between body weight and osteoarthritis. Baillière's Clinical Rheumatology 11(4):671–681

Felson D T, Zhang Y, et al 1997 Risk factors for incident radiographic knee osteoarthritis in the elderly: the Framingham Study. Arthritis and Rheumatism 40(4):728–733

Fisher N M, Pendergast D R 1994 Effects of a muscle exercise program on exercise capacity in subjects with osteoarthritis. Archives of Physical Medicine and Rehabilitation 75(7):792–797

Friedrich M, Cermak T, et al 1996 The effect of brochure use versus therapist teaching on patients performing therapeutic exercise and on changes in impairment status. Physical Therapy 76:1082–1088

Gabriel S E, Crowson C S, et al 1997 Direct medical costs unique to people with arthritis. Journal of Rheumatology 24(4):719–725

Harvey R 1991 Making it better: strategies for improving the effectiveness and quality of health services in Australia. Department of Health, Housing, and Community Services: 3–107

Hoffman C, Rice D, et al 1996 Persons with chronic conditions: their prevalence and costs. JAMA 276:1478–1479

Hopman-Rock M, de Bock G H, et al 1997 The pattern of health care utilization of elderly people with arthritic pain in the hip or knee. International Journal for Quality in Health Care 9(2):129–137

Jackson L D 1994 Maximizing treatment adherence among back-pain patients: an experimental study of the effects of physician-related cues in written medical messages. Health Communication 6(3):173–191

Jette A M, Rooks D, et al 1998 Home-based resistance training: predictors of participation and adherence. Gerontologist 38(4):412–421

Jette A M, Lachman M, et al 1999 Exercise – it's never too late: the Strong-for-Life Program. American Journal of Public Health 89:66–72

Keller B K, Morton J L, et al 1999 The effect of visual and hearing impairments on functional status. Journal of the American Geriatrics Society 47(11):1319–1325

King A C 1994 Community and public health approaches to the promotion of physical activity. Medicine and Science in Sports and Exercise 26(11):1405–1412

Lopez A D, Murray C L 1996 The global burden of disease, Volume 1. A comprehensive assessment of mortality and disability from disease, injuries and risk factors in 1990 and projections to 2020. Harvard University Press, Cambridge, MA

Mathers C, Vos T, et al 1999 Burden of disease and injury in Australia. Australian Institute of Health and Welfare, Canberra

McGinnis M J 1995 The public health burden of a sedentary lifestyle. Medicine and Science in Sports and Exercise 24:S196–S200

Minor M A, Reid J C, et al 1998 Development and validation of an exercise performance support system for people with lower extremity impairment. Arthritis Care Research 11(1):3–8

Nutbeam D, Wise M, et al 1993 Goals and targets for Australia's health in the year 2000 and beyond. A J Law, Canberra

Paffenberg R S, Kampert J B, et al 1994 Changes in physical activity and other lifeway patterns influencing longevity. Medicine and Science in Sports and Exercise 26:857–865

Philbin E F, Ries M D, et al 1996 Osteoarthritis as a determinant of an adverse coronary heart disease risk profile. Journal of Cardiovascular Risk 3(6):529–533

Rantanen T, Era P, et al 1997 Physical activity and the changes in maximal isometric strength in men and women from the age of 75 to 80 years. Journal of the American Geriatrics Society 45:1534–1535

Ries M D, Philbin E F, et al 1996 Improvement in cardiovascular fitness after total knee arthroplasty. Journal of Bone and Joint Surgery (Am) 78(11):1696–1701

Ries M D, Philbin E F, et al 1997 Effect of total hip arthroplasty on cardiovascular fitness. Journal of Arthroplasty 12(1):84–90

Sashika H, Matsuba Y, et al 1996 Home program of physical therapy: effect on disabilities of patients with total hip arthroplasty. Archives of Physical Medicine and Rehabilitation 77(3):273–277

Schneiders A G, Zusman M, et al 1997 Exercise therapy compliance in acute low back pain patients. Tenth Biennial Conference, Melbourne Convention Centre, Melbourne, Manipulative Physiotherapists Association of Australia

Shumway Cook A, Gruber W, et al 1997 The effect of multidimensional exercises on balance, mobility, and fall risk in community-dwelling older adults. Physical Therapy 77(1):46–57

Smith A D, Park D C, et al 1998 Age differences in context integration in memory. Psychology and Aging 13(1):21–28

Smith J R, Owen N, et al 1999 Active for life: physical activity patterns and health impacts in Victoria 1998. Department of Human Services, Melbourne, Victoria

Steinberg A M, Donald K J, et al 1998 Are older Australians being marginalised by technology? Veterans' Health (63):18–19

Terpstra S J, de Witte L P, et al 1992 Compliance of patients with an exercise program for rheumatoid arthritis. Physiotherapy Canada 44(2):37–41

Uitenbroek D G 1993 Seasonal variation in leisure time physical activity. Medicine and Science in Sports and Exercise 25:755–760

US Department of Health and Human Services 1996 Physical activity and health: a report of the Surgeon General. National Center for Chronic Disease Prevention and Health Promotion, Atlanta, GA

Victorian Department of Human Services 2000 The burden of disease in Victoria, 1996. Volume 1. The mortality burdens of disease, injury and risk factors and projections to 2016. Department of Human Services, Melbourne

Weiss B D, Reed R L, et al 1995 Literacy skills and communication methods of low-income older persons. Patient Education and Counselling 25:109–119

Whiting W L T, Smith A D 1997 Differential age-related processing limitations in recall and recognition tasks. Psychology and Aging 12(2):216–224

Wolf S L, Barnhart H X, et al 1996 Reducing frailty and falls in older persons: an investigation of Tai Chi and computerized balance training. Journal of the American Geriatrics Society 44:489–497

Wolfson L, Whipple R, et al 1996 Balance and strength training in older adults: intervention gains and Tai Chi maintenance. Journal of the American Geriatrics Society 44:498–506

World Health Organization 1996 World health report 1996. World Health Organization, Geneva

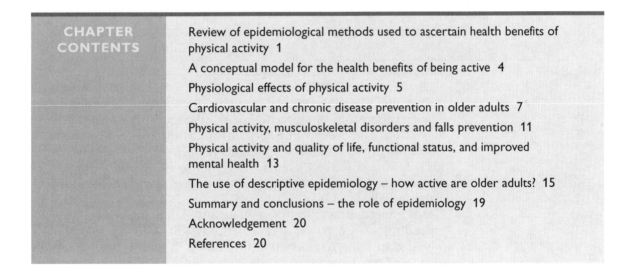

1

Health benefits of physical activity for older adults – epidemiological approaches to the evidence

Adrian Bauman

CHAPTER CONTENTS

Review of epidemiological methods used to ascertain health benefits of physical activity 1

A conceptual model for the health benefits of being active 4

Physiological effects of physical activity 5

Cardiovascular and chronic disease prevention in older adults 7

Physical activity, musculoskeletal disorders and falls prevention 11

Physical activity and quality of life, functional status, and improved mental health 13

The use of descriptive epidemiology – how active are older adults? 15

Summary and conclusions – the role of epidemiology 19

Acknowledgement 20

References 20

Review of epidemiological methods used to ascertain health benefits of physical activity

This chapter describes the evidence that physical activity (PA) may be beneficial to the health of older adults. This extends previous generic discussions of the benefits of being active for adult populations (Bauman and Owen 1999, USSG 1996). The discipline underpinning this chapter is epidemiology, which is the study of the 'distribution and determinants of health in populations' (Lawson and Bauman 2001).

The objectives of this chapter are to review the evidence for the health-promoting and disease prevention benefits of being active for adults aged at least 50 years. There are different groups of older adults, from the 'young-old', to the frail 'old-old' (>85 years of age) and health benefits may differ across groups. This is identified through description of the populations which were studied.

Figure 1.1 The generic research question of central interest.

Study factor/risk factor	Contributes to causes	Outcome factor
Physical activity (PA) Cardiorespiratory fitness Muscle strength Balance	⟶	Health/disease state

Table 1.1 Definitions of 'study factors' used in this chapter

Term used	Definition*	Types/context
Physical activity (PA)	Any large muscle movement that expends energy (usually isokinetic muscle contraction, using oxygen (aerobic training)); this includes all forms and settings where energy is expended	■ Categorized by type, intensity, duration, frequency ■ Settings include purposive leisure time (LTPA), transport-related, occupational, domestic, workplace
Exercise	Exercise is PA which is planned, structured and repetitive which has the goal of increasing or maintaining physical fitness (aerobic training)	Physical fitness usually implies cardiorespiratory fitness, but also could include muscle strength, power, balance, flexibility, body composition
Resistance training	Training designed to increase muscle strength and power	Requires different types of activity – weight training, repetitive muscle strengthening actions

*Adapted from US Department of Health and Human Services (1996), Caspersen et al (1985).

The central epidemiological question is to examine whether factors (known variously as 'study factors' or as 'risk factors or protective factors') are related or associated with specific health outcomes or disease states. Essentially, a constellation of different types of 'physical activity' are the study factors of interest. This is shown in Figure 1.1, and illustrates the generic form of the research question examined in this chapter, for populations of older adults.

It is important here to differentiate and define the various ways of expending energy, which may enhance health. A list of definitions is provided in Table 1.1, including the context in which they are usually found and researched. In addition, other domains of 'physical activity' investigated in elderly people include balance training, flexibility and proprioception, which also may have a role in disease prevention.

The epidemiological principles used in appraising the quality of evidence are summarized in Table 1.2. The best evidence emanates from experimental designs, usually described as randomized controlled designs (RCTs) in epidemiology. Studies which combine the results of many RCTs to provide a pooled quantitative average effect often use the technique known as meta-analysis.

However, much of the evidence is from well-designed observational studies, as populations cannot easily be randomly allocated to become physically active or not. This is similar to tobacco smoking, where the scientific evidence for ill-health effects comes from good quality observational studies. The best of these are cohort (longitudinal) studies, where large populations are followed for many years, and the relationship between exposure and outcome is assessed. Less powerful designs

Table 1.2 Epidemiological criteria for 'evidence' of health benefits

Research design used
■ Experimental (randomized controlled trials)
■ Observational studies

Measurement used
■ Reliability and validity of measurement of study factor (physical activity, fitness, strength), and of outcomes (e.g. cardiac disease, fractured femur)

Selection effects
■ Threats to external validity (representative of general population)
■ Threats to internal validity – loss of people, drop-outs, refusals

Issues in analysis
■ Appropriate statistical analysis, presentation
■ Adjust for confounders
■ Explore mediators and moderators

Criteria for 'causality'
■ Strong association, better research design, dose-response, findings replicated in other studies plausibility (possible physiological or bio-behavioural mechanisms or exploration described)

Adapted from Lawson and Bauman (2001).

include case-control studies, which are still used to assess the relationships between physical activity and rare disease outcomes, such as the risk of cancer.

Measurements of exposure (physical activity or fitness measures) need to be reliable and valid; measures used in physical activity assessment are reviewed elsewhere (Bauman and Merom 2002). Other epidemiological issues include having representative samples under study, so that results can be extrapolated to populations, and used for public policy development. It is important not to lose too many people in a follow-up study – otherwise the observed results may be due to the characteristics of the people who remain in the study; this is known as selection bias. Approaches to analysis of data are important, so that extraneous influences can be controlled for, and mediators and moderators sought (Bauman et al 2002). Finally, criteria for 'a causal relationship' require experimental evidence, but this may not be possible, as discussed above. Other criteria which strengthen the likelihood that an association is 'causal' include the strength of the statistical associations between physical activity and the health outcomes of interest, replication of similar findings across studies, and bio-physiological or psychological mechanisms which might explain how the health effects occur (Hill 1984, Lawson and Bauman 2001). The measures of association are usually expressed as relative risks (RR) or odds ratios (OR), which are measures of the likelihood of an outcome in one group, compared with another. For example, physical activity might double the likelihood of positive well-being (OR = 2) and reduce the likelihood of developing diabetes by 30% (OR = 0.7). For further descriptions, see introductory public health or epidemiological texts (e.g. Beaglehole et al 2000).

Table 1.3   Examples of research designs in studies of physical activity and health in elderly people

	Research design	Example from this chapter
Best scientific evidence	Meta-analysis	Kelley and Sharpe-Kelley (2001) – pooled synthesis of all RCTs showing that PA influenced blood pressure in older adults
	Multiple parallel RCTs	Schechtman and Ory (2001) – eight centres, each part of the FICSIT study – trials of PA to prevent falls, injury in frail elderly people
	Single RCT	Penninx et al (2002) – RCT of different PA programmes for older adults with osteoarthritis
	Well-designed population-based cohort study	Fried et al (1998) – cohort of 6000 elderly in California, followed for 5 years association between risk factors (inactivity, smoking, hypertension) and mortality
	(Population based) case-control study	Carpenter et al (1999) – 2027 postmenopausal women examined association between LTPA and breast cancer risk (compared with controls)
	Cross sectional surveys (from representative samples)	(Kritz-Silverstein et al 2001) – association shown cross-sectionally between PA and depression in a population sample of older Californians
Least convincing scientific evidence	Case series	As part of a review paper, four 'case studies' of active older adults described (Chodzko-Zajko 2000)

LTPA, leisure time physical activity; PA, physical activity; RCT, randomized controlled trial

Table 1.3 illustrates research designs, from the best scientific evidence, to the weakest scientific evidence. Specific examples from the epidemiology of physical activity in elderly people are shown in the right-hand column, to illustrate the different research designs. A key part of understanding evidence is to seek the best design possible for answering a specific research question. However, for many research questions, a well-designed cohort or case-control study may provide good observational data, which if repeated, could provide strong evidence. Even among intervention studies and trials, the RCT is not always feasible – for example, studies of strength training among very elderly people with small sample sizes can still be informative (MacRae et al 1996), even though only using a 'before after' (uncontrolled) intervention design.

The next sections of this chapter use these epidemiological principles to assess the evidence with respect to different health outcomes. First, physiological effects of PA are reviewed, followed by the protective role in reducing risks of chronic disease (cardiovascular disease, diabetes, some cancers). The final sections relate to quality of life, functional status and mood, all of which are important health benefits of PA for elderly people.

A conceptual model for the health benefits of being active

There are diverse health outcomes and benefits which might be associated with an active lifestyle. For elderly people, these range from disease prevention through to functional, psychological and social benefits. These are portrayed on a continuum in Figure 1.2, which enables a

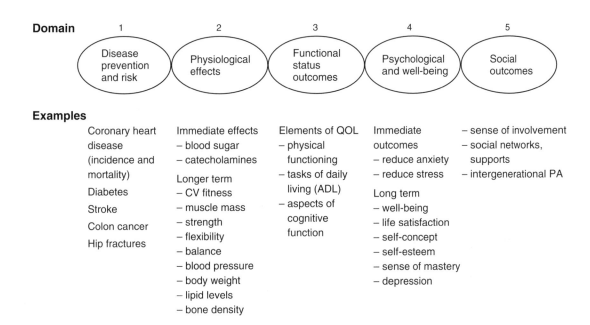

Figure 1.2 Conceptual model of health benefits of PA in older adults. Adapted, in part, from WHO (1997).

schematic classification system to be used for describing these health benefits. Some of these are adapted from the World Health Organization (1997) consensus statements on physical activity and health in elderly adults. Other schemata exist – a useful framework for the quality of life (QOL) components has been proposed by Stewart and King (1994, adapted in Rejeski and Mihalko 2001, WHO 1997), which divides QOL into 'functional outcomes' (physical, social and cognitive) and 'well being outcomes' (psychological, emotional).

Figure 1.2 shows biomedical outcomes on the left-hand side, with psychosocial and functional categories of outcomes on the right. Within these categories, short-term (immediate) and longer-term potential benefits are shown. Although the list of outcomes is not meant to be comprehensive, any additional outcomes for further study could be added to this schema.

Evidence is reviewed for each of these domains, starting with the biomedical and physiological effects of activity. The fifth domain, social outcomes, has the least evidence from an epidemiological perspective, but is researched and described in other disciplines, especially research in sociology and gerontology.

Physiological effects of physical activity

Before commencing a detailed discussion of the health outcomes influenced by PA, it is worth considering the antecedent physiological effects of PA for older adults. Note that some of these effects require vigorous (aerobic) levels of PA, but many are influenced by regular moderate-intensity PA carried out on most days of the week. In addition, there are other physiological outcomes achieved through resistance and strength training as well as balance and flexibility-oriented programmes.

The physiological outcomes discussed here include cardiorespiratory fitness, blood pressure, lipid levels, effects on muscle, joint flexibility, obesity and energy expenditure.

There is extensive evidence of the relationship between vigorous (aerobic) physical activity and increases in cardiorespiratory fitness and endurance. For older adults, aerobic training can slow or prevent age-related declines in cardiorespiratory endurance. A very active 70-year-old adult will have similar VO_{2max} (cardiorespiratory fitness) levels to a sedentary adult aged 30–40 years (US Department of Health and Human Services 1996, p. 76). This has implications for the delay in declines in VO_{2max} which might occur through lifelong physical activity participation.

Controlled trials in Finland have shown that active commuting to work (walking or cycling) can increase cardiorespiratory fitness (Oja et al 1991), and even regular walking on a golf course can have a small training effect in older adults (Parkkari et al 2000).

Effects of physical activity on lipid levels are similar in younger and older adults, with a beneficial effect on high density lipoprotein (HDL) cholesterol. However, the long-term health consequences of improving lipid profiles in older adults is less clear. There is some evidence of a positive effect of physical activity on haemostatic factors (such as fibrinogen, blood viscosity and platelet count), with beneficial effects seen even at light to moderate levels of PA (Wannamethee et al 2002). This is important for older adults, as it may provide one of the biological mechanisms through which physical activity is associated with reduced risks of cardiovascular diseases.

There is consistent RCT evidence that moderate PA is associated with small but significant reductions in systolic and diastolic blood pressure in adults (Halbert et al 1997). A recent meta-analysis examined this question for older adults, pooling data from seven controlled trials in subjects older than 50 years (Kelley and Sharpe-Kelley 2001). This study found an average reduction of 2 mmHg in systolic blood pressure across studies, which was significant, but a smaller (and not significant) reduction in diastolic blood pressure. This was consistent with other reviews, that there were small effects on blood pressure for older adults who engaged in regular physical activity (ACSM 1998).

There is a loss of muscle strength in humans after the fifth decade of life, with a decline of 5–10% per year (diPietro 2001). This is associated with decreased muscle power, increased (joint) stiffness, decreases in cartilage strength, and an increased risk of injury, especially falls. There are also changes in connective tissue elasticity with age. Thus the purpose of resistance training is especially important for older adults, to slow down these age-related changes. The health consequences of being active will reduce the risk of falls, and maintain musculoskeletal mobility. This latter characteristic can contribute to maintained functional status in older adults. Finally, an unrelated function of muscle is to promote the uptake of glucose – hence a decrease in muscle mass can change insulin resistance, and increase the risk of developing type 2 diabetes.

There are many studies showing that it is possible to increase muscle strength through progressive resistance training. Even among frail nonagenarians, programmes of strength training may be beneficial (Fiatarone et al 1990, 1994).

Because physical activity is an integral part of daily energy expenditure, it is important in obesity prevention. There is an increase in obesity with age, exacerbated by decreased muscle mass (which increases the relative proportion of body fat). Ageing is typically associated with decreased total energy expenditure (Starling 2001). Physical activity (moderate or vigorous) maintains energy expenditure, and may prevent the expected declines in the resting metabolic rate (RMR) seen with advancing age. A very active 60-year-old may have the RMR level of a sedentary person two decades younger (Starling 2001). However, efforts at increasing energy expenditure through vigorous intensity physical activity programmes among elderly adults may have little impact on net daily energy expenditure – there is some evidence that those who participate in vigorous programmes have 'compensatory sedentariness' at other times during the day, with reduced energy expenditure in domestic settings (Starling 2001). This highlights the concept of energy balance in obesity control, not just episodic physical activity.

In summary, the physiological benefits of all forms of physical activity have important benefits for older adults, especially related to preventing age-related changes in muscle strength and functioning. PA has benefits on blood pressure, lipids and fitness levels which are similar to those seen among younger adults (Mensink et al 1999). Physical activity of any form (endurance or resistance training) needs to be maintained in order to observe the benefits discussed above. Thus, maintenance of activity and muscle strength is important throughout the lifespan, and also for frail elderly people.

Cardiovascular and chronic disease prevention in older adults

Cardiovascular diseases

There is substantial epidemiological evidence that a sedentary lifestyle is a major risk factor for coronary heart disease (CHD), and the population risk attributable to inactivity appears to be similar to the risks posed by smoking, lipid levels or hypertension (Bauman 1998, 1999, US Department of Health and Human Services 1996). Evidence from a meta-analysis in 1990 indicated that those who are sedentary have nearly twice the risk of developing or dying from coronary heart disease (Berlin and Colditz 1990). Much of the research evidence explores effects of physical activity in the primary prevention of heart disease, and mostly reports data from well-designed population-based cohort studies. The benefits accrue particularly for promoting physical activity among those who are currently inactive, compared with those who participate in regular activity. These studies have typically investigated middle-aged

Figure 1.3 Review of the relationship between physical activity and cardiovascular disease outcomes among older adults.

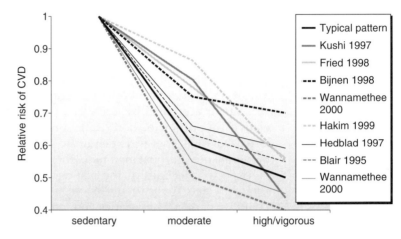

adults, but the evidence suggests that similar or even stronger associations are present for older adults (Talbot et al 2002). Further, inactivity can influence health costs and morbidity, not just mortality risk (LaCroix et al 1996).

The data from studies of physical activity and cardiovascular outcomes in older adults are summarized in Figure 1.3. This figure shows the relative risk of incident or fatal cardiovascular disease outcomes, across levels of physical activity or fitness. These studies examined populations that were middle-aged or older, usually at least 50 years of age, and were followed for several years to decades. The studies come from diverse populations and samples.

A Dutch study investigated 802 men aged 65 years or more in Zutphen (Bijnen et al 1998, in Figure 1.3); these were followed for 6 years, and risks of cardiovascular (CVD) death assessed. The pattern of risk is shown in the figure, but the authors concluded that 15% of all CVD deaths among older Dutch men were attributable to physical inactivity.

Other research summarized in Figure 1.3 shows very similar relationships between physical activity and cardiovascular disease. A large cohort of 40 000 postmenopausal women in Iowa showed a similar dose–response relationship between self-reported activity levels and CHD (Kushi et al 1997). Fried et al (1998) observed a similar relationship in four US communities in the older adults enrolled in the Cardiovascular Health Study. Wannamethee et al (2000) have used the British Regional Heart Study to recruit cardiac patients, and followed them to examine the same relationship. This study reported data from 5934 males, and risk estimates were adjusted for disease severity. Hakim et al (1999) reported data from the Honolulu Heart Health programme, following 2678 elderly males for 4 years, and examining CHD incidence. Hedblad et al (1997) examined the 1914 birth cohort in Malmo, Sweden, and examined the moderator effects of PA on the relationship between smoking and mortality. The final two studies in the figure examined changes in physical activity and subsequent changes in CHD or all-cause mortality.

These include the Dallas ACLS cohort study (Blair et al 1995) and the British study referred to above (Wannamethee et al 2000).

All of these show a consistent pattern – data extrapolated from the studies in the figure show that the greatest risk reduction occurs in moving the most sedentary to at least moderately active, with sometimes evidence of further benefit in further increments in activity levels. The pattern is reasonably consistent across studies, and is similar to that seen with younger adults (US Department of Health and Human Services 1996). A summary of the relationship, shown as the 'typical pattern' for this epidemiological relationship, is shown in bold. The 'adoption of PA' evidence (Blair et al 1995, Wannamethee et al 2000) reinforces the notion that the cardiac benefits of becoming more active can be derived at all ages, and reinforces the maxim that it is 'it is never too late to start being active'.

This relationship between moderate intensity PA and CHD outcomes is interesting, as some of the health benefit appears at levels of PA below that required for aerobic (cardiorespiratory) training (US Department of Health and Human Services 1996). These protective effects also appear to be independent of the additional influences of PA on lipid levels, hypertension and other CVD risk factors. Using epidemiological data such as these, the recommended levels of PA (for cardiovascular disease prevention) have been summarized as 'accumulating half an hour of at least moderate-intensity PA on most days of the week' (Commonwealth Dept of Health: National Australian Physical Activity Guidelines 1999, US Department of Health and Human Services 1996).

Physical activity has some benefits for patients with established coronary artery disease. This is seen in evaluations of the effects of cardiac rehabilitation programmes, which generally reduce the risk of subsequent cardiac events or mortality for those who participate in them (O'Connor 1989). However, the unique effects of the exercise components are difficult to disentangle from the overall programme benefits. Exercise-related benefits include increased fitness, improved oxygen consumption, and decreases in ischaemic responses for those who become active.

The mechanism for the cardiac health benefits of PA are gradually being elucidated. There is experimental evidence that sustained vigorous activity can lead to some regression of atherosclerosis, and improvements in cardiac endothelial cell functioning (Hambrecht et al 2000, 1993). This explains the epidemiological observation that only recent or current physical activity reduces cardiac risk, and not physical activity or fitness levels as an adolescent or young adult (Sherman et al 1999). The policy implications are that PA should be maintained, and it is the continuous or recent activity which may contribute to cardio-protection.

Stroke and other vascular disease

Existing data are less clear for a protective association between regular moderate physical activity and stroke (Lee and Paffenbarger 1998). There are two main types of stroke, ischaemic and haemorrhagic, and physical activity appears to be associated with a greater reduction of risk for the ischaemic type. The mechanism may be to reduce the risk of thrombus formation, or the effects of physical activity may be mediated indirectly through reducing blood pressure levels. Several epidemiological studies have suggested decreased risk of ischaemic stroke with increasing physical activity levels (Ellekjaer et al 2000, Shinton and Sagar 1993). A study from the Dallas ACLS cohort has reaffirmed this observation, with a one-third reduction in risk in the middle tertile, compared to the most sedentary third of the population. Additional stroke mortality risk reduction is noted for those in the most fit third of the population (Lee and Blair 2002).

A recent study has suggested that leg atherosclerosis may be reduced for those who are regularly active. A cohort of men born in Malmö, Sweden in 1914 were followed from age 55 to age 68 years, with measures of ankle blood pressures, as an index of lower limb vascular perfusion; those who were active showed better perfusion, suggesting lower rates of lower limb atherosclerosis (Engstrom et al 2001).

Diabetes

A central part of the primary prevention of diabetes is the promotion of physical activity (Ivy et al 1999). It has been estimated that a third to a half of all new cases of type 2 diabetes mellitus could be prevented by appropriate levels of physical activity. Both moderate and vigorous physical activity reduces the risk of type 2 diabetes in men, women and in different population groups (Folsom et al 2000, Hu et al 1999, Okada et al 2000). The relationship seems no different for older adults, where the incidence of diabetes is greatest. A typical finding is that the risk reduction is maximal for increasing activity among the most sedentary, moving them to at least moderate regular PA; this evidence is very similar to the CHD–physical activity relationship. For diabetes, the risk reduction is independent of relative body weight, skinfold values or adiposity.

A key study, published in 2002, was the Diabetes Prevention Program (DPP). This was a multicentre trial in the USA, which recruited 3234 adults at risk of developing diabetes, and randomly allocated them to a lifestyle intervention, to pharmacological therapy (metformin), or to a control group (DPP 2002). The lifestyle intervention was a 16-session intensive programme targeting weight loss, and achieving 150 minutes of moderate-intensity physical activity each week. The study was stopped after 2.8 years when the incidence of diabetes was reduced by 58% in the lifestyle group, compared with the controls. This study, and a similar Finnish one (Tuomilheto et al 2001) provide good experimental evidence that PA is a central component of primary and secondary diabetes prevention. In addition, for those with established diabetes, regular activity at least 3–4 times per week promotes muscle uptake of glucose, and helps with diabetes control.

Cancer prevention

There is some evidence that participation in physical activity may prevent some forms of cancer. There are now 48 studies which have examined the relationship between physical activity and colon cancer risk

(Colditz et al 1997, Thune and Furberg 2001), and most show a 30–70% risk reduction in the most active groups compared with those who are sedentary. The quantum of physical activity for cancer prevention may be more than that recommended for cardiovascular prevention; for cancer prevention, more sustained or more vigorous activity may be needed, with recommendations up to an hour per day of activity.

Many studies report a reduction in the risk of breast cancer among physically active women (Gammon et al 1998, Latikka et al 1998, Verloop et al 2000), but this appears to be strongest among older and post-menopausal women (Thune and Furberg 2001). There is some research regarding other cancers, but the evidence is inconclusive. Such research has examined physical activity in relation to cancers of the prostate, lung, ovary and uterus, but there are too few studies to enable clear policy statements for these cancers.

Physical activity, musculoskeletal disorders and falls prevention

Physical activity, in different forms, has a role to play in falls prevention, the risks of developing back pain, and in managing arthritis (Gardner et al 2000, Gregg et al 2000, Hopman-Rock and Westhoff 2000). These share, in part, common causal pathways in relation to inactivity. As age increases, mobility and muscle strength and power decrease. This leads to a decline in functional status, and an increased risk of injury, joint stiffness, and reduced independence (Buckwalter and Lane 1997). This is partly preventable and reversible, and even adults aged over 90 years can benefit from strength and flexibility training, through exercise and resistance training programmes (Fiatarone et al 1990, 1994).

Arthritis, back pain and bone loss

With respect to back pain, physical activity may help to prevent low back pain in the population, but is not clearly evidence-based in the management of acute back pain (Vuori 2001). This has implications for a role for PA in primary, rather than tertiary prevention (Lawson and Bauman 2001). The term 'primary prevention' implies strategies applied to well populations without disease, to reduce disease risk; 'secondary' prevention is to reduce risk in high risk groups – for example, secondary prevention programmes for occupations at risk of back injury. 'Tertiary prevention' refers to the role of physical activity in improving health outcomes for those with established chronic disease, such as physical activity to rehabilitate people with established back pain.

There is no evidence that physical activity prevents osteoarthritis (Vuori 2001), but it may do no harm for those already with the condition. Even for acute flare-ups of rheumatoid arthritis requiring hospitalization, programmes of muscle strengthening and cardiovascular training had no adverse impacts on joint swelling, pain or disease activity (van den Ende et al 2000). PA may have a role in joint protection through muscle strengthening. A case-control study examining the 'wear and tear' hypothesis failed to show that lifelong regular PA led to an increased risk of osteoarthritis (Sutton et al 2001).

Vigorous and high-intensity high-impact activity may increase the risk of injury or osteoarthritis (Vuori 2001), so that moderate intensity PA may be more useful for people with arthritis. This further reinforces the notion that activities such as regular walking, which have a much lower rate of injury than sports participation, may be the most useful for older adults (Hootman et al 2001).

The risks for hip and other bone fractures increase with age, and are costly to the health system. Part of the aetiology is bone demineralization, which occurs throughout adult life, especially increasing among postmenopausal women. Physical activity increases bone density in adolescents, but the reversibility of later age-related changes is less clear. Cross-sectionally and longitudinally, there is some evidence that bone mineral density (BMD) is associated with inactivity (Gregg et al 2000, Nguyen 1998, Ringsberg et al 2001), and interventions based on aerobic or resistance training may increase BMD by 2–5%, compared with controls. A meta-analysis of studies examining bone loss in post-menopausal women suggested that PA may prevent some bone loss, particularly in the lower spine, but that it had no effects on lower or upper limb bone loss (Berard et al 1997); and it is lower limb (femoral) bone loss that contributes to the most costly injury to the health system, namely fractured hips.

Falls prevention

Falls and fractures contribute substantially to health costs, and it is generally considered that physical activity has a role in reducing the rate of falls in the population (Campbell et al 1997, 1999). Individual observational studies have shown that leisure time physical activity participation is usually associated with a significant reduction in injurious falls. This has been noted in a review of only randomized trials, where a pooled sample size of 4933 people over aged 60 years was assembled. These showed that exercise programmes of various types were associated with fewer falls (Gardner et al 2000). One of the areas where clear answers are lacking is in defining the type of programme which leads to these benefits; for example, some falls prevention projects are multi-component integrated strategies, whereas others focus only on exercise, or on strength or balance training. Some studies use health professionals, and home-based exercise programmes (Robertson et al 2001), and others focus on strength and balance training (Lord 1995), yet all studies reported a significant reduction in falls. An attempt to disentangle effective intervention components was carried out through a pre-planned meta-analysis of the multicentre FICSIT project, which showed that balance training may make the most important contribution (Province et al 1995). Finally, many studies assess older adults in the community, and less is known, apart from some small studies, about those living in retirement and residential settings.

The data on falls are more abundant than data on the risk of specific fractures. Many intervention studies have too few subjects to detect reduced fracture incidence, although a plethora of case-control studies show inactivity to be a risk factor for hip fractures (Gillespie et al 2002,

Meyer et al 1993). Another systematic review has shown that moving from being sedentary to at least moderately active can reduce the risk of hip fractures by 20–40% (Gregg et al 2000). Overall, this has public health promise, but the components of interventions, for institutionalized and community-living elderly, remain to be defined.

Physical activity and quality of life, functional status, and improved mental health

Quality of life and functional status

The concept of quality of life (QOL) has many meanings (Rejeski and Mihalko 2001). It is usually used to imply a sense of well-being, or a cognitive judgement of satisfaction with one's life, or as a measure of functional status concerned with physical abilities or activities of daily living (ADL). Both of these definitional areas are important in the health of older adults, as they reflect the concept of 'successful ageing', with values emphasizing 'adding life to years not just years to life' (motto of the American Gerontological Society). The aim of interventions is to improve functional status during the ageing years, while reducing years with disability or impairment.

Studies of physical activity and quality of life tend to show consistently positive relationships, especially for those with impaired or reduced QOL. Further, researchers are describing different modes of activity; researchers have examined the impact of physical activity, strength training, tai chi, yoga and fitness programmes on a range of QOL outcomes in various population groups (Spirduso and Cronin 2001). Consistently, there appears to be an association between PA and perceived health, life satisfaction, decreased mood disturbance and life enjoyment (Menec and Chipperfield 1997, Mihalko and McAuley 1996, Rejeski and Mihalko 2001). These relationships appear across ages, initial physical activity levels and after adjustment for the baseline health status of participants. However, the dose–response relationship for physical activity and QOL outcomes is not clear, and defining the threshold requires further research (Spirduso and Cronin 2001). Physical activity, in the few studies that have examined it, appears to be associated with social relations among older adults (McAuley et al 2000) and with positive mood states (Blissmer et al 2000, Wanatabe et al 2001).

Using the SF-36 QOL measures, the FICSIT group conducted a pre-planned meta-analysis of the effects of different PA programmes on a range of QOL outcomes (Schechtman and Ory 2001). This analysis pooled 1733 older adults from RCTs in four FICSIT sites, and observed no effects on general health or pain scales, but significant effects of low intensity and flexibility exercise programmes on emotional health and social health dimensions of QOL.

Physical activity is associated with reduced functional limitations. A cohort study noted that the incidence of any functional limitation was reduced by 50% for those who were moderately active, compared with the sedentary, in a 6-year follow-up of 5000 people aged over 50 years (Huang et al 1998). Intervention studies show that aerobic and strength training can improve functional outcomes in Californian adults aged over 65 years (King et al 2000). Even hand grip strength (in 3000 Hawaiian seniors) was prospectively associated with reduced functional limitations and improved self-care tasks as well as walking speed (Rantanen et al 1999), suggesting that grip strength was a proxy measure for muscle strength.

Finally, the issue of cognitive function and physical activity has been widely researched, although conclusions are tenuous at this stage. Khatri et al (2001) reported a RCT of 84 depressed older adults, and allocated them to aerobic training or to antidepressant medication. The exercise group increased their fitness levels, and improved some areas of cognitive functioning, such as memory and executive functioning. Cohort studies have produced mixed findings. A US cohort of 5900 women, followed for 8 years, showed that those with increased activity levels had a slightly reduced risk of cognitive decline. A Quebec cohort (Laurin et al 2001) showed that at 5 years follow-up, the physically active group had a 31% lower risk of developing dementia, or Alzheimer's disease, but that PA had no effect on cognitive function in the absence of dementia.

Depression and mental health

Physical activity has a generally positive impact upon mood states (Arent et al 2000), which appears to be maximal for interventions comprising cardiovascular (aerobic) training or resistance training. The effect size from a meta-analysis (average intervention effect on positive or negative mood states) appears greater if fitness changes are observed, and appears greater for short-term follow-up measurements (Arent et al 2000). A similar concept, psychological well-being, has been explored in an older Finnish cohort, where well-being was related to even modest activity levels (Ruuskanen and Ruoppila 1995). Physical activity has also been related to increases in self-esteem and confidence (Biddle et al 2000).

Much of the research in this area has examined population level associations between PA and depression. Several studies have reported a cross-sectional association, where more active people have lower depression rates (Dunn et al 2001). A southern Californian cohort observed similar cross-sectional associations, but these were not seen at 8-year follow-up (Kritz-Silverstein et al 2001). A Finnish cohort did report some longitudinal effects, where those who had become less active had also become more depressed (Lampinen et al 2000).

Further research has provided clinical trial information of PA for depressed patients, and some studies of clinical anxiety. Studies have shown that moderately depressed patients can benefit from aerobic training. In a controlled trial of 156 depressed elderly patients, Blumenthal et al (1999) compared aerobic exercise with antidepressant medication; at the end of the trial, half of those in the exercise group were assessed as non-depressed, which was similar to the medication effects (Blumenthal et al 1999). However, a methodological limitation in this paper was the rapid reduction of depression symptoms in all groups, suggesting natural variation in symptoms, as antidepressant medication may take weeks for maximal effects.

This kind of research suggests that PA may help to normalize depressed mood in those with high initial depression scores. Research into non-depressed adults has found less clear effects of PA on mood (Lennox et al 1990). Other researchers have shown that resistance training has an effect on mild depression among older adults (mean age 71 years), with maintenance of improved depression scores at 10–20 weeks and at 26 months post programme (Singh et al 2001). This study showed resistance training to be similar to the effects of standard antidepressant medication or psychological counselling. Thus, different modes of activity may be beneficial; however, one study noted that aerobic activity, and not resistance training produced an antidepressant effect (Penninx et al 2002). Much of the intervention research is derived from small studies, with volunteer subjects, and population effects are not yet clear.

The use of descriptive epidemiology – how active are older adults?

Introduction and methods

This section demonstrates an example of the use of descriptive epidemiology in understanding physical activity participation among older adults. Other cross-sectional descriptive population research has identified the large proportion of elderly adults in the USA and UK that are inactive (Dallaso et al 1988, Drewnowski and Evans 2001). Data from the Netherlands suggest that older adults decrease their physical activity by 30 minutes per day, over a decade of follow-up (Bijnen 1998). Exploring the prevalence, of, and factors associated with, physical activity, and identifying population groups at risk of inactivity are important components of policy-relevant research.

The data used here come from three representative Active Australia (AA) national physical activity surveys, collected in November 1997, 1999 and 2000. Data from these three surveys are pooled, to provide a larger sample size in order to examine PA levels among older age groups, compared with younger adults.

Methods of these three surveys have been described previously, as well as the AA physical activity questions used (Armstrong et al 2000, Bauman and Merom 2002). The AA questions asked about reported time spent undertaking physical activities over the previous week, asking specifically about walking, moderate leisure time activities, vigorous leisure time activities, and 'vigorous yard work or gardening'. Algorithms were developed to classify the population as 'sufficiently physically active' (accumulating 150 minutes of at least moderate intensity activity per week and over at least five sessions in the previous week), or 'insufficiently active' (defined as sedentary, or reporting some activity but not meeting the threshold). Additional questions were asked about knowledge and understanding of the moderate physical activity message and recommendations, behavioural intention (to be more active), confidence in being active (self-efficacy, three items), and two 'social support for physical activity' items. The key stratification variable for this analysis was the age groups used, which examined older non-institutionalized adults in more detail than previous analyses (Armstrong et al 2000). The age groups reported here were younger adults (18–44 years), and three groups of older adults, namely those aged 45–54 years, 55–64 years and 65–75 years respectively. No adults older than 75 years were surveyed.

Results – activity patterns of older Australians

The three population surveys reported response rates from 65 to 74%. Data used here were unweighted sample data, from 12 256 survey responders. Physical activity participation is shown in Table 1.4. Data include the 'vigorous gardening and yard work' question, which was not included in previous PA estimates (Armstrong et al 2000). There are clear gender differences, with a greater proportion of older males reporting more moderate and vigorous activity, and gardening and yard work than age-matched females. Vigorous activity showed a strong age gradient, with decrements in time spent in vigorous activity with increasing age. Moderate activity and walking were lowest among middle age and late middle-aged adults, who showed lower levels than the youngest and the oldest groups. For total minutes of activity, there was a middle-aged 'slump' in activity for males 45–64 years, but this increased 'post retirement'. However, for females, total minutes declined again after age 65 years.

Table 1.4 Pooled data from the three surveys: minutes of physical activity in the previous week, by age group (mean minutes ± standard errors shown)

Age group and gender	Walking (min)	Moderate PA (min)	Vigorous PA (min)	'Chores and gardening' (min)	Total (sum of all categories – min)
18–44 years (n = 6328)					
Male	118.2 (3.2)	61.4 (2.5)	122.3 (3.6)	93.4 (3.4)	394.9 (6.9)
Female	135.5 (2.7)	33.2 (1.6)	73.5 (2.3)	59.3 (2.2)	301.7 (5.1)
45–54 years (n = 2317)					
Male	113.8 (5.2)	53.8 (4.2)	65.1 (4.3)	106.4 (5.8)	343.2 (4.2)
Female	135.9 (4.5)	33.8 (2.9)	45.4 (3.2)	76.3 (4.4)	291.9 (8.4)
55–64 years (n = 1719)					
Male	139.2 (6.8)	86.7 (5.1)	33.1 (3.4)	124.5 (7.9)	383.5 (13.8)
Female	132.7 (5.2)	75.3 (4.2)	33.1 (3.3)	85.4 (5.3)	317.2 (10.5)
65–75 years (n = 1759)					
Male	144.5 (2.4)	68.8 (2.1)	31.4 (3.8)	117.4 (7.9)	394.2 (14.2)
Female	124.8 (5.0)	43.3 (1.4)	17.9 (2.0)	67.9 (4.7)	298.7 (3.7)

The data in Figure 1.4 indicate that absolutely sedentary rates increased with age. Overall 'sufficiently active' rates were highest among younger adults, and lowest for males in the 45–54 age group, but declined throughout age groups for women. This suggests different patterns in physical activity participation by gender for populations at each decade of age from age 45 to 75 years.

Additional analyses examined behavioural 'intention to be more active', and also asked survey responders to rate statements about understanding of the recommended moderate physical activity message. Results, by age group, are shown in Table 1.5. Intention to be more active was much more prevalent among younger adults, and showed a clear decline with age, especially after age 65 years ($P < 0.001$). The confidence that they could be more active, reflected in a validated continuous measure of self-efficacy, also showed a clear decline with age ($F_{3,4733} = 14.0, P < 0.001$). Among the knowledge items, the proportions of people who thought that 'generally being more active', or a half hour brisk walk was beneficial did not change by age group; however, the perception that regular vigorous activity was essential for health was more often reported by younger adults, and showed a linear decline in agreement with age ($P < 0.001$). Agreement with the notion of 'accumulation of physical activity in blocks of 10 minutes' was more frequently reported by older adults ($P < 0.01$).

Trends in physical activity prevalence rates among older adults across surveys, using the age groups above, are shown in Figure 1.5. The sample sizes, within age groups, were too small to stratify by gender. Overall, the substantial declines in activity prevalence between 1997 and 1999 observed for the younger adults were less marked for middle-aged and older age groups, with no change at all for the 45–54 and 65–75 year old age groups. This suggests that the influences on trends in physical activity may be different for older adults.

Figure 1.4 Proportions who are completely sedentary and those meeting the recommendations for 'sufficiently active' of at least 150 minutes and 5 sessions per week, by age group and gender.

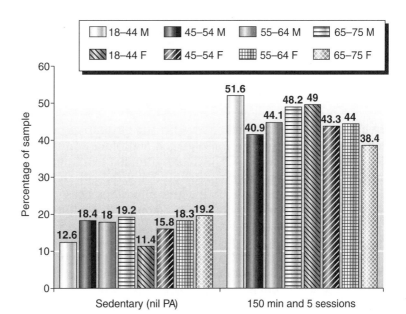

Table 1.5 Behavioural intention, self-efficacy measures and knowledge of current physical activity recommendations, by age group

Age group	Behavioural intention [Per cent who do not intend to be more active (%)]	Self-efficacy[†] [Mean score (SE)]	Statements about physical activity (% who agree)*				
			Generally being more active is healthy (%)	Brisk walk, half an hour daily is beneficial (%)	Vigorous exercise three times per week is necessary for health (%)	Activity benefits can be accumulated in blocks of 10 minutes (%)
18–44 years	31.6	7.5 (0.06)	87.4	92.2	63.6	75.4
45–54 years	41.1	7.3 (0.11)	87.2	92.7	58.3	78.3
55–64 years	50.1	7.1 (0.12)	87.2	91.0	53.7	80.8
65–75 years	61.5	6.6 (0.11)	85.0	90.7	48.0	85.7

*Rated from strongly agree to strongly disagree, on a five-point Likert scale; recoded into the percentage who 'strongly agreed or agreed'.
[†]Sum of three items from Sallis 1985 Self-efficacy for physical activity scale (in Armstrong et al 2000).

Figure 1.5 Trends in physical activity among older Australians 1997–2000.

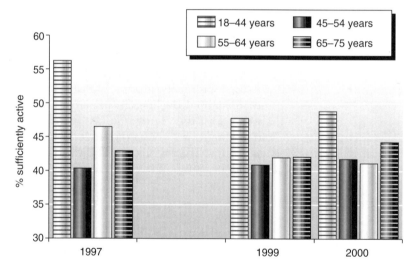

Relevance of population monitoring using survey data

This section has provided examples of population-level, representative data on middle-aged and older adults, from national physical activity surveys. The data are limited to adults no older than 75 years, and only sampled non-institutionalized elderly; nonetheless, they provide some preliminary insights into differences in the patterns of physical activity and its correlates among older adults. Strictly speaking, older adults require more specific physical activity survey questions, which are tailored to the cognitive profile, and types and intensity of activity performed. The Physical Activity Scale for the Elderly (PASE) and the Yale measure are two examples of specific measures for older adults (Washburn et al 2000), but have not yet been widely incorporated into population surveillance. Despite the acknowledged need for elderly-specific PA surveys, these preliminary data from a generic adult PA survey do show some differences by age, and these have policy and planning implications in terms of developing population-wide approaches to increasing levels of physical activity among older adults. Additional research issues include the epidemiological challenge of assessing activity patterns in all older adults, including those in institutional care, and of measuring other dimensions of PA, strength training behaviour, and balance and gait. Some of these may not be possible through routine population monitoring surveys, but require expensive research protocols, using objective assessments and complex sampling frames.

Summary and conclusions – the role of epidemiology

This chapter has reviewed the role of epidemiological research in understanding and monitoring physical activity among older adults. The health benefits associated with physical activity in elderly people are part of 'successful ageing', which is concerned with disease prevention, but more importantly among older adults, with delaying the declines in age-related function (Chodzko-Zajko 2000, Wagner et al 1992). The World Health Organization has concluded that 'physical activity is the single most useful thing that individuals can do to maintain their health and function and quality of life' (WHO 1997).

The evidence is strongest for cardiovascular disease, especially coronary heart disease, where moving the population from inactive to moderately active levels can reduce the risks of incident and fatal CHD by around 40–50%. The evidence is also good for diabetes, across all levels of prevention. The physiological benefits are diverse, but most notable are significant impacts on reducing blood pressure, and increases in muscle strength (Wagner et al 1992). The latter has an impact on the risk of injurious falls, as well as being related to functional outcomes and the performance of daily tasks. The psychological benefits include self-esteem and a sense of mastery, improved mood, and reduced depression for those who had initially high levels. There are also policy-relevant benefits on healthcare costs and morbidity (Perkins and Clark 2001). This provides a rationale for community-wide interventions to encourage activity among older adults. Finally, the social benefits, although least researched, are important. These include the potential for greater empowerment of older adults, better integration into communities, the formation of social networks and connections, and increased engagement with others (WHO 1997).

The previous section reviewed the descriptive epidemiology of physical activity participation among older Australians, using population surveys. These kinds of data are used to describe the differences in participation and PA correlates among different age groups. It is recognized that PA surveillance is particularly difficult among elderly people, due to the complexities of representative sampling, and of measuring all the domains of PA required for health in this diverse group, who range from mostly community-living adults in their 50s to mostly institutionalized frail elderly people in their 90s or older.

Finally, there is no simple final recommendation that fits all health outcomes, for all ages of older adulthood. The most pragmatic public health recommendation is that all older adults at all ages should be encouraged to move more, and increase aspects of physical activity in their lives; this may be balance and posture, strength training, or moderate and vigorous intensity activities, but it is important to maintain a regular habit throughout older years. Specific targets should be tailored to the capacity, motivation, expectations and confidence of older individuals, in all societies and demographic groups.

Acknowledgement

I thank the Australian Institute of Health and Welfare for access to national data sets analysed in the section on 'The use of descriptive epidemiology – how active are older adults?'

References

American College of Sports Medicine (ACSM) 1998 Guidelines – Exercise and physical activity for older adults. Medicine and Science in Sports and Exercise 30:992–1008

Arent S M, Landers D M, et al 2000 The effects of exercise on mood in older adults: a meta-analytic review. Journal of Aging and Physical Activity 8(4):407–430

Armstrong T, Bauman A, et al 2000 Physical activity patterns of Australian adults. AIHW Catalogue CVD 10. Australian Institute of Health and Welfare, Canberra

Bauman A 1998 The use of population attributable risk (PAR) in understanding the health benefits of physical activity. British Journal of Sports Medicine 32:279–280

Bauman A 1999 Encouraging physical activity: an under-recognised method of improving the health of older Australians. Veterans' Health 64:10–13

Bauman A, Merom D 2002 Measurement and surveillance of physical activity in Australia – An introductory guide. Australasian Epidemiologist 9(2):2–5

Bauman A, Owen N 1999 Physical activity of adult Australians: epidemiological evidence and potential strategies for health gain. Journal of Science in Medicine and Sport 2:30–41

Bauman A E, Sallis J F, et al 2002 Towards a better understanding of the influences on physical activity; the role of determinants, correlates, causal variables, mediators, moderators and confounders. American Journal of Preventative Medicine 23(2S):5–14

Beaglehole R, Bonita R, et al 2000 Basic epidemiology. World Health Organization, Geneva

Berard A, Bravo G, et al 1997 Meta-analysis of the effectiveness of physical activity for the prevention of bone loss in postmenopausal women. Osteoporosis International 7:331–337

Berlin J, Colditz G A 1990 A meta analysis of physical activity in the prevention of coronary heart disease. American Journal of Epidemiology 132:612–628

Biddle S, Fox K, et al 2000 Physical activity, aging and psychological well being. Routledge, London

Bijnen F C, Caspersen C J, et al 1998 Physical activity and 10-year mortality from cardiovascular diseases and all causes: the Zutphen Elderly Study. Archives of Internal Medicine 158:1499–1505

Blair S N, Kohl H, et al 1995 Changes in physical fitness and all-cause mortality. A prospective study of healthy and unhealthy men. JAMA 273:1093–1098

Blissmer E B, Katula J, et al 2002 Physical activity, self-esteem, and self-efficacy relationships in older adults: a randomized controlled trial. Annals of Behavioral Medicine 22(2):131–139

Blumenthal J A, Babyak M A, et al 1999 Effects of exercise training on older patients with major depression. Archives of Internal Medicine 159:2349–2356

Buckwalter J A, Lane N E 1997 Athletics and osteoarthritis. American Journal of Sports Medicine 25(6):873–881

Campbell A J, Robertson M, et al 1997 Randomised controlled trial of a general practice programme of home based exercise to prevent falls in elderly women. British Medical Journal 315:1065–1069

Campbell A J, Robertson M, et al 1999 Falls prevention over 2 years: a randomized controlled trial in women 80 years and older. Age and Ageing 28:513–518

Carpenter C L, Ross R K, et al 1999 Lifetime exercise activity and breast cancer risk among post-menopausal women. British Journal of Cancer 80:1852–1858

Caspersen C J, Powell K E, Christenson G M 1985 Physical activity, exercise, and physical fitness: definitions and distinctions for health-related research. Public Health Reports 100(2):126–131

Chodzko-Zajko W 2000 Successful aging in the new millennium: the role of regular physical activity. Quest 52:333–343

Colditz G A, Cannuscia C C, Frazier A L 1997 Physical activity and reduced risk of colon cancer. Cancer Causes and Control 8:649–667

Commonwealth Department of Health and Aged Care 1999 National Physical Activity Guidelines for Australians. Australian Government Publishing Service, Canberra

Dallaso H M, Morgan K, et al 1988 Level of customary physical activity among the old and very old living at home. Journal of Epidemiology and Community Health 42:121–127

Diabetes Prevention Program Research Group 2002 Reduction in the incidence of type 2 diabetes with lifestyle intervention or metformin. New England Journal of Medicine 346:393–403

DiPietro L 1996 The epidemiology of physical activity and physical function in older people. Medicine and Science in Sports and Exercise 28(5):596–600

DiPietro L 2001 Physical activity in aging: changes in patterns and their relationship to health and function. Journals of Gerontology Series A. Biological Sciences Medical Sciences S2:13–22

Drewnowski L, Evans W J 2001 Nutrition, physical activity, and quality of life in older adults: summary. Journal of Gerontology 56A(special issue):89–94

Dunn A L, Trivedi M H, O'Neal H A 2001 Physical activity dose–response effects on outcomes of depression and anxiety. Medicine and Science in Sports and Exercise 33(6 Suppl):587–597

Ellekjaer H, Holmen J, et al 2000 Physical activity and stroke mortality in women – ten year follow up of the Nord-Trondelag Health Survey 1984–86. Stroke 31:14–18

Engstrom G, Ogren M, et al 2001 Asymptomatic leg atherosclerosis is reduced by regular physical activity. Longitudinal results from the cohort. European Journal of Vascular and Endovascular Surgery 21:502–507

Fiatarone M A, Marks E C, et al 1990 High-intensity strength training in nonagenarians. Effects on skeletal muscle. JAMA 263(22):3029–3034

Fiatarone M A, O'Neill E F 1994 Exercise training and nutritional supplementation for physical frailty in very elderly people. New England Journal of Medicine 330(25):1769–1775

Folsom A, Kushi L H, et al 2000 Physical activity and incident diabetes in postmenopausal women. American Journal of Public Health 90:134–138

Fried L P, Kronmal R A, et al 1998 Risk factors for five year mortality in older adults – the Cardiovascular Health Study. JAMA 279(8):585–592

Gammon M D, Schoenberg J B, et al 1998 Recreational physical activity and breast cancer risk among women under age 45 years. American Journal of Epidemiology 147(3):273–280

Gardner M M, Robertson M C, et al 2000 Exercise in preventing falls and fall related injuries in older people: a review of randomised controlled trials. British Journal of Sports Medicine 34:7–17

Gillespie L D, Gillespie W J, et al 2002 Interventions for preventing falls in elderly people (Cochrane Review). Cochrane Library. Issue 2. Update Software, Oxford

Gregg E W, Pereira M A, et al 2000 Physical activity, falls, and fractures among older adults: a review of the epidemiologic evidence. Journal of the American Geriatrics Society 48(8):883–893

Hakim A A, Curb J D, et al 1999 Effects of walking on coronary heart disease in elderly men: the Honolulu Heart Program. Circulation 100(1):9–13

Halbert J A, Silagy C A, et al 1997 The effectiveness of exercise training in lowering blood pressure: a meta-analysis of randomised controlled trials of 4 weeks or longer. Journal of Human Hypertension 11:641–649

Hambrecht R, Niebauer J, et al 1993 Various intensities of leisure time physical activity in patients with coronary heart disease: effects on cardiorespiratory fitness and progress of coronary atherosclerotic lesions. Journal of the American College of Cardiology 22:468–477

Hambrecht R, Wolf A, et al 2000 Effect of exercise upon coronary endothelial function in patients with coronary artery disease. New England Journal of Medicine 342:454–460

Hedblad B, Ogren M, et al 1997 Reduced cardiovascular mortality risk in male smokers who are physically active. Results from a 25-year follow-up of the prospective population study men born in 1914. Archives of Internal Medicine 157(8):893–899

Hill A B 1984 A short textbook of medical statistics, 11th edn. Hodder and Stoughton, London

Hootman J M, Macera C A, et al 2001 Association among physical activity level, cardiorespiratory fitness and risk of musculoskeletal injury. American Journal of Epidemiology 154(3):251–258

Hopman-Rock M, Westhoff M H 2000 The effects of a health education and exercise program for older adults with osteoarthritis of the hip or knee. Journal of Rheumatology 27(8):1947–1954

Hu F B, Sigal R J, et al 1999 Walking compared with vigorous physical activity and risk of type 2 diabetes in women. JAMA 282(15):1433–1439

Huang Y, Macera C A 1998 Physical fitness, physical activity, and functional limitation in adults aged 40 and older. Medicine and Science in Sports and Exercise 30:1430–1435

Ivy J, Zderic T, et al 1999 Prevention and treatment of non-insulin-dependent diabetes mellitus. Exercise and Sport Sciences Reviews 27:1–36

Kelley G A, Sharpe-Kelley K 2001 Aerobic exercise and resting blood pressure in older adults: a meta-analytic review of randomized controlled trials. Journal of Gerontology 56A:298–303

Khatri P, et al 2001 Effects of exercise training on cognitive functioning among depressed older men and women. Journal of Aging and Physical Activity 9:43–57

King A C, Pruit L A, et al 2000 Comparative effects of two physical activity programs on measured and perceived physical functioning and other health-related quality of life outcomes in older adults. Journal of Gerontology 55:M74–83

Kritz-Silverstein D, Barrett-Connor E, Corbeau C 2001 Cross-sectional and prospective study of exercise and depressed mood in the elderly – the Rancho Bernardo Study. American Journal of Epidemiology 153:596–603

Kushi L H, Fee R M, et al 1997 Physical activity and mortality in post-menopausal women. JAMA 277:1287–1292

LaCroix A Z, Leveille S G, et al 1996 Does walking decrease the risk of cardiovascular disease hospitalizations and death in older adults? Journal of the American Geriatrics Society 44:113–120

Lampinen P, Heikkinen R L, et al 2000 Changes in intensity of physical exercise as predictors of depressive symptoms among older adults: an eight-year follow up. Preventive Medicine 30:371–380

Laurin D, Verreault R, et al 2001 Physical activity and risk of cognitive impairment and dementia in elderly persons. Archives of Neurology 58:498–504

Latikka P, Pukkala E, et al 1998 Relationship between the risk of breast cancer and physical activity. An epidemiological perspective. Sports Medicine 26(3):133–143

Lawson J S, Bauman A E 2001 Public Health Australia – an introduction. McGraw-Hill, Sydney

Lee C D, Blair S N 2002 Cardiorespiratory fitness and stroke mortality in men. Medicine and Science in Sports and Exercise 34(4):592–595

Lee I M, Paffenbarger R S 1998 Physical activity and stroke incidence – the Harvard Alumni Health Study. Stroke 29:2049–2054

Lennox S S, Bedell J R, et al 1990 The effect of exercise on normal mood. Journal of Psychosomatic Research 34(6):629–636

Lord S 1995 The effect of a 12 month exercise trial on balance, strength and falls in older women. Journal of American Geriatrics Society 43:1198–1206

MacRae P G, Asplund L A, et al 1996 A walking program for nursing home residents: effects on walk endurance, physical activity, mobility, and quality of life. Journal of the American Geriatrics Society 44:175–180

McAuley E, Blissmer B, et al 2000 Social relations, physical activity, and well-being in older adults. Preventive Medicine 31:608–617

Menec V H, Chipperfield J G 1997 Remaining active in later life; the role of locus of control in seniors' leisure activity participation, health and life satisfaction. Journal of Aging and Health 9:105–125

Mensink G B, Ziese T, et al 1999 Benefits of leisure-time physical activity on the cardiovascular risk profile at older age. International Journal of Epidemiology 28:659–666

Meyer H E, Tverdal A, et al 1993 Risk factors for hip fracture in middle-aged Norwegian women and men. American Journal of Epidemiology 137(11):1203–1211

Mihalko S L, McAuley E 1996 Strength training effects on subjective well being and physical function in the elderly. Journal of Aging and Physical Activity 4:56–68

Nguyen T V, Sambrooke P N, et al 1998 Bone loss, physical activity and weight change in elderly women: the Dubbo Osteoporosis Epidemiology Study. Journal of Bone and Mineral Research 13(9):1458–1467

O'Connor G T, Buring J E, et al 1989 An overview of randomized trials of rehabilitation with exercise after myocardial infarction. Circulation 80:234–244

Okada K, Hayashi T, et al 2000 Leisure time physical activity at weekends and risk of type 2 diabetes in Japanese men – the Osaka Health Survey. Diabetic Medicine 17:53–58

Oja P, Manttari A, et al 1991 Physiological effects of walking and cycling to work. Scandinavian Journal of Medicine and Science in Sports 1(3):151–157

Parkkari J, Natri A, et al 2000 A controlled trial of the health benefits of regular walking on a golf course. American Journal of Medicine 109(2):102–108

Penninx B, Rejeski W J, et al 2002 Exercise and depressive symptoms: a comparison of aerobic and resistance exercise effects on emotional and physical function in older persons with high and low depressive symptomatology. Journal of Gerontology 57B(2):P124–132

Perkins A J, Clark D O 2001 Assessing the association of walking with health services use and costs among socioeconomically disadvantaged older adults. Preventive Medicine 32:492–501

Province M A, Hadley E C, et al 1995 The effects of exercise on falls in elderly patients – a preplanned meta-analysis of the FICSIT trials. JAMA 273(17):1341–1357

Rantanen T, Guralnik J M, et al 1999 Midlife hand grip strength as a predictor of old age disability. JAMA 281(6):558–560

Rejeski W J, Mihalko S L 2001 Physical activity and quality of life in older adults. Journal of Gerontology 56A:23–35

Ringsberg K A, Gardsell P, et al 2001 The impact of long-term moderate physical activity on functional performance, bone mineral density and fracture incidence in elderly women. Gerontology 47:15–20

Robertson M C, Devlin N, et al 2001 Effectiveness and economic evaluation of a nurse delivered home exercise programme to prevent falls 1: randomised controlled trial. British Medical Journal 322:1–6

Ruuskanen J M, Ruoppila I 1995 Physical activity and psychological well-being among people aged 65 to 84 years. Age and Ageing 24(4):292–296

Schechtman K B, Ory M G 2001 The effects of exercise on the quality of life of frail older adults: a preplanned meta-analysis of the FICSIT trials. Annals of Internal Medicine 23(3):186–197

Sherman S E, D'Agostino R B, et al 1999 Comparison of past versus recent physical activity in the prevention of premature death and coronary artery disease. American Heart Journal 138:900–907

Shinton R, Sagar G 1993 Lifelong exercise and stroke. British Medical Journal 307:231–234

Singh N A, Clements K M, et al 2001 The efficacy of exercise as a long term antidepressant in elderly subjects: a randomised controlled trial. Journal of Gerontology 56A(8):M497–504

Spirduso W, Cronin D L 2001 Exercise dose–response effects on quality of life and independent living in older adults. Medicine and Science in Sports and Exercise 33(6):598–608

Starling RD 2001 Energy expenditure and aging: effects of physical activity. International Journal of Sport Nutrition, Exercise Metabolism (Suppl): S208–217

Stewart A L, King A C 1994 Conceptualizing and measuring quality of life in older populations. In: Abeles R P, Gift H C, et al (eds) Aging and quality of life. Springer Publishing, New York

Sutton A J, Muir K R, et al 2001 A case-control study to investigate the relation between low and moderate levels of physical activity and osteoarthritis of the knee using data collected as part of the Allied Dunbar National Fitness Survey. Annals of the Rheumatic Diseases 60(8):756–764

Talbot L A, Morrell C H, et al 2002 Comparison of cardiorespiratory fitness versus leisure time physical activity as predictors of coronary events in men aged ≤65 years and >65 years. American Journal of Cardiology 89:1187–1192

Thune I, Furberg A S 2001 Physical activity and cancer risk: dose–response and cancer, all sites and site-specific. Medicine and Science in Sports and Exercise 33 (6 Suppl):530–550

Tuomilehto J, Lindstrom J, et al 2001 Prevention of type 2 diabetes mellitus by changes in lifestyle among subjects with impaired glucose tolerance. New England Journal of Medicine 344:1343–1350

United States Department of Health and Human Services 1996 The Surgeon General's Report on Physical Activity and Health. US Government Printing Office, Washington, DC

van den Ende C H, Breedveld F C, et al 2000 Effect of intensive exercise on patients with active rheumatoid arthritis: a randomised clinical trial. Annals of the Rheumatic Diseases 59(8):615–621

van der Bij A K, Laurant M G H, et al 2002 Effectiveness of Physical Activity Interventions for Older Adults. American Journal of Preventative Medicine 22(2):120–133

Verloop J, Rookus M A, et al 2000 Physical activity and breast cancer risk in women aged 20–54 years. Journal of the National Cancer Institute 92(2):128–135

Vuori I M 2001 Dose–response of physical activity and low back pain, osteoarthritis, and osteoporosis. Medicine and Science in Sports and Exercise 33(6 Suppl):551–586

World Health Organization 1997 Heidelberg guidelines for promoting physical activities among older persons. Journal of Aging and Physical Activity 5:2–8

Wagner E H, LaCroix A Z, et al 1992 Effects of physical activity on health status in older adults I: observational studies. Annual Review of Public Health 13:451–468

Wannamethee S G, Shaper A G, et al 2000 Physical activity and mortality in older men with diagnosed coronary heart disease. Circulation 102(12):1358

Wannamethee S G, Lowe G D O, et al 2002 Physical activity and hemostatic and inflammatory variables in elderly men. Circulation 105:1785–1790

Washburn R, Heath G, et al 2000 Reliability and validity issues concerning large scale surveillance of physical activity. Research Quarterly for Exercise and Sport 71:104–113

Watanabe E, Takeshima N, et al 2001 Effects of increasing expenditure of energy during exercise on psychological well-being in older adults. Perceptual and Motor Skills 92:288–298

2

Grandmothers on the move: benefits, barriers and best practice interventions for physical activity in older women

Wendy J Brown and Christina Lee

CHAPTER CONTENTS

Why promote physical activity among older women? 27

Physical activity and healthy older women 30

Understanding physical activity among older women 32

Effectiveness of physical activity interventions for older women 33

Conclusions 35

References 35

One of the best-established gender differences in health is that women's life expectancy, worldwide, averages 3 years more than men's; in developed societies the difference is 8 years (Population Reference Bureau 2000). In Australia, average life expectancy for women is about 6 years longer than for men, with women on average living to 82, compared with 76 for men (Gibson et al 1999). Women therefore comprise the majority of our older population. While 56% of people aged 65–69 are women, this proportion increases to 65% for the over eighties (Gibson et al 1999). Hence many women have the advantage of longer life, but as a result they are more likely than men to suffer from disability and to experience multiple health problems as they age. Moreover, because men tend to die at an earlier age, women are more likely to live alone in old age.

Because women can expect to live longer than men, they are at greater risk of experiencing a number of debilitating conditions in older age. The main contention of this chapter is therefore that it is particularly important for women to maintain functional capacity as they age, and to remain independent and active for as long as they can. Physical activity in young and middle adulthood can help them to achieve this. It can also alleviate or help to control many of the chronic conditions which are typically experienced after the age of sixty (American College of Sports Medicine 1998). Despite this, women are less likely than men to be involved in physical activity at all life stages, and often lack the skills and resources to take up physical activity in older age. We argue that the best strategy for promoting physical activity among older women is to encourage the adoption and maintenance of physical activity in the middle years. Maintaining an existing pattern of behaviour is easier than attempting to develop a new one when one is already experiencing illness or disability, and women who are already physically active have lower rates of disability as they age (O'Brien and Vertinsky 1991). Canadian researchers have suggested that while regular physical activity could halve the level of age-related decline in physical and psychological functioning in older women, there are many barriers which make physical activity problematic in this age group (O'Brien and Vertinsky 1991).

Why promote physical activity among older women?

The most obvious reason for promoting physical activity among older women is that evidence now demonstrates clearly that women can obtain the same health benefits as men from regular physical activity. The major causes of premature death and disability in developed countries – cardiovascular disease, cancer, mental health problems, diabetes, injury, respiratory diseases and musculoskeletal problems – are as prevalent, and in some cases more prevalent, among women than men. Hence women have the same capacity to benefit from preventive measures as do men.

The importance of physical inactivity as a risk factor for the chronic diseases which are now endemic in Western countries is summarized in the US Surgeon General's Report on Physical Activity and Health (US Department of Health and Human Services 1996). This report highlights the evidence which confirms physical inactivity as a risk factor for all cause mortality, and for premature death due to cardiovascular disease, and outlines the compelling evidence for links between physical inactivity and reduced rates of diabetes, cancer, osteoporosis and depression.

The US Surgeon General's report does, however, rely largely on evidence drawn from studies which included only men. This is because the early epidemiological studies in this field, which focused predominantly on physical activity and the prevention of heart disease, included only male subjects. Examples are the early cohort studies of London transport workers and civil servants in the UK, and of the Harvard alumni and San Francisco longshoremen in the US (Morris et al 1966, 1973; Paffenbarger et al 1977, 1984). Indeed, women comprised only 3% of the participants in research relating to the role of physical activity in the prevention of cardiovascular disease that was cited in the US Surgeon General's report.

There is now good evidence to suggest that a graded inverse association exists between physical activity and premature death in women.

This evidence has come from several large US cohort studies, most notably the Iowa Women's Health Study (Kushi et al 1997) and the Nurses' Health Study (Hu et al 2000, Rockhill et al 2001), the results of which have been published since the release of the US Surgeon General's report. The findings of these studies confirm those which were reported earlier for men, indicating a 30–40% reduction in risk of death from heart disease and a 30–50% reduction in risk of stroke, with activity equating to 30 minutes of moderate intensity movement on 5 or more days each week (Hu et al 2000, Kushi et al 1997, Rockhill et al 2001). It is worth noting that the measures of physical activity used in the earlier (largely male) cohort studies tended to focus on somewhat 'male-centred' activities such as organized sport, city blocks walked and stair-climbing at work, or on other activities that are not particularly relevant to older women (Kushi et al 1997, Sesso et al 1999).

The evidence relating to the beneficial role of physical activity in the prevention of diabetes and some forms of cancer has also been strengthened by findings from these US women's cohort studies. Most notably, the Nurses' Health study found that the risk of type 2 diabetes is reduced by 40–50% in women who do more than 30 minutes of daily moderate intensity physical activity (Folsom et al 2000) and that the risk of breast cancer is reduced by 20% in women who report at least 7 hours of moderate intensity activity each week (Rockhill et al 1999).

There are also beneficial effects of physical activity for women in relation to degenerative conditions of the bones and joints. Women have somewhat higher levels of arthritis than men, but the particular risk for older women results from reduced bone mineral density. Low levels of oestrogen in postmenopausal women affect the rate of calcium resorption from bone, leading to reductions in bone mineral density and eventually to osteoporosis, which is responsible for considerable morbidity and mortality, particularly when falls lead to fracture of the hip, wrist and spine (Riggs and Melton 1986). The long-term effects of musculoskeletal disorders have a major impact on women's life expectancy, their quality of life and their ability to live independently. Although physical activity throughout childhood and adult life plays an important role in determining bone mineral density at menopause, the rate of bone loss after menopause can also be reduced by regular weight-bearing activity (Smith et al 1990).

Physical activity is also important for maintaining strength and balance, and thus reducing the risk of falls. When falls occur in women with reduced bone mineral density, they are highly likely to result in fractures, which are more common among older women than older men (National Health and Medical Research Council 1994). Falls are the leading cause of injury-related death and hospitalization for people aged over 65 years, can lead to placement in residential care, and may also lead to low self-esteem, loss of confidence, and avoidance of normal social and physical activities, which in turn can lead to isolation and loneliness (Lilley et al 1995).

There is now good evidence from the Baltimore study of ageing (Gregg et al 1998) and from three population studies in Denmark

(Høidrup et al 2001) that older women who maintain higher levels of energy expenditure, through activities such as walking and gardening, are 30–40% less likely to experience hip fracture than those who are sedentary. The Baltimore study also shows a 37% increase in risk of fracture among older women who spend more than 8 hours each day sitting down.

Physical activity is also an important factor in the alleviation and prevention of conditions that, although minor, can contribute significantly to quality of life. Minor symptoms including backache, headache, joint pain, tiredness, constipation, sleeping problems, and chronic pain are more commonly reported by women than by men (Emslie et al 1999), and all can be relieved by physical activity. Baseline data from the older cohort of the Australian Longitudinal Study of Women's Health (also known as the Women's Health Australia project), which is described in greater detail later in this chapter, show cross-sectional associations between physical activity and all of these symptoms, as well as with urinary incontinence and hypertension (Brown et al 2000).

A further rationale for the promotion of physical activity among older women is its relationship with emotional well-being. It is well established that physical activity is associated positively with emotional well-being and negatively with anxiety and depression, both in research focusing on the acute effects of a single bout of activity and in that dealing with the relationship between regular physical activity and emotional well-being in general (Biddle 2000). A number of physiological mechanisms by which exercise might cause positive mood states and emotional well-being have been proposed. There is a strong suggestion that physical activity improves mental health by improving the body's ability to deal with the physiological effects of stress (Salmon 2001). The evidence suggests that women, and older women in particular, have higher levels of depression and emotional distress than do men, and thus the psychological benefits of activity may be more significant for women than for men.

In general, research on the relationship between physical activity and emotional well-being has focused on young to middle-aged participants, used small and self-selected samples, and focused on people with a lifetime history of physical activity or on groups with identified psychological distress. But work with the older cohort of the Women's Health Australia project (Lee and Russell 2003) has shown that physical activity is associated with higher levels of emotional well-being, even when physical health and other confounders are controlled for.

The links between physical activity and health in older women are clearly illustrated in this cohort by exploration of the relationship between physical activity index and scores on the Short Form 36 Medical Outcomes Survey (SF-36, Ware and Sherbourne 1992), which are shown in Table 2.1. The figures were calculated after exclusion of women who reported 'needing help with daily activities', and thus exclude those who are unable to exercise because of existing disability. The data have been adjusted for potential confounders such as smoking, alcohol consumption, body mass index, country of birth, and area of residence.

Table 2.1   SF-36 physical and mental component summary scores for older participants (70–75 years) in the Australian Longitudinal Study on Women's Health who reported different levels of leisure time physical activity at baseline in 1996 (from Brown et al 2000)

SF-36 Summary score	Physical activity score			
	<5	5 to <15	15 to <25	⩾25
Physical component				
Mean	47.9	50.8	52.0	54.2
(95% CI)	(47.2–48.5)	(50.1–51.4)	(51.4–52.6)	(53.5–54.9)
Mental component				
Mean	48.4	50.0	50.3	50.6
(95% CI)	(47.7–49.0)	(49.4–50.7)	(49.7–51.0)	(49.8–51.4)

Among these older women, it is evident that increasing physical activity is associated with increasing self-reported health, and that there is a larger difference in SF-36 scores between women in the lowest two categories of physical activity than between women in the highest two categories. These data suggest that efforts to activate the most sedentary women will result in a greater population health gain than encouraging those who are already active to do more (Brown et al 2000).

Although there are no consistent sex differences for the risk of dementia, its strong relationship with age means that a higher number of women than men will develop Alzheimer's disease and related dementias. Recent results from the Baltimore study of ageing, and from Canada, show that, compared with those doing the lowest amounts of activity, women in the highest quartile of physical activity have 30–40% reduced risk of significant cognitive decline in their 60s and 70s (Laurin et al 2001, Yaffe et al 2001).

Physical activity and healthy older women

Until now this chapter has addressed a number of reasons why the promotion of physical activity is of particular importance among older women. Before moving on to address physical activity prevalence, it is worth reiterating that most of the health problems which can be alleviated or prevented by physical activity are chronic in nature. Moreover, there is good evidence that health behaviours in the younger and middle years predict longevity and well-being. Thus, we argue that the best way to enhance physical activity levels among older women in future will be to provide opportunities for women to be physically active in young and middle adulthood, and to develop the skills they need to adapt patterns of physical activity to their changing health and life circumstances as they age.

Levels of physical activity among older Australian women

Given the accumulating evidence of the benefits of physical activity for older women, it is interesting to reflect on levels of physical activity among older women in Australia. The most recent data from the Active Australia national physical activity survey show that older women are the least likely of any population group to be adequately active for good health (Armstrong et al 2000). Interestingly, these data show that the proportion of men who obtain sufficient physical activity to benefit their health appears to increase after retirement, whereas for women it does not.

In 1996, the Women's Health Australia research team collected data from three cohorts of women who were then aged 18–23 ($n = 14\,502$), 45–50 ($n = 13\,609$) and 70–75 ($n = 11\,421$). The women were randomly sampled from the Medicare database, with over-sampling of women from rural and remote areas of Australia. They are largely representative of Australian women in the general population (Brown et al 1998). A physical activity index ranging from 0 to 80 was derived from habitual frequency of participation in moderate and vigorous physical activity. On this scale, a score of 3 or 5 was assigned to each weekly session of moderate or vigorous activity, and a score of 15 (which equates with participation in moderate activity five times weekly, or participation in vigorous activity three times a week) was set as the threshold for sufficient physical activity to obtain health benefits. After exclusion of all women who reported needing help with daily care, 55.7% of the young women, 41.7% of the mid-age women, and 43.3% of the older women reached the threshold score of 15 (Brown et al 2000). Figure 2.1 shows the distribution of scores for each cohort. The median scores for the young, mid-age and older women were 15.5, 8 and 7.5 respectively, with first and third quartiles of 8 and 27.5 for the young women, 3 and 20 for the mid-age women, and 3 and 20 for the older women. Hence one quarter of the mid-age and older women were almost completely sedentary (score less than 3). While the data clearly demonstrate a decrease in

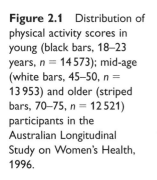

Figure 2.1   Distribution of physical activity scores in young (black bars, 18–23 years, $n = 14\,573$); mid-age (white bars, 45–50, $n = 13\,953$) and older (striped bars, 70–75, $n = 12\,521$) participants in the Australian Longitudinal Study on Women's Health, 1996.

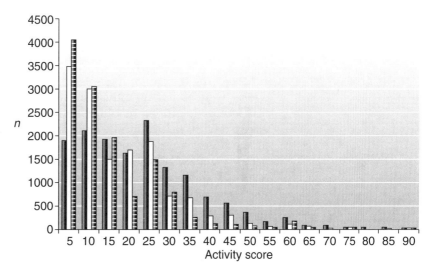

activity with increasing age, the largest difference is between young and mid-age women, rather than between mid-age and older women. The findings of this study have implications for targeting physical activity promotion, suggesting that it is important to develop and introduce promotion strategies at a younger age, to try to prevent the decline in physical activity levels during early adulthood and particularly motherhood, and encourage maintenance of physical activity, if women are to be physically active in older age (Brown et al 2000).

Understanding physical activity among older women

In light of the well-documented health benefits of physical activity, there is a clear need to develop public health strategies which will increase levels of physical activity among older women. While we have already argued that it would be most effective to encourage women to adopt higher levels of activity at an early age, and to maintain these into older age, there is also a clear need to encourage women who are already in their 60s and 70s to be more active. In order to do this, we need to understand more about older women's attitudes to activity, and their perceptions of the barriers to, and benefits of, being more active.

Until recently, women, particularly older women, were somewhat neglected in research on physical activity and its promotion (King et al 1997, Whiteley and Winett 2000) at least in part because of social stereotypes suggesting that exercise is inappropriate or unsafe for older women (O'Brien Cousins, 2000). However, in Australia, the development of a media campaign to promote physical activity for older people, in association with the International Year of Older Persons in 1999, provided an opportunity to learn more about older people's understanding of and preferences for physical activity, through a series of focus groups conducted with older men and women in Newcastle, New South Wales (Brown et al 1999).

The most common activities among the women in these groups were walking, gardening and housework, though many participated in organized activities such as golf, dancing, and lawn bowls and in individual recreational activities such as swimming. Both women and men saw community work and caring for grandchildren as important opportunities for physical activity. Health, social support, 'doing something useful', enjoying the environment, and avoiding the negative stereotypes of ageing were the main motivations for physical activity. Barriers to physical activity identified by older women included poor health, no-one to exercise with, inappropriate or unsafe environments and facilities, and lack of interest. Providing and receiving social support, through being active together, was seen by many of the women as a motivation for activity ('*The social contact means you are using your mind as well as your muscles … contact is important for older people*'), and lack of someone to exercise with was seen as one of the most important barriers. This was especially true for women who had been recently widowed: '*We did a lot of walking … once he died I did not have the time or the inclination to go and do it.*' In addition to loss of a husband, death of the family dog was also cited as an initiator of sedentariness: *'I used to walk my dog every day but when he died I stopped'* and one suggestion for promoting more physical activity was *'to forget the television and buy everyone a dog'*.

The beliefs about benefits and risks of physical activity which were raised in these focus groups with Australian women are similar to those reported by O'Brien Cousins (2000) for a sample of older Canadian women. In her study, O'Brien Cousins found that most older women recognized the broad health benefits of different types of physical activity, but many reported medical reasons why they personally should be excused from 'fitness-promoting' exercise. In some instances, the fear that being more active might be dangerous stemmed from real fragility or medical problems. There was, however, more often a lack of experience with physical activity, concern about 'looking foolish', and a fear of accidents or being assaulted or robbed while out walking. Most of these concerns were also shared by the women in the Australian focus group study (Brown et al 1999).

As the perceived risks of physical activity are very real for older women, any attempt to promote physical activity to this group must acknowledge and address the perceived risks, and must not blame women who have been sedentary during their adult lives for remaining sedentary in older age. Widespread dissemination of information about the small risk of injury and harm, as well as of the benefits of even small increases in physical activity, may help to allay women's fears about becoming more physically active.

Effectiveness of physical activity interventions for older women

Two recent reviews of the effectiveness of interventions to promote increased physical activity among older adults found that many of the studies had important methodological problems (King et al 1998, van der Bij et al 2002). For example, because of the nature of the research, the vast majority of the participants in research studies are already at the stage of motivational readiness to make changes to their activity levels. Few studies have focused on pre-contemplators or those with very low levels of activity. Moreover, few studies have included participants from disadvantaged backgrounds, such as those with low income, or from culturally and linguistically diverse populations, and most interventions have been offered for only 6 months to 1 year, with little long-term follow-up (King et al 1998).

To date, the only study to demonstrate very long-term compliance to a physical activity programme was a randomized control trial of walking, conducted with relatively well-educated, postmenopausal white women in the Pittsburgh area of the USA (Pereira et al 1998). At 10-year follow-up, the median values for time spent walking were significantly higher in the intervention group compared with controls. Although the sample size was small, the authors suggested that there may have been some impact on heart disease, hospitalizations, surgeries and falls among the walking group, though the differences were not statistically significant (Pereira et al 1998).

Data from intervention studies with older women (and men) suggest that home-based, group-based and educational interventions can result in increased levels of physical activity, but that changes are small and short-lived, especially for education-only interventions. Participation rates tend to decline with increased duration of intervention, and longer-term adherence (up to 6 months) appears to be higher in structured classes, or group-based activities. The majority of effective programmes have used a combination of behavioural and/or cognitive tools (such as goal-setting, self-monitoring, feedback, support, and relapse prevention training; King et al 1998).

In the CHAMPS project (Community Healthy Activity Model Program for Seniors), trained staff assisted participants to develop and maintain a regimen that they would be capable of 'sticking with and could participate in throughout their lives' (Stewart et al 2001, p. M466). Not surprisingly, individually tailored choices seem to be most effective in encouraging people to adhere to activity programmes. There would, after all, be little point in trying to get older women to attend a water aerobics programme if they (as some of O'Brien Cousins' participants did) expressed concerns about 'being seen in bathing suit', 'getting water in my ears', or 'a fear of water'. In the CHAMPS project, each participant had the opportunity to attend ten group workshops, in addition to receiving help with their individual programmes. After 1 year, weekly energy expenditure levels were increased by about 500 kcal expended in moderate or more vigorous activities, which is equivalent to adding a 20-minute brisk walk five times a week to baseline levels of activity (Stewart et al 2001).

In our early work with women from non-English-speaking European backgrounds in the Hunter region of New South Wales, we used this approach of combining individually tailored walking programmes with group classes which included exercises for improving strength, balance, agility and flexibility (Brown and Lee 1994, Brown et al 1996). It is likely that interventions of the intensity used in this project (and in the CHAMPS project), with a combination of individual and group-based formats, may be required if long-lasting behaviour change is to be achieved.

In their review, King et al (1998) proposed that home-based or home-plus group-based interventions with telephone reminder strategies for encouraging physical activity show particular promise in terms of behaviour change. In 12 randomized control trials which have used a telephone supervised programme, there is evidence of success in promoting various types of activity, with maintenance of enhanced activity levels for up to 2 years (King et al 1998). They also suggest that alternatives to traditional classes, and more training and supervision of community members who can deliver interventions, will be needed if we are to see changes in population levels of activity in this age group.

While the optimal level of physical activity for health among older women has yet to be defined, results of two of the FICSIT (Frailty and Injuries – Cooperative Studies Intervention Techniques) projects suggest that activities such as tai chi and walking can improve balance and reduce the risk of falling better than any other forms of activity (Buchner et al 1997, Wolff et al 1996). However, in terms of 'best buys' for overall health benefit, there is a general consensus that comprehensive programmes which combine moderate intensity endurance activities with other forms of strength, flexibility and balance training, and tailoring of activities to individual needs and preferences, will be most successful in terms of health benefit (American College of Sports Medicine 1998).

Conclusions

There is now a plethora of evidence to show that regular participation in moderate intensity physical activity will prevent or reduce the declines in functional capacity which accompany ageing, and will help to prevent or control a wide range of chronic diseases. However, levels of physical activity among older women in Western societies are currently very low, and attempts to improve them will require fairly intensive and sustained efforts from a range of stakeholders. A combination of individually tailored and group-based approaches, which incorporate various cognitive behaviour change strategies, shows most promise in terms of sustainable behaviour change. Social support for being more active is also likely to be essential in effecting behaviour change in older women, as exemplified by one of the Women's Health Australia participants:

I have had the same GP for 27 years. Every time I see him he tells me I should do more physical activity. He has been telling me that for 27 years – but I never did anything. Three weeks ago my friend came and picked me up and took me to an exercise class. I have been going now for three weeks and have never felt better – I should have done it earlier – but it was the fact that my neighbour came and picked me up and took me with her. I think the way to get people exercising is to have those who already do it take someone else with them. This will work much better than getting doctors to talk about it.

For optimal physical and mental health benefits, it is likely that programmes which include opportunities for moderate intensity aerobic activity (such as walking), as well as activities designed to improve strength, flexibility and balance, will be required. Regular participation in such activities has the potential to improve functional capacity and quality of life for older women, who are currently the fastest growing, but most sedentary people in Western societies.

References

American College of Sports Medicine 1998 ACSM position stand on exercise and physical activity for older adults. Medicine and Science in Sports and Exercise 30:992–1008

Armstrong T, Bauman A, et al 2000 Physical activity patterns of Australian adults: results of the 1999 National Physical Activity Survey. Australian Institute of Health and Welfare, Canberra

Biddle S 2000 Exercise, emotions, and mental health. In: Hanin Y L, et al (eds) Emotions in sport. Human Kinetics, Champaign, IL, p 267–291

Brown W J, Lee C 1994 Exercise and dietary modification with women of non-English speaking background: a pilot study with Polish-Australian women. International Journal of Behavioral Medicine 1:185–203

Brown W J, Lee C, et al 1996 Exercise and dietary modification with women of non-English speaking background: a heart health program for Greek-Australian women. International Journal of Health Promotion 11:117–125

Brown W J, Bryson L, et al 1998 Women's Health Australia: recruitment for a national longitudinal cohort study. Women and Health 28:23–40

Brown W J, Fuller B, et al 1999 Never too late: older people's perceptions of physical activity. Health Promotion Journal of Australia 9:55–63

Brown W J, Lee C, et al 2000 Leisure-time physical activity in the lives of Australian women: relationship with well-being and symptoms. Research Quarterly for Exercise and Sport 71:206–216

Buchner D M, Cress M E, et al 1997 A comparison of the effects of three types of endurance training on balance and other fall risk factors in older adults. Aging 9:112–119

Emslie C, Hunt K, et al 1999 Gender differences in minor morbidity among full time employees of a British university. Journal of Epidemiology and Community Health 53:465–475

Folsom A R, Kushi L, et al 2000 Physical activity and incident diabetes mellitus in postmenopausal women. American Journal of Public Health 90:134–138

Gibson D, Banham C, et al (eds) 1999 Older Australia at a glance. Australian Institute of Health and Welfare & the Office for Older Australians, Canberra

Gregg E W, Cauley J A, et al 1998 Physical activity and osteoporotic fracture risk in older women. Annals of Internal Medicine 129:81–88

Høidrup S, Sørensen T I A, et al 2001 Leisure-time physical activity levels and changes in relation to risk of hip fracture in men and women. American Journal of Epidemiology 154:60–68

Hu F B, Stampfer M J, et al 2000 Trends in the incidence of coronary heart disease and changes in diet and lifestyle in women. New England Journal of Medicine 343:530–537

King A C, Kiernan M 1997 Physical activity and women's health: issues and future directions. In: Gallant S J, et al (eds) Health care for women: psychological, social, and behavioral influences. American Psychological Association, Washington, DC, p 133–146

King A C, Rejeski W J, et al 1998 Physical activity interventions targeting older adults: a critical review and recommendations. American Journal of Preventive Medicine 15:316–333

Kushi L H, Fee R M, et al 1997 Physical activity and mortality in postmenopausal women. JAMA 277(16):1287–1292

Laurin D, Verreault R, et al 2001 Physical activity and risk of cognitive impairment and dementia in elderly persons. Archives of Neurology 58:498–504

Lee C, Russell A 2003 Effects of physical activity on emotional well-being among older Australian women: cross-sectional and longitudinal analyses. Journal of Psychosomatic Research 54:155–160

Lilley J, Arie T, et al 1995 Accidents involving older people: a review of the literature. Age and Ageing 24:346–365

Morris J N, Kagan A, et al 1966 Incidence and prediction of ischaemic heart disease in London busmen. Lancet ii:553–559

Morris J N, Chave S P W, et al 1973 Vigorous exercise in leisure time and the incidence of coronary heart disease. Lancet i:333–339

National Health and Medical Research Council 1994 Falls and the older person. (Series on clinical management problems in the elderly 6.) Canberra: Commonwealth of Australia

O'Brien Cousins S J 2000 My heart couldn't take it: older women's beliefs about exercise benefits and risks. Journal of Gerontology Series B 55:283–294

O'Brien S J, Vertinsky P A 1991 Unfit survivors: exercise as a resource for aging women. Gerontologist 31:347–357

Paffenbarger R S, Hale W E, et al 1977 Work-energy level, personal characteristics, and fatal heart attack: a birth-cohort effect. American Journal of Epidemiology 105:200–213

Paffenbarger R S, Hyde R T, et al 1984 A natural history of athleticism and cardiovascular health. JAMA 252:491–495

Pereira M A, Kriska A M, et al 1998 A randomized walking trial in postmenopausal women. Archives of Internal Medicine 158:1695–1701

Population Reference Bureau 2000 World Population Datasheet. PRB, Washington, DC (http://www.prb.org/)

Riggs B L, Melton L J 1986 Involutional osteoporosis. New England Journal of Medicine 314:1676–1686

Rockhill B, Willett W C, et al 1999 A prospective study of recreational physical activity and breast cancer risk. Archives of Internal Medicine 159:2290–2296

Rockhill B, Willett W C, et al 2001 Physical activity and mortality: a prospective study among women. American Journal of Public Health 91:578–583

Salmon P 2001 Effects of physical exercise on anxiety, depression, and sensitivity to stress: a unifying theory. Clinical Psychology Review 21:33–61

Sesso H D, Paffenbarger R S, et al 1999 Physical activity and cardiovascular disease risk in middle-aged and older women. American Journal of Epidemiology 150(4):408–416

Smith E L, Smith K A, et al 1990 Exercise, fitness, osteoarthritis, and osteoporosis. In: Bouchard C J, Shephard R J, et al (eds) Exercise, fitness, and health: a consensus of current knowledge. Human Kinetics, Champaign, IL, p 517–528

Stewart A L, Verboncoeur C J, et al 2001 Physical activity outcomes of CHAMPS II: A physical activity promotion program for older adults. Journal of Gerontology: Medical Sciences 56A:M465–470

US Department of Health and Human Services 1996 Physical activity and health: a report of the Surgeon General. US Department of Health and Human Services, Centers for Disease Control and Prevention, National Center for Chronic Disease Prevention and Health Promotion, Atlanta, Georgia

van der Bij A K, Laurant M G H, et al 2002 Effectiveness of physical activity interventions for older adults: a review. American Journal of Preventive Medicine 22:120–133

Ware J E, Sherbourne C D 1992 The MOS 36-item Short-Form Health Survey (SF-36): I. Conceptual framework and item selection. Medical Care 30: 473–483

Whiteley J A, Winett R A 2000 Gender and fitness: enhancing women's health through principled exercise training. In: Eisler R M, et al (eds) Handbook of gender, culture, and health. Lawrence Erlbaum Associates, Mahwah, NJ, p 343–373

Wolff SL, Barnhart H X, et al 1996 Reducing frailty and falls in older persons: an investigation of tai chi and computerized balance training. Journal of the American Geriatrics Society 44:489–497

Yaffe K, Barnes D, et al 2001 A prospective study of physical activity and cognitive decline in elderly women. Archives of Internal Medicine 161:1703–1708

3

Assisting health professionals to promote physical activity and exercise in older people

Colette Browning, David Menzies
and Shane Thomas

CHAPTER CONTENTS

Models of health behaviour change 40

Self-management 49

Promoting physical activity and exercise adherence in older people in clinical and community settings 51

Designing physical activity interventions for older adults 56

Conclusion 58

References 59

Despite the now substantial evidence that physical activity can improve health in later life through risk factor modification, promoting physical activity as an important health behaviour for older people has not had the focus it deserves (Minkler et al 2000). Inactivity contributes to 200 000 deaths per year in the USA (Sallis 2001) and in Australia physical activity is the second most important area for risk factor reduction with regard to the overall burden of disease (Bauman and Smith 2000). The concept of healthy ageing, while discussed in the academic literature for some time, has only recently provided a point of focus in ageing policy (Browning and Kendig 2003). The role of physical activity in promoting healthy ageing has been discussed by Bauman in this book and elsewhere (Bauman and Smith 2000). If we accept that physical activity and exercise interventions can postpone or reduce the burden of disability and illness in old age, then the role of health professionals in promoting physical activity is central in achieving the goal of healthy ageing for older people.

The aim of this chapter is to provide health professionals working with older people with information and guidelines about facilitating behaviour change as it pertains to initiating or increasing levels of physical activity and exercise in their older clients. The focus is on clinical and community settings rather than on mass media health promotion programmes. The chapter illustrates the major issues for health professionals in changing client behaviour and provides guidelines for the design of physical activity interventions in the community or clinic.

Health professionals working with older people have the opportunity to promote physical activity and exercise in their clients not only as a prescription for specific medical conditions or injuries but also as a way of promoting healthy ageing in the community. For many older clients, increasing physical activity will contribute significantly to their health. For the older person with arthritis, improving function and pain management may require the client to adopt new behaviours such as increased physical activity and relaxation techniques. Older people with hypertension need to manage medication and increase their levels of physical activity. Following fracture people are prescribed therapeutic exercises that may not be part of their behavioural repertoire. People with diabetes are required to monitor their diet and engage in physical activity. At the population level, one of the goals for health promotion practitioners is to reduce inactivity and promote physical activity in everyday life.

In promoting physical activity and exercise, health professionals attempt to elicit behaviour change. This may involve encouraging older people to increase the amount of activity in their everyday life through walking and other moderate activities, prescribing specific exercises to improve strength and balance (Bauman and Smith 2000) or prescribing specific exercises for rehabilitation after injury.

Promoting behaviour change is not an easy task for health professionals who often work in contexts where resources, particularly time resources, are scarce. Many clinicians are finding that their caseloads have an increasing proportion of older adults with chronic illnesses. The impact of this on general medical practitioners (GPs), for example, is an increasing requirement to provide disease-specific interventions as well as general lifestyle advice (Eakin 2001). For allied health professionals, such as physiotherapists, occupational therapists and podiatrists, older people may be referred to therapy for a specific condition or injury yet present with other co-morbidities that need to be considered in their health management plan. Despite some exceptions, the training of health professionals often does not pay detailed attention to the complexities of human behaviour and how the practitioner can work with the patient to achieve behaviour change.

A prescription of 'You need to loose weight. Cut down on the fat in your diet and do more exercise' assumes that behaviour change is the responsibility of the person alone and that the authority of the practitioner is sufficient to effect these changes. Health professionals, especially GPs, may be credible sources of information about exercise for older adults (Booth et al 1997). Many other factors, however, influence the propensity to change. Health practitioners need to examine their role in these communications and view the solution to a patient problem as an opportunity to work in a partnership. As Rollnick et al (2000, p. 7) noted 'Behaviour change, or the lack of it, is not just the patient's problem.' The relatively recent concept of self-management of chronic disease (based largely on behaviour change principles), while assuming that clients can be enabled and desire to take control of their illness, also assumes a central role for the practitioner in training specific disease management and lifestyle skills in older people.

In order to set the context for achieving behaviour change in health settings, it is necessary to examine the underlying models that inform behaviour change practice. The literature on self-management and the role of the practitioner in training and supporting self-management behaviours for particular chronic illnesses in older people will also be examined. Finally, examples of physical activity interventions for older people will be presented and a summary of the principles and practices that need to be incorporated in physical activity interventions for older people will be included.

Models of health behaviour change

A fundamental task for health professionals working with older people is to promote behaviour change. Whether working with older patients with chronic illnesses or disabilities or those who are relatively healthy, in order to promote health and well-being, the practitioner needs to understand the prescribed therapy/intervention in terms of how to assist the person to adopt new behaviours.

As pointed out by Rollnick et al (2000) it is not sufficient simply to give people advice and expect that the authority of the health professional will translate into behaviour change. In order to promote behaviour change, the health practitioner needs to be familiar with the underlying models about how health behaviours, attitudes and the social contexts are linked in bringing about change. It is not appropriate to provide a lengthy treatise on all of the models. The reader is referred to Conner and Norman (1995), Norman et al (2000) and Prochaska and Velicer (1997) for a more detailed discussion of the various models of behaviour change. However, several models usefully inform the present discussion. These include the health belief model, the theory of planned behaviour, health locus of control/self-efficacy and the stages of change model.

Health belief model

The health belief model asserts that whether people will take preventive action to avoid or modify the effects of illness depends upon several factors (Becker and Maiman 1975, Harrison et al 1992, Janz and Becker 1984, Rosenstock et al 1988). These include:

- the person's perceived seriousness of the health problem, and
- the person's perceived susceptibility to the health problem.

According to the health belief model, these two factors are combined to form a judgement about the perceived threat of the illness or injury. In other words, if you consider an illness not to be serious or unlikely to occur, it is unlikely that you will invest in a major effort to avoid it.

Moderating the decision to take preventive health actions is the person's perception of the costs (the negative utility or barriers) associated with the behaviour required to avoid or moderate the illness and the perceived benefits that would be accrued if an action was taken. These costs might include a large amount of effort, loss of enjoyment or monetary expense. Benefits might include improving mobility, feeling healthier and reducing healthcare costs. In a later version of the model health motivation or how ready an individual is to be concerned about health matters was added (Conner and Norman 1995). Thus under the health belief model, the person makes an individual decision concerning the balance between the perceived benefits, the perceived threat (susceptibility and severity) and the barriers to action. Perceived susceptibility, perceived severity, health motivation, perceived benefits and perceived barriers are all influenced by demographic variables (age, gender, etc.) and personal characteristics (e.g. personality, response to peers, etc.). The health belief model further asserts that cues to action such as mass media publicity campaigns, exposure to the negative consequences of illness, health worker advice and so on can initiate preventive actions.

Figure 3.1 shows how the health belief model can be applied to an older woman who is overweight and at risk for diabetes. She has been

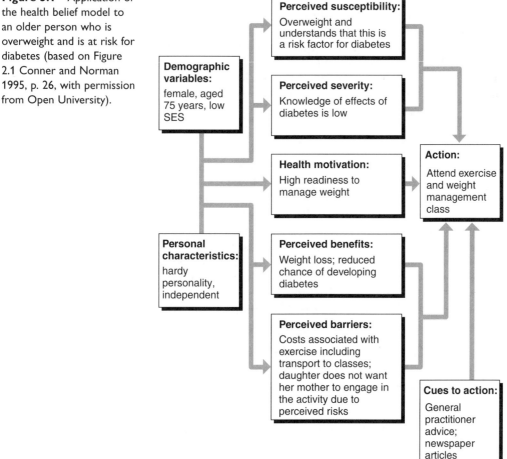

Figure 3.1 Application of the health belief model to an older person who is overweight and is at risk for diabetes (based on Figure 2.1 Conner and Norman 1995, p. 26, with permission from Open University).

advised by her GP (cue to action) to attend a weight management and exercise class (action). She read an article in the local newspaper about the benefits of physical activity for older people (cue to action). The woman understands that being overweight is not healthy and that reducing her weight would reduce her risks for diabetes (perceived susceptibility) but has low knowledge of the effects of diabetes (perceived severity). Her daughter has expressed negative views (fear of injury to the mother) about her mother exercising and the woman is not sure how she will get to the exercise classes (perceived barrier). In this case, the health practitioner would need to help the woman understand the effects of diabetes, that is, increase her knowledge about the perceived severity of the condition. Additional social support would need to be provided to counter the lack of support for the activity from the woman's daughter. Barriers related to access to the exercise programme would need to be addressed.

Therefore, in the context of the health belief model, the health professional wishing to induce behaviour change should provide information about the severity of the problem and the person's susceptibility to disease or disability, provide cues to action by providing information about the negative consequences of the disease (or not engaging in the health behaviour), provide information about the positive consequences of preventive actions (benefits), and address barriers to action.

This cognitive model provides a common sense approach to behaviour change and has contributed to a range of interventions over the last 30 or so years. However, a criticism of the model is that it does not take into account social and emotional influences on behaviour or distinguish between direct and indirect cognitive influences on behaviour (Conner and Norman 1995).

The theory of reasoned action/ planned behaviour

Ajzen and Fishbein's model, the theory of reasoned action, asserts that the person's intention to perform a particular action is the best predictor of whether they will perform that action. In other words, what you intend to do, you are likely to do (Ajzen and Fishbein 1980). This assumption is really a restatement of the definition of an attitude. An attitude is an intention to behave in a certain predisposed manner. So it is hardly a controversial statement to claim that intentions precede actions as proposed by this theory.

The theory of reasoned action assumes that people's intentions to perform actions are determined by two attitudes:

- the attitude concerning the intrinsic value of the action to the person (attitude towards the behaviour), and
- attitudes about the social appropriateness of the action (the subjective norm).

A later development of the model, the theory of planned behaviour, incorporated perceived behavioural control as an added component (Ajzen 1991). Control beliefs are influenced by factors that may inhibit or enhance the target behaviour, for example, skills, information, opportunities and barriers.

Thus, if the person believes that exercise is a good thing to do because it is likely to lead to health benefits and the person's friends and family themselves exercise and they believe that they have access to resources/opportunities to perform the target behaviour successfully, then it is likely that they will form a behavioural intention to exercise. If, on the other hand, the person holds the beliefs that the health benefits of exercise are not evident, that it is not the social norm to exercise, or that they do not have the resources to perform the behaviour, then they may not do so. A behaviour change programme based on this model would attempt to change these beliefs perhaps by presenting information to challenge them.

Figure 3.2 shows how the theory of planned behaviour could be applied to an older person who has experienced falls in the previous year and has been advised by a physiotherapist to take up strength training to improve lower limb strength and balance. In this example, the older person holds a negative attitude to strength training. The older person's children also express negative social norms about strength training. However, the older person believes that they can access the weight-training programme offered in the community. The physiotherapist would need to challenge negative attitudes and demonstrate that strength training will improve strength and balance and assist in falls management.

The theory of planned behaviour, like the health belief model, has been subject to extensive empirical testing (Ajzen 1991, Sheppard et al 1988). Criticisms of the theory include the focus on perceived control rather than actual control and the neglect of the influence of broader social and structural influences on behaviour (Conner and Norman 1995).

Figure 3.2 Application of the theory of planned behaviour to an older person who is a faller and needs to do strength training to improve lower limb strength and balance.

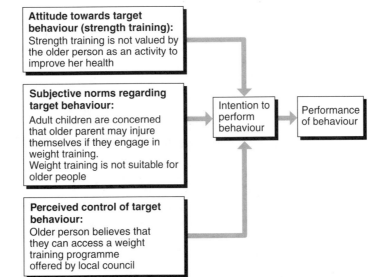

Health locus of control and self-efficacy

Other models of health behaviour change are based on the related concepts of health locus of control and self-efficacy.

The health locus of control model was developed by Wallston and Wallston (see Wallston and Wallston 1984). It was based on Rotter's earlier work on general locus of control. This model assumes that people's beliefs about whether they can control what happens to them through their own actions influences behaviour.

People with high internal health locus of control tend to believe that their destiny (health) is controlled by their own actions. In other words, people with high internal locus of control believe that they can determine their own health outcomes through their own actions. People with high external locus of control tend to believe their health is determined by forces outside their control. These forces may include other people, fate, genetics, divine intervention and so on. Individuals with high external health locus of control may be less motivated to change their behaviour or to take preventive health actions because they believe that it is likely to be ineffective. Why worry when you can't change things?

The health locus of control construct is quite similar to the theoretical construct of self-efficacy (Bandura 1994) with one important difference. Health locus of control is assumed to be generalized, like a personality trait. On the other hand, efficacy is content specific. People with high self-efficacy in a particular domain believe that they can effectively do whatever is required of them to enhance that specific domain. Thus, within the self-efficacy framework, high self-efficacy beliefs are associated with a propensity to change specific health behaviours and take action whereas low self-efficacy beliefs are not.

It does not make sense to state that a person has high or low self-efficacy without stating which particular actions and beliefs are under consideration. It is efficacy with respect to specific actions, rather than a 'general' efficacy. Wallston (1992) revised his health locus of control model to match more closely the domain-specific underpinnings of the self-efficacy model, after research showed that general locus of control measures were poor predictors of specific health actions.

Health behaviour change interventions based on the health locus of control and the self-efficacy models should focus on convincing the person that they have the personal resources required to act in the required manner. In other words, effort should be put into convincing the person that they can change and that it will make a difference to their health. To improve an older person's self-efficacy with respect to exercise, behaviour change needs to be managed in small steps (behavioural shaping). A method of managing behaviour change is to ask the person what they are 100% confident of achieving in a given week (self-efficacy). In the case of a sedentary older person behavioural contracting could be used to successively approximate the target behaviour and improve self-efficacy. For example, if the target behaviour is walking for 30 minutes on most days of the week, in the first week the target may be to walk for 10 minutes three times per week. This would be negotiated with the older person in a way that ensured that for the target behaviour in that week, the older person was 100% certain that he/she could achieve the goal. Initial targets need to be lowered until the person is 100% confident that they can achieve the target behaviour. In the second week, the person's self-efficacy should be improved based on successfully achieving their goals from the previous week. At this point the exercise goal for the second week can be increased. This procedure is repeated over successive weeks. Using this technique is a form of behavioural contracting where the older person makes a commitment to achieve set goals each week.

The stages of change model

The transtheoretical model of behavioural change proposed by Prochaska and Di Clemente has four central tenets (Prochaska and Di Clemente 1984, Prochaska and Velicer 1997).

The first tenet is that people vary in the speed of adoption of health-related behaviours. The sequence of changes proposed by the model is:

- pre-contemplation (the person is not practising nor planning to practise the target health behaviour)
- contemplation (the person is not practising but is considering the practice of the target health behaviour)
- preparation (the person is preparing actively to initiate the behaviour)
- action (the person adopts the target health behaviour)
- maintenance (the person maintains the target health behaviour for an extended period).

The second tenet of the stages of change model is that ten processes (five experiential and five behavioural) can be identified that therapists and other people use to achieve behaviour change (Burkholder and Nigg 2002, Prochaska and Di Clemente 1984). *Consciousness-raising* may involve, for example, obtaining information about the problem behaviour to assess its impact (e.g. the impact of sedentary behaviour on heart disease). *Dramatic relief* occurs when one has an emotional response to an event (e.g. knowing someone who had a heart attack due to lack of physical fitness). *Environmental re-evaluation* occurs when the person assesses the impact of the behaviour on his or her environment (e.g. the person may not be able to play sport with their children due to being unfit). *Self-re-evaluation* occurs when the person considers the impact of the behaviour on himself/herself (e.g. being unfit makes the person feel tired and unhappy). *Social liberation* involves recognition of the changes in societal norms with respect to the behaviour (e.g. recognizing the increased advertising regarding the promotion of healthy lifestyles by government and private industry). *Counter-conditioning* involves substituting the problem behaviour with the target behaviour (e.g. watching television after dinner is replaced with going for a walk). *Helping relationships* describes the process of seeking social support for the target behaviour (e.g. joining a group exercise programme). *Reinforcement management* involves setting up a reward system to reinforce the target behaviour (e.g. engaging in a favourite activity at the end of each week after walking for 30 minutes on most days during the week). *Self-liberation* involves making a commitment to change (e.g. telling your spouse that you are going to commence an exercise programme). *Stimulus control* involves altering the environment to provide cues for the target behaviour (e.g. placing exercise bike in the television room).

Prochaska and Di Clemente (1984) proposed that different processes are used at the various stages and that this enables interventions to be tailored for the individual. For example, at the pre-contemplation stage all processes are used less often, at the contemplation stage *consciousness-raising, self-re-evaluation* and *dramatic relief* are used to move to the preparation stage and at the action stage, *stimulus control, reinforcement management, counter-conditioning* and *self-liberation* are used (Burkholder and Nigg 2002).

The third main tenet of the model is the notion of decisional balance. Balance is assumed to be the sum of the positive and negative features of the target health behaviour. To assess decisional balance, a person is asked a series of questions that identify the positive (e.g. 'I feel better if I exercise') and negative (e.g. 'I would feel self-conscious if people saw me exercising') aspects of the target behaviour. In the action and maintenance stages of the model it is assumed that the decisional balance is positive (i.e. positive features of the target behaviour outweigh the negative features). For the pre-contemplation and contemplation stages the balance is negative. Self-efficacy is the fourth component of the model and incorporates confidence in maintaining the new behaviour and resisting the temptation to relapse.

Progress through the stages of the model may occur in both forward and reverse directions. The model is useful in identifying the motivational readiness of the person to adopt a new behaviour. The type of intervention required depends on where in the sequence of changes the person is situated (i.e. what is their motivational readiness to change). For contemplators, it would be important to help the person evaluate the costs and benefits associated with physical activity while for those who are already engaged in sufficient physical activity, the intervention would need to address behavioural strategies to enhance maintenance. For example, maintenance could be enhanced by increasing social support, developing a reward system or using stimulus control (Burkholder and Nigg 2002).

Figure 3.3 shows how the stages of change model can be used to describe the stages an older person may go through in order to increase her physical activity levels. To use this model the practitioner needs to first identify at what stage the older person is in the stages of change. Various short, easy-to-use questionnaires are available in the literature that can be used for this identification process (Nigg and Riebe 2002). The practitioner would also need to identify the processes that the person uses with respect to physical activity habits. For example, does the person read articles to learn more about physical activity (*consciousness raising*)? Does the person believe that physical activity will make then healthier (*self-re-evaluation*)? Does the person use a calendar to schedule physical activity time (*stimulus control*)? The practitioner would then tailor the intervention to move the person to the next stage (e.g. contemplation to preparation) by incorporating experiences (processes of change)

Figure 3.3 Application of the stages of change model to an older person who needs to increase her level of physical activity.

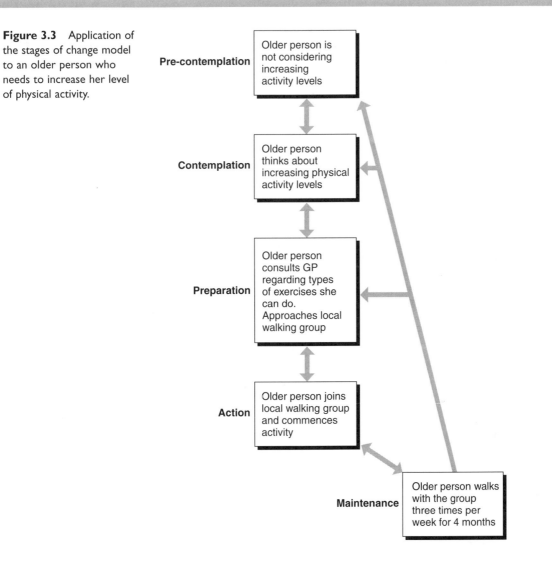

that affect physical activity habits. Nigg and Reibe (2002) provide a questionnaire that identifies the person's processes of change associated with physical activity.

The stages of change model has been used in a wide range of settings. Prochaska et al (1992), in a major review of behaviour change studies using their model, concluded that most people fail in their attempts to change health behaviours and that the great majority at any one time are not engaged with health service providers.

In conclusion, if health professionals want to assist their patients to change attitudes and behaviour, it is important that they are informed by knowledge of the underlying theories of behaviour change. Table 3.1 summarizes the implications for physical activity interventions of each for the models.

Rollnick et al (2000) provide a comprehensive guidebook for practitioners who want to learn more about behaviour change in health

Table 3.1 Summary table of implications of health behaviour models for physical activity interventions

Health behaviour model	Assumptions of model	Strategies required in behaviour change programme
Health belief model	Person takes health actions on basis of assessment of ■ perceived seriousness of health problem ■ perceived susceptibility to health problem ■ perceptions of costs of health actions ■ health motivation	■ emphasize serious consequences of disease ■ ensure person understands at risk groups and concepts ■ emphasize ease of preventive actions
Theory of planned behaviour	Person takes health actions based on assessment of ■ attitudes concerning intrinsic value of health action ■ perceptions of social appropriateness of the action ■ perceived control beliefs	■ emphasize benefits of health actions ■ emphasize other influential figures who undertake these actions (e.g. appeal to authority)
Health locus of control/self-efficacy	Person takes health actions based on assessment of ■ whether the health consequences are alterable by one's own behaviour ■ whether the person can perform the required actions	■ include case studies of improved health through preventive actions ■ promote self-efficacy through case studies ■ used staged behaviour change approach to increase self-efficacy
Prochaska and Di Clemente model of stages of change	Behaviour change goes through the following stages ■ pre-contemplation ■ contemplation ■ preparation ■ action ■ maintenance	The following are adapted from Dunlap and Barry (1999) and Jordan and Nigg (2002) ■ identify stage of change and incorporate stage-specific *processes* ■ elicit positive and negative aspects of target behaviour(s) and provide simple information (*consciousness raising, dramatic relief*) ■ motivate and elicit commitment ■ enhance self-efficacy ■ identify classes for older people (*social liberation*) ■ identify goals and plan start date and type of physical activity ■ use social support (*helping relationships*) ■ use *stimulus control* ■ review goals and suggest coping strategies for fatigue, discomfort, lack of motivation, etc. ■ praise high self-efficacy ■ use *reinforcement management, counter-conditioning and stimulus control* ■ review coping strategies and reassess goals and physical activity type

settings. The book uses the stages of change model and focuses on two influences on readiness to change, namely the importance of the behaviour change to the person being treated and the confidence of the person in changing their behaviour. One of the roles of the practitioner is to increase the person's motivation to change. Although a general guide for practice, the methods are appropriate for use with older clients to increase physical activity and promote therapeutic exercise compliance. Burbank and Riebe (2002) also provide a practical overview of promoting exercise in older people using the stages of change model. One of the chapters in that book (Jordan and Nigg 2002) specifically addresses how to tailor physical activity interventions for older adults at different stages of motivational readiness.

Behaviour change is also fundamental to the concept of self-management of disease and disability that has its origins in the important role of patient education in health care (Holman and Lorig 2000). Older clients are likely to present with at least one chronic illness or disability (Hoffman et al 1996) and it is therefore important for the health professional to understand the principles of self-management and how they apply to promoting physical activity and exercise.

Self-management

Self-management is recognized as a common model for managing chronic disease and changing health behaviours (Battersby et al 2002) and Jayasuriya et al (2001a) provide a comprehensive review of the chronic disease self-management literature. Physical activity is a significant component of many self-management programmes, especially in the older adult population where those over 65 have at least one chronic health condition such as diabetes, cardiovascular disease, musculoskeletal problems or decreased mental health (Australian Institute for Health and Welfare 2000, World Health Organization 2002). Each of these conditions can be attenuated through the effects of physical activity, resulting in improved management of the condition and delayed loss of physical function (Battersby et al 2002). Health professionals can make use of the concepts of chronic disease self-management and apply them to their older clients, especially in the realm of physical activity.

There are numerous definitions of self-management and there is still some contention over what constitutes best practice for chronic illness (Brown 1999). Gruman and Von Korff (1996, p. 1) stated that self-management can be defined as 'engaging in activities that protect and promote health, monitoring and managing of symptoms and signs of illness, managing the impacts of illness on functioning, emotions and interpersonal relationships and adhering to treatment regimes'. Ruggiero et al (1997) describe self-management as a process of using a number of behaviours and skills to manage illness. Others emphasize the role of partnerships between the client and the health practitioners involved in their care (Von Korff et al 1997).

Many self-management programmes have focused on educational interventions and knowledge outcomes, with little attention paid to incorporating behaviour change models in the design of the intervention. Yet many commentators have argued that behaviour change models are important in self-management programmes (Jayasuriya et al 2001b). Von Korff et al (1997) emphasized the importance of collaboration between the client, their family and the health professional in setting goals and planning actions to achieve these goals. The client must have correct knowledge about their condition and the value of the behaviours that they will engage in. They also need to be educated in the skills to implement self-management behaviours and ongoing support should be provided. Jayasuriya et al (2001b) point out that the adoption of new health behaviours and self-management skills is a process rather than a single event. The health and circumstances of an older person may change over time and ongoing monitoring and follow-up is needed to maintain change. This observation is consistent with the stages of change model discussed earlier in the chapter.

The necessity for older people to feel some sense of control in their own health care is also a consistent theme throughout the self-management literature. A number of studies have focused on patient empowerment, and the issue of control is a consistent element when addressing health behaviour change (Anderson et al 1997, Feder et al 2000). However, as shown by Paterson (2001) in an investigation of the self-care decision-making of people with diabetes, practitioners may discount the knowledge gained by the experienced client and not create the consultative setting conducive to informed decision-making. For older adults who have grown up in a period where consumer participation in health was not promoted, difficulties may arise in accepting control of their own health. Health professionals need to be sensitive to these potential cohort differences.

The importance of chronic illness management as a concern for health policy makers is illustrated by some recent initiatives in Australia. In Australia, the Federal Government have committed funds to a trial of several chronic disease self-management projects that incorporate general practitioners and allied health professionals working in partnership with their clients to manage various chronic illnesses such as arthritis, diabetes and heart disease (Department of Health and Aged Care 2000). All projects incorporate behaviour change principles and use models such as the stages of change model and Lorig's chronic disease self-management model (Lorig et al 1993). Eight demonstration projects targeting people aged 50 years and over with cardiovascular disease, diabetes, arthritis, osteoporosis, or respiratory disorders have been funded. In Victoria 'The Good Life Club' recruits older people with diabetes and a co-morbidity of cardiovascular disease. General practitioners initiate a care plan and participants are allocated to a 'coach' whose task is to help the clients learn self-management skills including blood sugar monitoring and management, healthy eating habits and increased physical activity. The intervention incorporates the stages of change model and coaches are trained in the skills necessary to identify stages and to assist clients to move through the stages. All demonstration projects are currently under evaluation and it is expected that initial outcomes will be available by 2004.

In summary, although personal responsibility is a key theme in self-management, health professionals have a central role to play in assisting older people to develop and maintain the skills needed for self-management (Holman and Lorig 2000). Collaboration between the person, their family and practitioner is an important element of self-management. Older people and practitioners need to recognize the importance of individualized programmes gained through personally living with the condition, and respect the insight of 'what works for me' in learning self-management skills (Price 1993). As such, health professionals need to overcome professional distance and value the perceptions of the older person. Finally, self-management programmes need to incorporate behaviour change principles and practices in order to maximize outcomes for older people.

The next section of the chapter examines physical activity interventions for older people that have included behaviour change principles in their design.

Promoting physical activity and exercise adherence in older people in clinical and community settings

So far the factors that influence health behaviours through an examination of the various behaviour change models have been discussed. It has been shown that the concept of self-management of chronic illness can incorporate behaviour change principles and that for many older clients physical activity prescription may be a central part of managing their chronic conditions. How can the health practitioner incorporate these ideas into their own practice with older people? First, the factors affecting the initiation and maintenance of physical activity will be examined. Second, the research literature that evaluates physical activity interventions in older adults will be presented. The setting for the majority of physical activity interventions for older adults reported in the research literature has been in primary care where a GP initiates the intervention and other health professionals may be involved. Finally the factors in the design of physical activity interventions that contribute most to successful outcomes will be drawn together.

Factors affecting initiation and maintenance of physical activity

The older adult is confronted with many barriers to the *initiation* of physical activity. These factors can be classified as individual, social and structural (Dunlap and Barry 1999). Individual factors include: disability due to chronic conditions, for example problems with communication due to hearing or visual impairments; negative beliefs about the benefits of activity and the amount of activity necessary for health benefits; low self-efficacy beliefs; perceptions that exercise is unpleasant and not enjoyable; not having engaged in physical activity for some time; and fears associated with injury caused by exercise (Dunlap and Barry 1999). For example, Bruce et al (2002) found that fear of falling was independently associated with low levels of physical activity in community-dwelling older women.

Social barriers include societal stereotypes regarding activity in older people, social isolation, lack of role models and negative attitudes of family, friends and health professionals. Booth et al (1997) found that support from family and friends was an important determinant of physical activity in older adults. Chogahara (1999) found that negative messages about physical activity from health professionals had detrimental effects on physical activity in older adults. Older people may be more vulnerable to negative advice from health professionals if their health is under threat (Chogahara 1999). Seeman (2000) also concluded that negative influences from family, friends and health professionals can have detrimental effects on the health of older people. Structural barriers are also important and include access to appropriate venues for activity, neighbourhood safety, transport and socio-economic disadvantage (Dunlap and Barry 1999). From the health professional's perspective, it is necessary to take all these factors into account when prescribing physical activity or specific exercises to the older client (Resnick 2001).

The factors associated with the *maintenance* of physical activity have also received attention in the research literature. Marcus et al (2000, p. 38) concluded that although 'Some behavioral strategies may be more important for the maintenance phase compared with the initiation phase ... it is critical that future studies provide information on the greatest barriers to the initiation of activity and short-term and long-term maintenance of physical activity behavior.' There are a number of factors that contribute to the lack of long-term maintenance of physical activity. Providing information about the benefits of physical activity or using authority to influence client behaviours does not directly address the barriers to maintenance. These approaches may trigger the client to commence a physical activity programme. However, once a specific behaviour is established, it may be necessary to change the reward structures to maintain that behaviour or introduce specific coping skills that address relapse. For example, in a study of women college students, those who had fewer coping mechanisms for dealing with stressful situations were more likely to drop out of exercise classes (Simkin and Gross 1994). Litt et al (2002), in a study of exercise behaviour in older women, found that maintenance of exercise at 12-month follow-up was associated with social support.

The type of physical activity programme has been shown to impact on long-term maintenance. King et al (1995) assigned people aged 50 to 65 years to one of three activity groups: a high-intensity structured exercise group conducted in a community setting, a high intensity home-based programme or a moderated intensity home-based programme. The home-based programmes were supervised via telephone support. At 1-year follow-up participants in the home-based programmes were more adherent than those in the community-based programme and at 2-year follow-up the high-intensity home-based group were more adherent than the moderate intensity home-based group. Those who showed less stress and were more unfit at baseline were more likely to be adherent at the 2-year follow-up.

In a review of rehabilitation interventions, Marcus et al (2000) concluded that exercise adherence (maintenance) was associated with staff contact, supervision of exercises, using moderate-intensity exercises and including behavioural principles in the design of the intervention. Jordan and Nigg (2002) point out that individuals who reach the maintenance phase of the stages of change model show very high levels of confidence in their ability to maintain physical activity. They suggest that at this stage older people need to be reminded of the strategies they used to resist relapse. The following techniques have also been highlighted by Jordan and Nigg (2002) as important in the maintenance phase:

■ *counter-conditioning* (if the person doubts their ability to maintain physical activity then suggest a relaxing activity)
■ *reinforcement management* (use personal rewards for good habits)
■ *helping relationships* (use family and friends as reinforcers of behaviour)
■ *stimulus control* (use lists of benefits of physical activity, pictures of role models in prominent places in the home).

Physical activity interventions for older adults

In this section, specific examples of physical activity interventions for older adults are examined. Most physical activity interventions for older adults that are reported in the research literature have occurred in general practice settings. General practitioners are in a key position to help older people to modify lifestyle risk factors such as physical activity, as they have a high rate of contact with the general public. In Australia 83% of the adult population visits a GP yearly (Bauman et al 2002). However, in a study of older community-dwelling adults in the USA, less than 50% had ever received advice to exercise from their physician (Damush et al 1999). Not only are general practitioners in an appropriate situation to provide such information, but they are regarded by patients as a confidant, respected for their knowledge and are often approached by those who are concerned about their lifestyle. The GP is seen as a credible and preferred source of health information and in particular physical activity information, especially amongst older patients (Booth et al 1997). However, although the GP may act as a 'gatekeeper' in the healthcare system, it is important that GPs form partnerships with other health professionals in assisting their patients to affect behaviour change.

Most physical activity interventions for older adults in healthcare settings involve providing advice and varying degrees of counselling with or without written materials (Eakin 2001). In a review of physical activity interventions in primary care settings Eakin et al (2000) concluded that advice and counselling results in relatively short-term increases in physical activity with little evidence of long-term maintenance. As indicated above, incorporating behavioural principles can strengthen the efficacy of the intervention.

Halbert et al (2000) conducted a randomized controlled trial of individualized physical activity advice given to patients aged 60 years and over recruited from two general practice settings. Both the intervention and control group received a 20-minute session with an exercise specialist. The intervention incorporated elements of the health belief model and the theory of planned behaviour. The intervention group received information about the benefits of physical activity and an exercise plan. Barriers to engaging in physical activity and strategies for overcoming barriers were discussed with each person. The exercise plan approach incorporated modest targets that would be increased over time. Members of the control group were given a pamphlet about nutrition. Follow-up at 3 and 6 months included a mail-out questionnaire and the intervention group was given the option of an interview. Interviews for all participants were conducted at 12-month follow-up. Halbert et al (2000) found that physical activity increased over a 12-month period in both the intervention and control group, with the greater increase in physical activity occurring in the intervention group.

The stages of change model has been used in a number of physical activity interventions. As discussed earlier in the chapter, the model allows stage targeting and stage tailoring (Nigg and Riebe 2002). People are assessed according to the stage of change they occupy and the intervention is tailored to account for the person's processes that support behaviour change, self-efficacy and decisional balance. Some examples of physical activity interventions that use this model are discussed below.

A non-randomized controlled trial of physician counselling to promote physical activity in healthy sedentary clients included 98 participants in an intervention group and 114 controls (Calfas et al 1996). The intervention participants received 3 to 5 minutes of counselling with a follow-up booster phone call from a health educator. The PACE (Physician-based Assessment and Counselling for Exercise) programme utilized in this study incorporated psychosocial factors from the health belief model and the theory of planned behaviour, and the self-efficacy concept. These factors include increasing social support to be active from family and friends, increasing self-efficacy, reducing barriers to activity and increasing knowledge of the benefits of activity. PACE also incorporates the stages of change model and involves the completion of a 'stages of change' assessment by the patient while in the waiting room. The patient answers 11 graded statements about physical activity (e.g. not active at the moment and do not intend to become active, through to physically active on a regular basis). This information is then used by the physician to tailor the counselling to one of three stages of change: pre-contemplation, contemplation or action. Measures of the stage of readiness to adopt physical activity and self-reported physical activity levels were taken at baseline and at 4- to 6-week follow-ups. Whereas the intervention group showed a mean increase in walking time of 37 minutes per week the control group only increased their walking time by 7 minutes per week. This brief structured behavioural change intervention was considered efficacious as it increased readiness to adopt physical activity in the intervention group. However, the intervention did not incorporate long-term follow-up to assess maintenance of change in walking.

Two other physical activity interventions are worthy of mention as they incorporate some key factors that appear consistently in the literature as leading to successful interventions and lend themselves to easy integration in primary care. These factors include tailoring of interventions to individual preferences, maximizing enjoyment and incorporating behaviour change principles in the intervention. The Community Healthy Activities Model Program for Seniors (CHAMPS) (Stewart et al 1998, 2001) and work by the Activity Counselling Trial (ACT) Research Group (King et al 1997, Activity Counselling Trial Research Group 2001) have led to sustained increases in physical activity in older adults.

CHAMPS is a community-based physical activity intervention for older people (aged 65 to 90 years) that incorporates individual tailoring of physical activity that is sensitive to the participant's health status, activity preference (and hence enjoyment) and ability. The focus is on physical activities that participants can do on their own as well as structured programmes available in the community. CHAMPS uses an initial interview and follow-up newsletters and telephone calls to provide ongoing support. Evaluation of CHAMPS showed improvements in caloric expenditure, and improvements in self-esteem (Stewart et al 1998, 2001). The importance of enjoyment as a factor in physical activity engagement was also confirmed by Stevens et al (2000). They concluded that enjoyment was the key causal variable in the maintenance of physical activity in the Groningen Active Living Model (GALM), a programme designed to increase physical activity in older adults, through enhancing self-efficacy, social support and enjoyment.

The ACT is a 2-year randomized clinical trial of two primary care physical activity behavioural interventions. Sedentary adults aged 35 to 75 years were randomly assigned to one of three groups: A, Standard Care; B, Staff-Assistance Intervention; or C, Staff-Counselling Intervention. In all groups patients received physician advice to increase their levels of physical activity as well as standard recommendations for engaging in physical activity for 30 minutes on most days. Behaviour change strategies were incorporated in groups B and C. The ACT interventions were based on theories of behaviour change and included enhancing self-efficacy by setting realistic goals and maximizing chances of success. Enjoyable activities were selected, problem solving was used to address barriers and participants were helped to identify the benefits of physical activity. The intervention incorporated the stages of change approach whereby participants were classified according to their stages of motivational readiness for change (i.e. contemplators, those in action stage, etc.). The intervention was tailored to the specific stage of change. Social modelling was used via video presentation of people engaged in physical activity. Goal-setting and problem solving skills were also incorporated into the intervention. Group B accessed staff input at physician visits via counselling sessions with a health educator, interactive mail, newsletters and telephone calls. An electronic step-counter was given to the participants to encourage self-monitoring. Group C received more intensive staff input, including ongoing telephone and face-to-face counselling and behaviour change classes. For group C, classes focused on goal setting, problem solving, social support and encouraging small achievable changes in behaviour. The main outcome measures were cardiorespiratory fitness and self-reported physical activity. For women, cardiovascular fitness was significantly higher in the staff assistance group and the staff counselling group than in the advice only group. For women, there was no difference between the assistance and counselling groups in cardiorespiratory fitness. For men there were no differences between the groups in cardiorespiratory fitness or total physical activity.

Looking to the future of providing physical activity interventions to the increasing numbers of older adults in the community, one cannot ignore the potential impact of computer technologies, E-health and technological advances in the delivery of information. These technologies have the potential to impact significantly on the delivery of health promotion interventions to individuals (Bock et al 2001). It has been postulated in an article on the future of physical activity in older adults that by the year 2010 increasing numbers of older adults will exercise as part of a therapeutic regime (Chodzko-Zajjko et al 1999). The internet can provide very fast feedback and knowledge on a daily basis to this population. With the advent of electronic health coaches, clients can have in-home expert systems that will guide and individually tailor programmes based on specific profiles and conditions. With the ability to connect exercise machines and devices that read physiological parameters to the internet, there now exists the potential for supervised physical activity without face-to-face intervention.

There are some examples in the literature of information technology (IT) interventions to promote physical activity. Bock et al (2001) found that an IT intervention resulted in slightly better maintenance of physical activity levels than the standard clinical intervention. The IT intervention was considered to be a low intensity intervention that reduced barriers and provided a low-cost individualized public health message. It provided more consistent intervention than a clinic-based strategy as it was subject to less disruption and fewer requirements for travel on the part of the participant than face-to-face interventions. The Diabetes Network Internet-based Physical Activity Intervention programme, a randomized pilot study of a physical activity intervention using the internet, also found an overall moderate improvement in physical activity levels in a cohort of people with diabetes (McKay et al 2001). The intervention utilized an online 'personal coach' (an occupational therapist) with access to an endocrinologist, a dietician and an exercise physiologist. The programme involved goal setting, individualized feedback and strategies to overcome barriers. The clients were also able to post and receive messages.

Designing physical activity interventions for older adults

This section of the chapter describes guidelines that will assist health practitioners in the design of physical activity interventions for older people. The guidelines focus on individual factors in behaviour change. However, health practitioners also need to be aware of the structural and cultural barriers to enhancing health and physical activity in older people. A full discussion of these issues is beyond the scope of this chapter. The reader is referred to Graham (2000).

A further point that should be noted is that health practitioners need to build evaluation into the design of their interventions. Health professionals are increasingly being called upon to use evidenced-based interventions and this evidence is reliant on the use of reliable and valid outcome measures that are linked to the objectives of the intervention. The development of appropriate outcome measures in itself is a major topic and beyond the scope of this chapter. The reader is referred to the following texts – Bowling (1997, 2001), Nolan and Mock (2000), Stewart and Ware (1992) – for a discussion of outcome measures in health settings.

Guidelines for physical activity interventions

The stages of change model is a very useful model that healthcare practitioners can use to identify the stage of readiness to change of their older clients and tailor interventions accordingly. Many of the examples of physical activity interventions given in this chapter have utilized this model with success.

It is therefore recommended that health practitioners utilize the stages of change model in their physical activity interventions. Specifically the intervention needs to:

- identify motivational readiness to change (i.e. pre-contemplation, contemplation etc.)
- incorporate a stage-matched intervention (see Jordan and Nigg 2002).

It is also recommended that the following behaviour change principles outlined earlier in this chapter in the discussion of the models be incorporated in physical activity interventions for older people (Booth et al 2000, Burbank and Riebe 2002, Dunlap and Barry 1999, King et al 1998, McAuley et al 2000, Marcus et al 2000, US Preventive Services Task Force 1996):

Health belief model

- Challenge incorrect health beliefs about the seriousness of and susceptibility to a health problem (pre-contemplation and contemplation stages).
- Change beliefs about the benefits of physical activity/exercise (pre-contemplation and contemplation stages).
- Provide cues to action for the initiation of physical activity/exercise (pre-contemplation and contemplation stages).
- Examine and reduce barriers to initiating and maintaining physical activity/exercise (all stages of readiness to change).
- Use social support and role models to reduce barriers and reinforce maintenance (all stages of readiness to change).

Theory of planned behaviour

- Challenge attitudes about the value of physical activity/exercise (pre-contemplation and contemplation stages).
- Challenge social norms about the appropriateness of physical activity/exercise for older people (pre-contemplation and contemplation stages).

- Use social support and role models to challenge and change negative attitudes and maintain positive attitudes (all stages of readiness to change).
- Enhance control beliefs by:
  - reducing barriers
  - providing correct information about physical activity/exercise benefits and time commitment required
  - providing enjoyable activities, and
  - enhancing access to programmes (all stages of readiness to change).

Self-efficacy

- Use a staged approach to promoting changes in physical activity/exercise behaviours (behavioural shaping) (preparation, action and maintenance stages).
- Ensure that the older person only commits to an activity that he/she is confident of achieving (contemplation, preparation, action and maintenance stages).
- Use behavioural contracting to enhance self-efficacy.
- Use reward strategies (including the client's self-determined rewards and telephone and personal follow-up by the health practitioner) to reinforce behaviours and enhance self-efficacy.
- Over time increase the demands of the activity as self-efficacy increases (action and maintenance stages).

Finally, the concept of self-management used in the chronic disease literature needs to be utilized by health practitioners working with older adults to assist their clients through partnerships to gain control of the management of their conditions, many of which can be improved through physical activity.

Conclusion

One of the most reliable findings with physical activities is that people feel better (Chodzo-Zajjko et al 1999). As a result, finding ways to increase the willingness of people to assume responsibility for their own health and not rely on a 'magic bullet' to cure their ills must be a priority. Self-management is essential in all aspects of life and taking control over physical activity is a major step towards overall control. Health professionals have an important role to play in the initiation and support of self-management behaviours in old age, and helping clients change their physical activity behaviours is central to improving function and quality of life.

From a policy perspective, older adults have been considered to be a special group, but what must be noted is that with the ageing of the baby-boomers, older people will comprise a significant proportion of the total population. In a world environment that will be dominated by older adults, promoting healthy or active ageing has become a focus for governments worldwide (Browning and Kendig 2003, World Health Organization 2002).

We are already seeing a shift from an acceptance of early retirement to a recognition that people will need to be more self-reliant economically in the future. It has been argued that eventually the economic benefits for government of self-responsibility for health will pervade the system (Chodzo-Zajjko et al 1999). In the interim, every effort must be made to promote physical activity in older adults through sound evidence-based interventions that involve partnerships between health professionals and their clients.

References

Activity Counselling Trial Research Group 2001 Effects of physical activity in primary care. The Activity Counselling Trial: a randomised trial. JAMA 286:677–687

Ajzen I 1991 The theory of planned behaviour. Organizational Behaviour and Human Decision Processes 50:179–211

Ajzen I, Fishbein M 1980 Understanding attitudes and predicting social behaviour. Prentice Hall, Englewood Cliffs, NJ

Anderson R M, Funnell M M, Arnold M S 1997 Using the empowerment approach to help patients change behaviour. In: Rubin R, Anderson B (eds) Practical psychology for diabetes clinicians. American Diabetes Association, p 163–171

Australian Institute of Health and Welfare (AIHW) 2000. Disability and ageing: Australian population patterns and trends. AIHW, Canberra

Bandura A 1994 Self-efficacy: thought control of action. Freeman, New York

Battersby M, Reece M, Higgins P, Markwick M 2002 What is self management? Flinders University Coordinated Care Training Unit. http://som.flinders.edu.au/FUSA/CCTU/SelfManage.htm

Bauman A E, Smith B J 2000 Healthy ageing: what role can physical activity play? Medical Journal of Australia 173(2):88–90

Bauman A, Bellew B, Vita P, Brown W, Owen N 2002 Getting Australia active towards better practice for the promotion of physical activity. National Public Health Partnership, Melbourne

Becker M H, Maiman L A 1975 Sociobehavioural determinants of compliance with health and medical care recommendations. Medical Care 13:10–24

Bock B, Marcus B, Pinto B 2001 Maintenance of physical activity following an individualized motivationally tailored intervention. Annals of Behavioural Medicine 23:79–87

Booth M L, Bauman A, Owen N, Gore C J 1997 Physical activity preferences, preferred sources of assistance, and perceived barriers to increased activity among physically inactive Australians. Preventive Medicine 26:131–137

Booth M L, Owen N, Bauman A, Clavisi O, Leslie E 2000 Social-cognitive and perceived environmental influences associated with physical activity in older adults. Preventive Medicine 31(1):15–22

Bowling A 1997 Measuring health: a review of quality of life measurement scales. Open University Press, Buckingham

Bowling A 2001 Measuring disease: a review of disease-specific quality of life measurement scales. Open University Press, Buckingham

Brown S A 1999 Interventions to promote diabetes self-management: state of science. The Diabetes Educator 25 (Suppl 6):S52–59

Browning C, Kendig H 2003 Healthy ageing: a new focus on older people's health and wellbeing. In: Liamputtong P, Gardner H (eds) Health care reform and the community. Oxford University Press, Sydney

Bruce D G, Devine A, Prince R 2002 Recreational physical activity levels in healthy older women: the importance of fear of falling. Journal of the American Geriatrics Society 50:84–89

Burbank P M, Riebe D 2002 Promoting exercise and behaviour change in older adults: interventions with the transtheoretical model. Springer Publishing Company, New York

Burkholder G J, Nigg C C 2002 Overview of the transtheoretical model. In: Burbank P M, Riebe D (eds) Promoting exercise and behaviour change in older adults. Springer Publishing Company, New York, p 85–146

Calfas K J, Long B J, Sallis J F, et al 1996 A controlled trial of physician counselling to promote the adoption of physical activity. Preventive Medicine 25:225–233

Chodzko-Zalko W, Beling J, Bortz W, et al 1999 The 1999 Albert and Elaine Borchard Symposium: the future role of regular physical activity in successful aging. http://www.isapa.org/borchard

Chogahara M 1999 A multidimensional scale for assessing positive and negative social influences on physical activity in older adults. Journals of Gerontology: Social Sciences 54B:S356–367

Conner M, Norman P (eds) 1995 Predicting health behaviour: research and practice with social cognition models. Open University Press, Maidenhead

Damush T M, Stewart A L, Mills K M, King A C, Ritter P L 1999 Prevalence and correlates of physician recommendations to exercise among older adults. Journals of Gerontology: Medical Sciences 54A:M423–427

Department of Health and Aged Care (DHAC) 2000. Annual Report. DHAC, Canberra

Dunlap J, Barry H 1999 Overcoming exercise barriers in older adults. http://www.physsportsmed.com/issues/1999/1010-15-99/dunlap.htm

Eakin E 2001 Promoting physical activity among middle-aged and older adults in health care settings. Journal of Aging and Physical Activity 9:29–37

Eakin E, Glasgow R E, Riley K M 2000 Review of primary care-based physical activity intervention studies: effectiveness and implications for practice and future research. Journal of Family Practice 49:158–168

Feder G, Griffiths C, Elridge S, Gantley M 2000 Patient empowerment and coronary heart disease. Lancet 356:1278

Graham H (ed) 2000 Understanding health inequalities. Open University Press, Buckingham

Gruman J, Von Korff M 1996 Indexed bibliography of behavioral interventions for chronic disease. Center for Advancement in Health, Washington, DC

Halbert J, Silagy C, Finucane P, Withers R, Hamdorf P 2000 Physical activity and cardiovascular risk factors: effect of advice from an exercise specialist in Australian general practice. Medical Journal of Australia 173:84–87

Harrison J A, Mullen P D, Green L W 1992 A meta-analysis of studies of the health belief model with adults. Health Education Research 7:107–116

Hoffman C, Rice D, Sung H 1996 Persons with chronic conditions: their prevalence and costs. Journal of the American Medical Association 276:1478–1479

Holman H, Lorig K 2000 Patients as partners in managing chronic disease. British Medical Journal 320:526–527

Janz N, Becker M H 1984 The health belief model: a decade later. Health Education Quarterly 11:1–47

Jayasuriya P, Roach S, Shaw E L B 2001a Self-management of chronic disease. Royal Australian College of General Practitioners. http://www.racgp.org.au/document.asp?id=3926

Jayasuriya P, Roach S, Bailey L, Shaw E 2001b Self-management for chronic disease. Australian Family Physician 30:913–916

Jordan P J, Nigg C R 2002 Applying the transtheoretical model: tailoring interventions to stages of change. In: Burbank PM, Riebe D (eds) Promoting exercise and behaviour change in older adults. Springer Publishing Company, New York, p 181–207

King A C, Haskell W L, Young D R, Oka R K, Stefanick M L 1995 Long-term effects of varying intensities and formats of physical activity on participation rates, fitness and lipoproteins in men and women aged 50–65 years. Circulation 91:2596–2604

King A C, Sallis J F, Dunn A L, et al 1997 Overview of the Activity Counselling Trial (ACT) intervention for promoting physical activity in primary health care settings. Medicine and Science in Sports and Medicine 29:1086–1096

King A C, Rejeski W J, Buchner D M 1998 Physical activity interventions targeting older adults: a critical review and recommendations. American Journal of Preventive Medicine 15:316–333

Litt M D, Kleppinger A, Judge J O 2002 Initiation and maintenance of exercise behaviour in older women: predictors from the social learning model. Journal of Behavioural Medicine 25:83–97

Lorig K, Mazonson P, Holman H R 1993 Evidence suggesting that health education for self-management in patients with chronic arthritis has sustained health benefits while reducing health care costs. Arthritis and Rheumatism 36:439–446

McAuley E, Blissmer B, Marquez D X, et al 2000 Social relations, physical activity and well being in older adults. Preventive Medicine 31:608–617

McKay H G, King D, Eakin E G, Seeley J R, Glasgow R 2001 The diabetes network internet-based physical activity intervention: a randomised pilot study. Diabetes Care 24:1328–1333

Marcus B H, Dubbert P, Forsyth L H, et al 2000 Physical activity behavior change: Issues in adoption and maintenance. Health Psychology 19:32–41

Minkler M, Schauffer H, Clements-Nolle K 2000 Health promotion for older Americans in the 21st century. American Journal of Health Promotion 14:371–379

Nigg C R, Riebe D 2002 The transtheoretical model: research review of exercise behavior and older adults. In: Burbank P M, Riebe D (eds) Promoting exercise and behavior change in older adults. Springer Publishing Company, New York, p 147–180

Nolan T, Mock V (eds) 2000 Measuring patient outcomes. Sage Publications, London

Norman P, Abraham C, Conner M (eds) 2000 Understanding and changing health behaviour: from health beliefs to self-regulation. Harwood Academic, London

Paterson B 2001 Myth of empowerment in chronic illness. Journal of Advanced Nursing 34:574–581

Price M J 1993 An experimental model of learning diabetes self-management. Qualitative Health Research 3:29–54

Prochaska J O, Di Clemente C C 1984 The transtheoretical approach: crossing traditional boundaries of change. Dorsey Press, Homewood, IL

Prochaska J O, Velicer W F 1997 The transtheoretical model of behaviour change. American Journal of Health Promotion 12:38–48

Prochaska J O, Di Clemente C C, Norcross J C 1992 In search of how people change: applications to addictive behaviours. American Psychologist 47:1102–1114

Resnick B 2001 Testing a model of overall activity in older adults. Journal of Aging and Physical Activity 9:142–160

Rollnick S, Mason P, Butler C 2000 Health behaviour change: a guide for practitioners. Churchill Livingstone, Edinburgh

Rosenstock I M, Strecher V J, Becker M H 1988 Social learning theory and the health belief model. Health Education Quarterly 15:175–183

Ruggiero L, Glasgow R, Dryfoos J M, et al 1997 Diabetes self-management. Self reported recommendations and patterns in a large population. Diabetes Care 20(4):586–587

Sallis J 2001 Progress in behavioural research on physical activity. Annals of Behavioural Medicine 23:77–78

Seeman T 2000 Health promoting effects of friends and family on health outcomes in older adults. American Journal of Health Promotion 14:362–370

Sheppard B H, Hartwick J, Warshaw P R 1988 The theory of reasoned action: a meta-analysis of past research and recommendations for modifications and future research. Journal of Consumer Research 15:325–339

Simkin L R, Gross A M 1994 Assessment of coping with high risk situations for exercise relapse among healthy women. Health Psychology 13(3):274–277

Stevens M, Lemmink K, de Greef M, Rispens P 2000 Groningen Active Living Model (GALM). Stimulating physical activity in sedentary older adults: first results. Preventive Medicine 31(5):547–553

Stewart A L, Ware J E 1992 Measuring functioning and well-being: the medical outcomes study approach. Duke University Press

Stewart A L, Mills K M, Sepsis P G, et al 1998 Evaluation of CHAMPS, a physical activity promotion program for older adults. Annals of Behavioral Medicine 19(4):353–361

Stewart A L, Verboncoeur C J, McLellan B Y, et al 2001 Physical activity outcomes of CHAMPS II: a physical activity promotion program. Journals of Gerontology: Biological Sciences and Medical Sciences 56:M465–470

US Preventive Services Task Force 1996 Guide to clinical preventive services, 2nd edn. Williams & Wilkins, Baltimore

Von Korff M, Gruman J, Schaefer J, Curry S, Wagner E 1997 Collaborative management of chronic illness. Annals of Internal Medicine 127:1097–1102

Wallston K A 1992 Hocus-pocus, the focus isn't strictly on locus: Rotter's social learning theory modified for health. Cognitive Behaviour Therapy and Research 16:1183–1199

Wallston K A, Wallston B S 1984 Social psychological models of health behaviour: an examination and integration. In: Sanders G, Suls J (eds) Social psychology of health and illness. Lawrence Erlbaum Associates, Hillsdale, NJ, p 65–95

World Health Organization (WHO) 2002 Active ageing: a policy framework. WHO, Geneva

4 Physical activity and health in an ageing workforce

John Carlson and Geraldine Naughton

CHAPTER CONTENTS

Physical inactivity 64

Injury 65

The workplace and physical activity 66

Successful workplace physical activity programmes 68

Conclusion 71

References 71

Workforce ageing is one of the emerging challenges for the 21st century. A key focus of health promotion programmes is to keep older workers physically active and injury free. In Australia, employees over the age of 35 years comprise 55% of the workforce and employees aged over 45 years comprise 30% of the workforce (Australian Bureau of Statistics (ABS) 1999). More than 80% of the projected growth in the labour force from 1998 to 2016 will be in people 45 years of age and over. In the European Union, it is estimated that the proportion of ageing workers aged 50–64 years will steadily increase in the next 15 years, and between 1995 and 2015, the numbers aged 50–64 years are expected to grow by more than 25%. In 2015 in European countries such as Germany, Finland, Belgium, Italy, the Netherlands and Austria, more than 30% of the workforce will be aged 50 and above (European Foundation for the Improvement of Living and Working Conditions 1999).

The physiological changes that occur with normal ageing can have a major influence on work performance. Changes can occur in the cardio-vascular, neurological, musculoskeletal, sensory and autonomic nervous systems (Spirduso 1996). The consequences of physiological ageing can be demonstrated in functional changes such as reduced strength and endurance (Shephard 1996) and loss of balance (O'Loughlin et al 1993). The rate and magnitude of change, however, vary between individuals and are influenced by diverse factors such as genetic predisposition and lifestyle practices and choices (Hansson et al 2001, Warburton et al 2001). The choice of a physically active lifestyle is related to increased function and delayed onset of cardiovascular disease (Mazzeo 1998, Powell et al 1987). With the number of older workers on the rise, the workplace is seen as an ideal environment where the promotion of physical activity may lead to increased health and well-being (Warr 1994).

The physical nature of work environments is predicted to change rapidly throughout the 21st century. Advances in technology and automation in industry will reduce the need for physically demanding jobs in the workforce. Decreasing the number and duration of manual tasks at work, together with insufficient physical activity during leisure time (Booth et al 1997), increases the likelihood of muscle weakness, osteoporosis and reduced aerobic capacity (Commonwealth Department of Health and Aged Care 2000).

Physical inactivity

According to Mathers et al (1999), physical inactivity is responsible for about 7% of the burden of all preventable illness and disabilities. Physical inactivity is second only to smoking as a cause of morbidity and premature mortality. Physical inactivity is also linked to the development of cardiovascular disease and the increasing incidence of musculoskeletal injuries observed in the workplace, such as low back pain (Straker 2000). Conversely, regular activity has been reported to be associated with increased physical and psychological self-sufficiency, as well as independence and quality of life in older workers (Biddle et al 2000, Biddle and Mutrie 2001).

The growing concern about physical inactivity presents an even greater challenge when applied to the ageing worker. The US Surgeon General's report on physical activity and health (Surgeon General 1996) and Canada's physical activity guide (Health Canada 2001) document the economic and health impacts of inactivity in the workplace. Well-established health benefits of a physically active workforce include absence or attenuation of coronary heart disease, a reduced incidence of musculoskeletal dysfunction, and improved management of diseases such as non-insulin-dependent diabetes mellitus, osteoporosis, obesity and hypertension (Blair et al 1989, Linnan and Marcus 2001, Mazzeo et al 1998, US President's Council on Physical Fitness and Sports 1997). Regular physical activity has also been shown to attenuate age-related reductions in muscle strength, functional capacity and cognitive performance (Pate et al 1995).

Health promotion programmes that encourage older workers to remain physically active can potentially optimize their performance during the final years of employment (Mockenhaupt 2001). Progressive and caring practices towards older workers can enable employers to make the most of their competencies, maturity and knowledge (Encel 2001).

Conversely, in workplaces that do not have health promotion policies for older workers, reduced workplace performance and increased illness and injuries have been reported (Linnan and Marcus 2001).

Injury

Worksite injuries are a major concern, especially as the workforce ages. In North America, older workers have been shown to experience a greater number of musculoskeletal injuries compared with middle-aged workers (Choi et al 1996). The disabilities arising from workplace injuries were more severe in older workers and their recovery was reduced compared with younger colleagues (Choi et al 1996). A large number of these injuries led to long periods of physical inactivity and consequent decline in health. In Australia, the total national economic cost of workplace injuries is approximately $A27 million per annum. In the USA workers' compensation costs amount to $US57 million (National Occupational Research Agenda 2003, National Occupational Health and Safety Commission 2001), while in Great Britain the cost of work-related injuries, ill health and non-injury accidents is between £12.42 and £17.74 billion (Health and Safety Executive Northern Ireland 2002).

Despite increasing technology in the workforce, manual handling and other tasks involving significant physical activity are still directly responsible for workplace injuries and trauma. Approximately 40% of all occupational injuries are related to the musculoskeletal system. Straker (2000) reported that work-related back pain is the largest workplace-related issue and is responsible for an estimated 25% of workplace health expenses. Advances in office computerization have also been associated with the repetitive office work of 'white collar workers', such as keyboarding being linked to growing sources of stress (Hinman et al 1997), neck and back pain (Worth 2000). Australian and US workers have more than a two in five chance of experiencing a serious work-related injury or disease during the course of their working life as a result of manual handling, repetitive movement or prolonged maintenance of abnormal postures (Worth 2000). A large proportion of occupational injuries are attributable to poor movement technique, reduced physical conditioning or inappropriate workplace design (Maher 2000).

Applied research at the worksite provides evidence that regular physical activity has the potential to reduce injury rates, prevent accidents and optimize recovery from trauma (Dishman et al 1998). For example, large corporate organizations in the USA and Canada with employee health and fitness programmes reported reductions in healthcare claims and absenteeism as well as increased health benefits in the form of reduced stress and reduced body weight (Goetzel and Ozminkowski 2000, Lechner et al 1997, Naas 1992, Pelletier 1996, Shephard 1996). A less desirable scenario is when older employees continue working despite untreated depression, muscle sprains or strains, fatigue or severe low back pain. This can compromise productivity and increase the risk of further injury (Goetzel and Ozminkowski 2000).

The workplace and physical activity

The 'ageing of workforces' in industrialized nations is of growing concern to both employers and employees. In progressive workplaces, employers acknowledge that older workers frequently have high levels of knowledge, skills, loyalty and reliability and low levels of absenteeism (Warr 1994). As a result, their health is viewed as paramount (Warr 1994). Other employers argue that older workers should make way for younger people who they perceive are more able to grasp new ideas and adapt to technology (Encel 2001). Currently no definitive evidence exists showing that older workers are less productive than younger adults.

The health and well-being of employees influences their contribution to the workplace. According to Hansson et al (2001) employers are striving to facilitate worker satisfaction in older employees by varying work schedules, providing assistance with manual work, by enabling job and tool redesign and by reducing reliance on the human performance element of many work tasks. A major motivation for employers to keep their workforce healthy is the payment of health insurance premiums when the employee becomes ill or injured (Drummond et al 1997, Katzmarzy et al 2000). Health insurance costs throughout industrialized nations are soaring due to increasing injury rates. Over 60% of workplace injury claims are related to musculoskeletal sprains and strains (Victorian Workcover Authority 2000). Many musculoskeletal disorders in ageing workers could be prevented with optimal physical activity and training programmes (Vuori 1995). Persistently high numbers of claims and increasing expenses of hospital treatment, pathology, diagnostic imaging, medications and rehabilitation maintain pressure on both the health insurance industry and employers. Increasing healthcare and health insurance costs can negatively impact on productivity and profitability (Health Canada 2001). Traditional industry sectors, such as the manufacturing industry, are under particular pressure to remain competitive in a global economy. As with other industries, they need to maximize work productivity and minimize loss of person hours due to injury, illness, work-related stress or absenteeism (Bureau of Labor Statistics 2001). A major challenge is for employers to fulfil their responsibilities to injured workers, contain rising health insurance costs, manage an ageing workforce, as well as cope with the increased incidence of musculoskeletal injuries.

Because employees spend up to eight hours a day at work, the workplace is an ideal setting for promoting physical activity and healthy life practices (King et al 1990, O'Connell 1997, Pronk et al 1995). Motivating factors for the adoption of physical activity and health promotion programmes are multidimensional. Key determinants include the presence of occupational health and safety regulations, good will and corporate incentives.

The USA embraced worksite wellness programmes in the 1970s. A review of these programmes suggests that well-designed programmes with an emphasis on physical activity yield modest health outcomes for workers across all age groups (Dishman et al 1998, Shephard 1996).

Nevertheless few rigorous studies have examined the financial return on investment of employee fitness and health programmes (Goetzel et al 1999). Goetzel et al (1999) estimated that the return may range from $US1.50 to $US13.00 per US dollar spent.

The expansion of worksite health promotion in Australia has closely paralleled the USA (Heaney and Goetzel 1997). Types of programmes offered to the workers are extensive and varied. At the worksite, the programmes offered to older workers have incorporated components of health promotion, health education, specific exercise interventions and environmental control of the job task (ergonomic design). Pencack (1991) identified three types of worksite programmes: (1) those that increased awareness of risks for injury and benefits of physical activity; (2) programmes on how to effect lifestyle change; and (3) environmental adaptation programmes. Dishman et al (1998) found that worksite physical activity programmes incorporated interventions such as behaviour modification, cognitive behaviour modification, health education, health risk appraisal and exercises.

If older workers require encouragement to maintain or increase their level of physical activity, the workplace ideals associated with a physically active and healthy workforce need to be made clear and agreed upon by all. The following discussion will outline some of the practices adopted in the workplace to increase physical activity.

Health promotion

Health promotion programmes provide information and advice on how workers can adopt healthy lifestyle choices, and what the benefits can be. Some health promotion programmes have targeted behavioural risk awareness (Emmons et al 1999). Others have provided information and materials, health and fitness screening, corporate exercise challenges, incentives for healthy lifestyle practices, health education and counselling, and different combinations of these components (Gomel et al 1993, Heaney and Goetzel 1997, Pencak 1991, Poole et al 2001). The adoption of physical activity is the most widely chosen intervention within the range of health promotion issues provided to workers (Grosch et al 1998).

Exercise and fitness programmes

Many workplaces have initiated exercise programmes at or near the worksite in an attempt to increase levels of fitness. Others subsidize memberships fees for gymnasiums, make time available during working hours for exercise, install facilities at the worksite such as gyms and aerobics rooms, mat work or cycle pathways around the worksite, or conduct supervised exercise classes at the worksite (Genaidy et al 1994, Horneij et al 2001). Some programmes have short-term interventions (Angoti et al 2000) whilst others have ongoing corporate fitness programmes within onsite facilities (Emmons et al 1999). Unfortunately, many of these have reported low attendance or a drop-off in attendance in short-term programmes after the initial period of interest (Emmons et al 1999, Grandjean et al 1996). Others have reported greater success

(Dishman et al 1998, Linnan and Marcus 2001, Shephard 1996) in terms of absenteeism, injuries, morale, productivity and health costs. An absence of scientific rigour in the research and design of health-related interventions in the workplace is, however, frequently noted (Heaney and Goetzel 1997, Linnan and Marcus 2001).

Injury prevention

Many workplace injuries are related to manual handling tasks and injuries increase proportionally with work demands. Because advanced age can be associated with muscle weakness and reduced range of movement in some individuals, injuries arising from manual handling are more severe in older workers (Hansson et al 2001). Manual handling hazard identification and hazard reduction are key injury prevention strategies. Programmes that encourage workers to take the initiative for identifying and reducing the risks of manual handling injuries have resulted in significant reductions in injury rates, especially for low back pain (Gerdle et al 1995, Grundewall et al 1993, Kellet et al 1991). Injury prevention strategies and adoption of early return-to-work programmes can substantially reduce costs and enhance productivity (Wellness Councils of America 2002).

Some physically demanding work tasks or work environments have the potential to predispose workers to injuries arising from physiological or psychological stress (National Occupational Health and Safety Commission 2001). Thus in addition to physical injuries such as muscle strains and joint sprains, workplace efficiency and productivity can be compromised by non-physical stress disorders, stress-related work dissatisfaction and stress-related early retirements (Victorian Workcover 2001). Physical activity programmes that maximize workplace performance and job satisfaction can help to minimize stress and absenteeism (Hansson et al 2001).

Successful workplace physical activity programmes

Although the benefits of regular physical activity are well established, many older workers either do not receive or ignore this message. According to Booth et al (2002) 'the barriers to increased participation can be real or perceived'. Such barriers can present major challenges for the uptake and maintenance of activity in older adults (Martin and Sinden 2001). Booth et al (1997) identified six perceived barriers to activity in active and inactive older adults; 'already active enough', 'have an injury or disability', 'poor health', 'too old', 'don't have enough time' and 'I'm not the sporty type'. Other barriers to participation in physical activity in older workers include environmental factors (e.g. weather, facilities), motivational and time issues and the presence of injuries that prohibit or restrict movement or function (Booth et al 1997, Chinn et al 1999, Clark 1999, Conn 1998).

The following sections summarize some of the key issues to address when implementing physical activity programmes for older workers (Harris et al 1999, King et al 1990, Shephard 1996).

Workplace leadership and commitment	High-level managerial support is an important element for 'driving' physical activity in the workplace. Demonstrated cooperation and commitment from leadership is pivotal to success. Examples of strong employer commitment include the provision of access to worksite or neighbouring physical activity facilities, allocation of time during work to exercise, and financial incentives based on health and lifestyle improvements.
Older worker involvement	Ideally, older workers show a commitment towards improving their own health. They should be encouraged to plan and evaluate progress towards their physical activity goals and be assisted in achieving them. Health promotion providers such as fitness leaders or exercise consultants might find it useful to ask older workers to identify the stage of behavioural change that best represents their current physical activity patterns (Prochaska and Marcus 1994). An example would be thinking about the benefits of different types of exercise before actually choosing to adopt an exercise programme. It can also be useful to ask older workers to identify their preferred physical activity modes and the ways in which their specific needs can be taken into account in order to increase activity and participation. A strong incentive is to minimize discomfort and stress. To be active in enjoyable physical activities and to participate at convenient times are additional considerations. An ideal scenario is when the needs of the older worker are matched with the desire of the organization for establishing a workplace physical activity programme.
Ensure a clear purpose for the physical activity programme	To increase physical activity in the workplace, home and community, the relevance of the activity must be apparent to the individual. Internal motivators for physical activity include such things as weight control, health concerns and self-esteem. External motivators are factors such as social interaction, partner encouragement, fun and competition. Most people do not adopt physical activity as a lifestyle choice without a clear purpose or goal (Biddle and Mutrie 2001). Managers could adopt policies that focus on the positive outcomes from valuing the contribution of physically active older workers to workplace productivity. Increased physical activity could also a be promoted as a way to improve enjoyment of family life away from work.
Promote team inclusiveness	Inclusiveness strategies require acceptance, commitment by management, employees and health promotion providers to the values of increasing physical activity in the workplace. Valuing physical activity in the older workers of a team can be approached in many ways. These include developing policies for the promotion of physical activity at work and home, increasing awareness of stress management activities at work and at home and the provision of incentives to enable early detection of injury risks by the workers themselves (Harris et al 1999).

Create social and environmental support structures for physical activity	Social support for physical activity programmes can be provided by the managerial team, through the provision of flexible working hours and recognition of active older workers who support efforts by other workers to increase health-related lifestyle improvements. Social support from friends, family and members of the community is a major way to maintain or increase activity levels. Health-related changes in the work environment require professional leadership and infrastructure. Examples of infrastructure changes include the provision of showers, bicycle storage spaces and change rooms, health promotion newsletters, and increasing awareness of resources for physical activity in the worksite neighbourhood that are low cost and convenient. The physical environment should also be regularly audited for physical hazards and stress levels.
Cultural context	In order to create a workplace culture that increases physical activity, there is a need to address the barriers provided by employers and workers. Employers often cite legal liability or the lack of evidenced based research as disincentives for establishing health promotion programmes. Employees can sometimes contribute to a 'negative activity culture' by citing lack of time, potential embarrassment in being seen performing exercises, cultural differences, or the lack of supportive environments to improve health-related choices. A successful culture is one in which both the employer and the worker feel empowered to remove barriers to physical activity for the benefit of both parties.
Increased opportunities for incidental physical activity	Opportunities to increase incidental physical activity in the workplace can assist workers to achieve their activity goals. Examples of how to increase incidental activity include signs to promote the use of stairs rather than elevators, parking or public transport zones at least 500 metres from the workplace, walking breaks to suggested destinations close to the workplace, posters depicting ergonomically sound stretches and the provision of drinking water fountains located a short distance from work stations. These are simple to implement yet the overall contribution to increasing physical activity can be marked.
Measure outcomes	To support workplace physical activity incentives, it is useful to evaluate changes in worker performance and compliance over time. In addition, in consultation with the older worker, the purpose of increasing physical activity levels should be clearly identified.
	Programmes to increase activity levels are ideally developed within each workplace by management together with the workers. Imposing an external model of health promotion and injury prevention is unlikely to be as effective as designing a programme tailored to the needs and environment of that workplace. Worksite incentives for health-related improvements in older workers are dependent on dynamic, respectful

and collaborative relationships within the specific workplace environment (Veitch et al 1997). Examples of successful programmes include walking, running, and swimming classes and tailored programmes for individuals (Dishman et al 1998). Health promotion campaigns can also be adopted within the workplace. International examples of health promotion activities suitable for the workplace include Heart Week, Healthy Bones Week, QUIT Week, Walk or Cycle to Work Days (Canada, Australia and UK) and enable participation on a more generic level.

Conclusion

The worksite presents an ideal yet challenging setting in which physical activity can be promoted in ageing workers. It could be argued that many programmes designed to increase physical activity only attract those who are already active or who are predisposed to being active. It may be that these programmes are not reaching the targeted 'at greatest risk' individuals who really need to increase physical activity. The challenge for the workplace is to increase physical activity amongst ageing workers who are currently not active and to continue to facilitate activity in workers who are habitually active.

References

Angoti C M, Chan W T, et al 2000 Combined dietary and exercise intervention for control of serum cholesterol in the workplace. American Journal of Health Promotion 15:9–16

Australian Bureau of Statistics 1999 Labour Force Australia, January 1999. Catalogue #6203.0, P27

Biddle S J H, Mutrie N 2001 Psychology of physical activity: determinants, well-being and interventions. Routledge, London

Biddle S J H, Fox K R, Boutcher S H (eds) 2000 Physical activity and psychological wellbeing. Routledge, London

Blair S N, Kohl H W, Paffenberger R S Jr, et al 1989 Physical fitness and all-cause mortality – a prospective study of healthy men and women. JAMA 281:327–334

Booth M L, Bauman A, Owen N, Gore C J 1997 Physical activity preferences, preferred sources of assistance and perceived barriers to increased activity among physically inactive Australians. Preventive Medicine 26:131–137

Booth M L, Bauman A, Owen N 2002 Perceived barriers to physical activity among older Australians. Journal of Aging and Physical Activity 10: 271–280

Bureau of Labor Statistics 2001 US Department of Labor 2000 OSH Summary Estimates. Retrieved March 2002 from http://www.bls.gov/iif/oshwc/osh/os/osch0022.pdf

Chinn D J, White M, Harland J, Drinkwater C, Raybould S 1999 Barriers to physical activity and socio-economic position: implications for health promotion. Journal of Epidemiology and Community Health 53:191–192

Choi B C K, Levitisky M, Lloyd R D, Stones I M 1996 Patterns and risk factors for sprains in Ontario Canada 1990: an analysis of the workplace health and safety agency database. Journal of Environmental and Occupational Medicine 38:379–389

Clark D O 1999 Physical activity and its correlates among primary care patients aged 55 years or older. Journal of Gerontology: Social Sciences 54B(1):41–48

Commonwealth Department of Health and Aged Care and The Australian Sports Commission 2000 The cost of illness attributable to physical inactivity in Australia. A preliminary study. Commonwealth of Australia. Retrieved. December 18, 2001, from http://www.health.gov.au/pubhlth/publicat/document/phys_costofillness.pdf

Conn V S 1998 Older adults and exercise: path analysis of self-efficacy related constructs. Nursing Research 47(3):180–189

Dishman R K, Oldenburg B, et al 1998 Worksite physical activity intervention. American Journal of Preventive Medicine 15(4):344–361

Drummond M F, Cooke J, Walley T 1997 Economic evaluation under managed competition: evidence from the UK. Social Science and Medicine 45(4):583–595

Emmons K M, Linnan L A, et al 1999 The Working Healthy Project: a worksite health-promotion trial targeting physical activity, diet, and smoking. Journal of Occupational Environmental Medicine 41(7):545–555

Encel S 2001 Working later in life. Australasian Journal of Ageing 20(3, Suppl 2): 69–73

European Foundation for the Improvement of Living and Working Conditions 1999 Active strategies for an ageing workforce. Office for Official Publications of the European Communities, Luxembourg

Genaidy A, Davis N, et al 1994 Effects of a job-simulated exercise programme on employees performing manual handling operations. Ergonomics 37(1):95–106

Gerdle B, Brulin C, Elert J, Eliasson P, Granlund B 1995 Effect of general fitness program on musculoskeletal symptoms, clinical status, physiological capacity and perceived work environment among home care service personnel. Journal of Occupational Rehabilitation 5:1–16

Goetzel R Z, Ozminkowski R J 2000 Disease management as part of total health management. Disease Management and Health Outcomes 8(3):12–128

Goetzel R Z, Juday T R, Ozminkowski R J 1999 What's the ROI? A systematic review of return on investment (ROI). Studies of Corporate Health and Productivity Management Initiatives. Proceedings Association for Worksite Health Promotion's Worksite Health Conference

Gomel M, Oldenburg B, Simpson J M, Owen N 1993 Worksite cardiovascular risk reduction: a randomised trial of health risk assessment, education, counselling and incentives. American Journal of Public Health 83:1231–1238

Grandjean P W, Oden G L, et al 1996 Lipid and lipoprotein changes in women following six months of exercise training in a worksite fitness program. Journal of Sports Medicine Physical Fitness 36(1):54–59

Grosch J W, Alterman T, Petersen M R, Murphy L R 1998 Worksite health promotion programs in the US: factors associated with availability and participation. American Journal of Health Promotion 13:36–45

Grundewall B, Liljequist M, Hansson T 1993 Primary prevention of back symptoms and absence from work. A prospective randomised study among hospital employees. Spine 18:587–594

Hansson R O, Robson S M, Linios M J 2001 Stress and coping in older workers. Work 17:247–256

Harris D, Oldenburg B, Owen N 1999 Australian National Workplace Health Project: strategies for gaining access, support and commitment. Health Promotion Journal of Australia 9(1):40–54

Health and Safety Executive Northern Ireland 2002 The cost of work related injuries. Ill health and non-injury accidents to the NI Economy. Report.

Retrieved January 2003 from http://www.hseni.gov.uk/pdfs/
Cost%20of%20Incidents/Cost%20of%20Incidents_E_Summary.pdf

Health Canada 2002 The business case for active living, an on-line evidence-based
resource (2001). Retrieved April 2002 from http://www.hc-sc.gc.ca/english/
index.html

Heaney C A, Goetzel R Z 1997 A review of health-related outcomes of
multicomponent worksite health promotion programs. American Journal
of Health Promotion 11(4):290–308

Hinman M, Ezzo L, et al 1997 Computerized exercise program does not affect
stress levels of asymptomatic VDT users. Journal of Occupational
Rehabilitation 7(1):45–51

Horneij E, Hemborg B, et al 2001 No significant differences between intervention
programmes on neck, shoulder and low back pain: a prospective randomized
study among home-care personnel. Journal of Rehabilitation Medicine
33(4):170–176

Katzmarzy P T, Gledhill N, Shephard R J 2000 The economic burden of physical
inactivity in Canada. Canadian Medical Association Journal 163(11):1435–1440

Kellet K, Kellet D, Nordholm L 1991 Effects of an exercise program on sick leave
due to back pain. Physical Therapy 71:283–293

King A C, Taylor C B, Haskell W L, DeBusk R F 1990 Identifying strategies for
increasing employee physical activity levels: findings from the Stanford/
Lockheed Exercise Survey. Health Education Quarterly 17(3):269–285

Lechner L, de Vries H, Adriaansen I, Drabbels L 1997 Effects of employee fitness
program on reduced absenteeism. Journal of Occupational and Environmental
Medicine 39(9):827–831

Linnan L A, Marcus B 2001 Worksite-based physical activity programs and older
adults: current status and priorities for the future. Journal of Aging and
Physical Activity 9:59–70

Maher C G 2000 A systematic review of workplace interventions to prevent low
back pain. Australian Journal of Physiotherapy 46:259–269

Martin K A, Sinden A R 2001 Who will stay and who will go? A review of older
adults' adherence to randomised controlled trials of exercise. Journal of Aging
and Physical Activity 9:91–114

Mathers C, Vos T, Stevenson C 1999 The burden of disease and injury in
Australia. Australian Institute of Health and Welfare, Canberra. AIHW Cat
No PHE 17

Mazzeo R S, Cavanagh P, Evans W J, et al 1998 American College of Sports
Medicine Position Stand: exercise and physical activity for older adults.
Medicine and Science in Sports and Exercise 30(6):992–1008

Mockenhaupt R 2001 Executive Summary. Journal of Aging and Physical
Activity 9:S3–4

Moore T M 1998 A workplace stretching program: physiologic and perception
measurements before and after participation. AAOHN Journal 46(12):563–568

Morris J N 1994 Exercise in the prevention of coronary heart disease: today's
best buy in public health. Medicine and Science in Sport and Exercise
26:807–814

Naas R 1992 DuPont links wellness program to reduced absenteeism. Business
and Health 10:19

National Health and Medical Research Council (NH&MRC) 1999 Paradigm
shift: injury from problem to solution. New research directions. Research
development committee. Commonwealth of Australia

National Occupational Health and Safety Commission 2001 Compendium of
Workers' Compensation Statistics, Australia, 1998–99. National OHS Research

Directions Statement, Canberra. Retrieved January 2002 from http://www.nohsc.gov.au/pdf/statistics/compendium98-99.pdf

National Occupational Research Agenda 2003 Social and economic consequences of workplace illness and injury, 1999. http://www.cdc.gov/niosh/nrsoce.html

Nichols J F, Wellman E, et al 2000 Impact of a worksite behavioural skills intervention. American Journal of Health Promotion 14(4):218–221

O'Connell M P 1997 Health impact of workplace health promotion programs and methodological quality of the research literature including commentary by Omenn G S and Chapman L S. Art of Health Promotion 1(3):1–8

O'Loughlin J L, Robitalle Y, Biovin J F, Suissa S 1993 Incidence of and risk factors for falls and injuries among community dwelling elderly. American Journal of Epidemiology 137:342–354

Pate R M, Pratt N, Blair S N, et al 1995 Physical activity and public health: a recommendation from the Centers for Disease Control and Prevention and the American College of Sports Medicine. JAMA 273:402–407

Pelletier K R 1996 A review and analysis of the health and cost-effective outcome studies of comprehensive health promotion and disease prevention programs at the worksite: 1993–1995. American Journal of Health Promotion 10(5):380–388

Pencak M 1991 Workplace health promotion programs: an overview. Nursing Clinics of North America 26:233–240

Pender N J, Smith L C, et al 1987 Building better workers: comparing corporate fitness center members' and non-members' levels of absenteeism, productivity, job-related strain and anxiety. AAOHN Journal 35(9):386–390

Pohjonen T, Ranta R 2001 Effects of a worksite physical exercise intervention on physical fitness, perceived health status, and work ability among home care workers: five-year follow-up. Preventive Medicine 32(6):465–475

Poole K, Kumpfer K, Pett M 2001 The impact of an incentive-based worksite health promotion program on modifiable health risk factors. American Journal of Health Promotion 16(1):21–26

Powell K E, Thompson P D, Caspersen C J, Kendrick J S 1987 Physical activity and the incidence of coronary heart disease. Annual Review of Public Health 8:253–287

Pritchard J E, Nowson C A, et al 1997 A worksite program for overweight middle-aged men achieves less weight loss with exercise than with dietary change. Journal of the American Dietetic Association 97(1):37–42

Prochaska J O, Marcus B H 1994 The transtheoretical model: applications to exercise. In: Dishman RK (ed) Advances in exercise adherence. Human Kinetics, Champaign, IL, p 161–180

Pronk S J, Pronk N P, et al 1995 Impact of a daily 10-minute strength and flexibility program in a manufacturing plant. American Journal of Health Promotion 9(3):175–178

Reardon J 1998 The history and impact of worksite wellness. Nursing Economics 16:5–15

Shephard R J 1996 Worksite fitness and exercise programs: a review of methodology and health impact. American Journal of Health Promotion 10:436–452

Spirduso W 1996 Physical dimensions of ageing. Human Kinetics, Champaign, IL

Straker L 2000 Preventing work-related back pain. In: Worth D L (ed) Moving in on occupational injury. Butterworth-Heinemann, Melbourne

Surgeon General 1996 Physical activity and health. US Department of Health and Human Services, Centers for Disease Control, Atlanta

US Centers for Disease Control and Prevention 2001 Increasing physical activity: a report on recommendations from the Task Force on Community Preventative Services. Morbidity and Mortality Weekly Report, Volume 50

US President's Council on Physical Fitness and Sports 1997. Physical fitness and the prevention of type II diabetes. Research Digest 2:10

Veitch J, Owen N, Burns J, Sallis J F 1997 Physical activity promotion for male factory workers: a realistic option? Health Promotion Journal of Australia l7(3):169–174

Victorian Workcover Authority 2001 Annual Report, Melbourne

Vuori I 1995 Exercise and physical health: musculo-skeletal health and functional abilities. Conference Notes International Scientific Consensus Conference, Quebec

Warburton E R, Gledhill N, Quinney A 2001 Musculofitness and health. Canadian Journal of Applied Physiology 26(2):217–237

Warr P B 1994 Age and job performance. In: Snel J, Cremer R (eds) Work and ageing. Taylor & Francis, London

Wellness Councils of America 2002 The cost benefit of worksite wellness. Retrieved April 2002 from http://www.24hourfitness.com/.html/corp_well/bottom_line/

Worth D R 2000 Moving in on occupational injury. Butterworth-Heinemann, Melbourne

5

Biomechanical and neuromuscular considerations in the maintenance of an active lifestyle

Bruce Elliott, David Lloyd and Tim Ackland

CHAPTER
CONTENTS

Introduction 76

Physical activity and osteoporosis 77

Physical activity and osteoarthritis 82

Physical activity pre- and post-surgery 89

Protection from falls 90

Summary 92

References 92

Introduction

In ancient times movement meant survival, whereas today it plays a large role in protecting a person from many chronic diseases and determining their quality of life. This statement is certainly true for elderly people where activity plays an essential role in both the physical and mental aspects of life. A comparison of the overall risk between sedentary and active individuals shows that those who choose to engage in moderate physical activity live longer than their sedentary peers through to about 90 years (Linsted et al 1991). MacRae et al (1994) showed that an exercise programme structured around everyday movements significantly reduced the rate of falls in elderly women. However, one must accept that the risk of musculoskeletal injury from activity increases with age, and that these dangers are appreciable if the person is untrained or is in the first few weeks of a programme (Pollock 1988).

In 1996 the World Health Organization identified ageing and health, particularly with respect to women, as a major world issue. Approximately 14% of Australians are over 65 years of age and, therefore, the role of exercise from a health perspective is obviously an area of great concern. While physical activity has clearly been linked to a feeling of well-being and other behavioural benefits (US Department of Health and Human Services 1996), the advantages addressed in this chapter relate to the biological responses to physical loading and to selected motor control and physical capacities related to protecting against a fall. The question that must be answered with reference to the quality of life of elderly people is how much activity is sufficient to have a positive influence on the body, without placing it under undue stress. It is well known that excessive loading is associated with injuries, as the majority of musculoskeletal injuries from a fall are the result of excessive impact loading (Whiting and Zernicke 1998). A distinction must then be drawn between activity levels that may lead to such diseases as osteoarthritis, and those that assist in reducing the risk of osteoporosis, improve body strength and control of movement following surgery, and are needed for the maintenance of a generally healthy life. Specificity of activity must be considered, as some activities originally thought to be of benefit in the fight against osteoporosis have now been shown to have no benefit at all. Specificity must also be considered from a neuromuscular perspective, as selected activities are of great benefit in improving strength and balance during everyday tasks performed by older people and thus protect against falls. The physical and behavioural modifications that are caused by a fall often lead to loss of functional independence and are extremely costly for the healthcare system.

This chapter will review the current literature on biomechanical and neuromuscular aspects of activity in older people from a functional perspective. While the role of various exercises in loading the body will be discussed, no attempt will be made to prescribe actual training programmes. Subsections deal with load response to activity (with particular discussion of osteoporosis, osteoarthritis and the need for movement following surgery – Figure 5.1) and physical activities that enable the elderly to improve the quality of their lives.

Physical activity and osteoporosis

Osteoporosis: a disease characterized by low bone mass and microarchitectural deterioration of bone tissue leading to enhanced bone fragility and a consequent increase in fracture risk.

Osteoporosis and associated fractures increase markedly with age and are a major cause of mortality and morbidity. The World Health Organization (1998) predicted the number of hip fractures worldwide in 2025 could be as high as 16 million, hence osteoporosis has a substantial and increasing economic significance. The frequency of osteoporotic fractures is higher in women than men due to their greater life expectancy and postmenopausal hormonal changes.

An optimal model for the prevention of osteoporotic fractures includes maximizing and maintaining bone strength, while at the same time not overloading the bone. Because the response of bone to mechanical load is specific to the bone under load (Swissa-Sivan et al 1989), therapeutic exercise programmes need to include general activities (walking, swimming, etc.) to improve mobility and coordination as well as high-resistance activities that target specific areas of the body.

Figure 5.1 Model for joint and tissue loading.

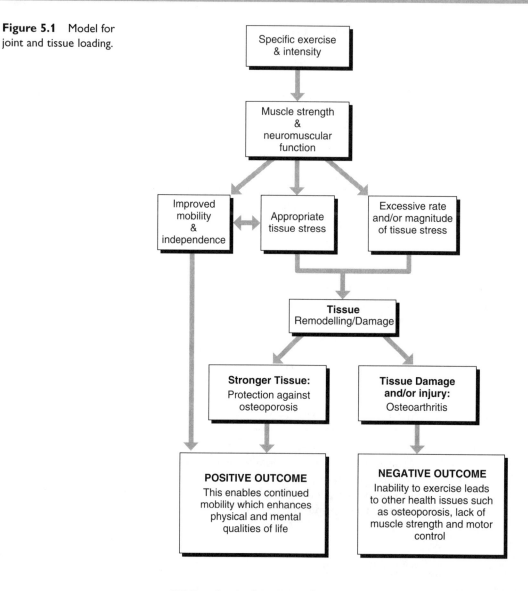

While physical activity through childhood and adolescence is geared to increase bone mass and strength (Chow et al 1987, Morris et al 1997), in elderly people, exercise is usually designed to reduce the rate of bone loss (Rikli and McManus 1990, Smith et al 1989). The absolute risk of osteoporosis varies between populations and is generally highest in countries where activity is reduced in the general structure of life (Law et al 1991, Rikli and McManus 1990, Smith et al 1989).

The human skeleton responds to mechanical stimuli resulting from physical activity. However, it is not simply the magnitude of load that is important. Biomechanics research demonstrates the importance of a number of factors related to the mechanical strain placed on bone, including:

- strain magnitude
- strain rate

- strain gradient
- strain frequency
- strain history.

The *mechanostat theory* relating *strain magnitude* to bone mass (as depicted by Forwood and Turner 1995) is a useful, though simplistic, start point for understanding the influence of load on bone modelling and remodelling. Provided all hormonal and other environmental factors are constant, bone will maintain mass with normal daily activities within the so-called 'physiological loading zone'. When skeletal loading diminishes through enforced bedrest, limb casting or space flight, for example, remodelling occurs such that bone resorption (osteoclastic activity) predominates over formation (osteoblastic activity). Conversely, when the skeleton is subjected to an overload, perhaps caused by a higher than usual level of training or exertion, bone remodelling occurs with formation predominating over resorption.

Marrying our knowledge of endocrinology to Frost's (1983) *minimum effective strain* theory helps us to explore the interaction of hormonal influences with mechanical strain. Here, the resultant effect on bone integrity is wrought by the opposing forces of endocrine drive (stimulating net resorption of bone) and mechanical drive (promoting net bone formation). This leads us to better understand the devastating effect to bone health of the female menopause, in which markedly reduced levels of oestrogen cause a general 1–2% reduction in bone mass per annum, even with no change in individual activity levels (Gallagher 1996). Similarly, we can now appreciate why some women endurance athletes (often those experiencing amenorrhoea) have low bone mass and suffer repeated stress fractures despite high levels of bone loading (Rutherford 1993).

The rate at which strain develops can also influence the adaptive response of bone. *Strain rate* can be related to the magnitude of strain because an increased rate of strain is needed to achieve higher loads within a constant time frame. However, this is not always so. Research by O'Connor et al (1982) showed strong correlations between bone remodelling, strain rate and strain magnitude. In contrast, Rubin and Lanyon (1984) showed that high static loads, with zero strain rate, do not protect bone from atrophy.

Strain gradient refers to the way strain is distributed through the bone cross-section. The *error strain distribution theory* (Lanyon 1996) states that the skeleton's structural competence is maintained by making architectural adjustments to reduce deviations from normal dynamic strain distributions. While repetitive strains caused by accustomed loading patterns such as in walking, running or swimming are useful, the loading caused by new exercises or unanticipated activities has a greater osteogenic effect. Modelling may occur at lower strain magnitudes if the distribution of strain across the bone is unusual.

Continuous exercises of an accustomed nature, such as walking or jogging, expose bone to a high number of loading cycles. However, the strain frequency appears to be of less importance than strain magnitude, rate and gradient. Though a minimum number of loading cycles must be achieved to provide the mechanical stimulus for bone formation, there appears to be a threshold above which no additional bone formation is accrued.

The concept of *strain history* incorporates the characteristics of mechanical strain (magnitude, rate, gradient and frequency) to which the body has become accustomed in recent times. People with low bone mass as a result of a sedentary lifestyle or enforced immobility have the greatest potential for increased bone formation. That is, they will achieve a greater bone modelling response to a new exercise programme than a fit, active individual with normal bone mass (Kerr et al 2001).

So how do we affect the mechanical strain on our skeleton through exercise? The skeleton is primarily subjected to load caused by gravity through weight bearing, and this is supplemented by the actions of muscles and other external forces. By these means, exercise causes compression, tensile, torsion, bending and/or shear forces on selected bones within the skeletal structure. However, not all exercises produce an osteogenic effect. Recent research by Kerr et al (1996, 2001) has demonstrated that resistance training can provide sufficient stimulus for bone modelling in a postmenopausal population, but the effect is site specific and dependent on strain magnitude and strain gradient.

In the study by Kerr et al (2001) calcium-replete subjects ($n = 127$) were randomly assigned to one of three groups; control, circuit training or strength training. All women were at least 4 years past the menopause, were able to commit to exercising for three 1-hour sessions per week, but none was on hormone replacement therapy. Bone density at various sites was measured using an Hologic QDR 4500 DEXA machine at baseline and 6-monthly intervals over the course of the 2-year training period. There were no differences between groups at baseline for body weight, body composition, bone mineral density, strength or aerobic capacity. The overall retention of subjects was 71% over the 2-year period. Both training groups performed a core of resistance exercises designed to stress the skeleton around the DEXA scan sites, with the strength group completing 3 sets × 8 repetitions while the load progressively increased throughout the study. The circuit group used light loads (3 sets × 25 repetitions) and this was supplemented with weight-supported aerobic activity. Naturally, the strength group experienced a significant improvement in 1 RM (one repetition maximum) strength compared with the circuit and control groups. Significant increases in bone mineral density were observed at the hip site for the strength group (Figure 5.2), though no differences were seen at the distal radius, lumbar or distal tibia sites. In contrast, an earlier study by Kerr et al (1996) had reported significant differences at the distal radius site between the strength-trained side of the body and the contralateral, untrained side.

When considered together, the studies by Kerr et al (1996, 2001) provide valuable information regarding the type of exercise programme one might prescribe to maintain bone mass in a healthy population, or increase bone mass in people with osteopenia (low bone mass). Clearly, any form of exercise will provide health benefits, such as improved cardiovascular output or falls prevention, for the older person. However,

Figure 5.2 The percentage change from baseline in bone mineral density (BMD) over the two years of the study (Kerr et al 2001) at the intertrochanteric hip scan site. The strength group was significantly different ($P < 0.05$) from the circuit and control groups at all time points after baseline. (Reproduced from Kerr et al Journal of Bone and Mineral Research 2001, 16: 175–177, with permission of the American Society for Bone and Mineral Research.)

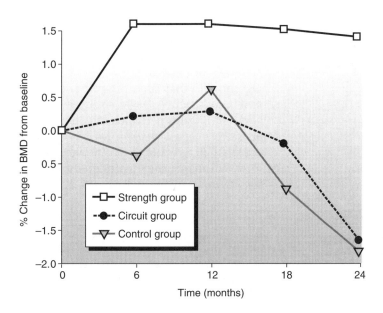

only certain exercise modalities that provide opportunities to load the skeleton with sufficient intensity and with novel strain distributions, will have an osteogenic effect.

Ackland (1998) proposed the following exercise regimes in four levels of intensity to provide general health benefits as well as a progression from a space awareness/falls prevention strategy to resistance training designed to maintain or increase bone formation.

1. Water activities – swimming and hydrotherapy. Water running, stretching and mobility exercises in a warm and weight-supported environment promote joint mobility, and improve cardiovascular circulation and muscle tone. Though not providing sufficient mechanical strain to produce an osteogenic effect, this exercise modality aids in the transfer to land-based exercises.
2. Body awareness/falls prevention – movement to music, dancing, tai chi and mobility training. These activities promote balance and stability, spatial awareness and movement confidence, all of which are important for reducing the risk of falling.
3. Low impact locomotion/low intensity resistance exercises – aerobic activity including walking, cycling and swimming, as well as light barbell, dumbbell and Theraband™ resistance exercises. This level of exercise requires closer monitoring of participants and should be performed in small groups, with an emphasis on maintaining correct posture. Nevertheless, with appropriate supervision, these activities can be suitable for individuals with osteopenia or osteoporosis (no current fracture), or those with a current fracture, who must exercise cautiously and require close supervision. If the activity provides an unusual strain on the bone, it may have an osteogenic effect despite the low magnitude of strain.

4. High loading resistance exercises – for example machine or free weight resistance exercises or rowing. Clearly, the skeleton must be loaded to a degree beyond that which is normally encountered in activities of daily living to obtain a therapeutic effect. Therefore, we recommend that such programmes are closely supervised by qualified personnel. A basic strength training protocol of 8–10 RM × 3 sets × 2–3 times per week may be followed, with loads reviewed and adjusted every 2 weeks. However, it is vital that the load increments are small (0.5–1.0 kg) and that participants are given plenty of variety. This will ensure they maintain their enthusiasm for exercise, and that the strain on the bone is varied.

Physical activity and osteoarthritis

Osteoarthritis is an 'organ failure' of an articular joint, where the disease affects the cartilage, bone and other periarticular structures of the major weight-bearing joints of the human body (Bailey et al 1997, 2001).

Arthritis is a debilitating disease affecting 5–10% of people and 44% of these have osteoarthritis (OA) (Access Economics 2001). OA is the most common rheumatic disease in the world and the knee joint is the weight-bearing joint most often affected (Felson et al 2000a).

While light and moderate activities do not appear to increase the risk of knee OA in elderly people, heavy physical activity has been shown to be an important risk factor (McAlindon et al 1999). Cheng et al (2000) supported this view, reporting that high levels of physical activity may be a risk factor for symptomatic OA among men under 50 years of age. It may therefore be prudent for adults to avoid sports/activities that involve high loading of the major joints (Kujala et al 1994), as Vingard et al (1993) reported a 4.5-fold increase in the risk of hip surgery among 50–70-year-old men who had played sports characterized by high loads. A variety of stresses (both sporting, such as cricket wicket keepers, and occupational, such as shoulder joints of pneumatic drillers) can predispose the participant to an increased incidence of OA (Panush and Brown 1987).

In contrast, aquatic exercises and locomotion (those with a low impact force at foot-strike) are excellent forms of activity for people with arthritis. Swimming is not a prerequisite skill, however, as activities may be performed while standing in the water, holding the side of the pool, or using flotation devices (McNeal 1990). The repeated impact forces associated with long distance running are not generally related to an increased incidence of OA (Lane et al 1987, 1993). Sohn and Micheli (1985) showed further that severe arthritic pain in the hips of people aged 57 years was similar (≈2%) for those who had engaged in swimming or running as a form of recreational activity.

However, the actual causative pathway to OA is still to be clearly defined. It is clear that a number of pathways can lead to the final, common malformation of the joint (Felson et al 2000a, 2000b). Increasing evidence suggests that OA is caused by an imbalance between the mechanical properties and integrity of bone, cartilage and other periarticular structures of the joint. It is important to appreciate that OA is a disease of all the articular structures, as this helps define how physical activity may be associated with the development of the condition, but also may help provide insight into how to prevent or reduce the symptoms. The following discussion will mainly focus on the knee joint, to which most research effort has been directed.

OA and the knee joint	The bone and articular cartilage of the joint are affected differently during the developmental stages of OA. The articular cartilage is the low friction surface that permits adjacent bones to articulate. Directly beneath the cartilage is the subchondral bone (cortical bone), and underneath that is cancellous or trabecular bone. Trabecular bone is the fastest of these tissues to remodel, then subchondral bone, and finally cartilage which is slow to remodel (Boyd et al 2000, Farkas et al 1987).

The diseased joint has highly remodelled bony structures; the most prominent being the presence of osteophytes (bony outgrowths at the margins of the joint) and sclerosis of the subchondral bone (bone of very high density). Osteophytes are thought to be produced by the body to increase articular area, buttress the joint, and to re-tension the lax ligaments of the OA joint. In advanced stages of OA, animal model studies have shown that trabeculae are thicker with a higher bone mass, compared to normal (Wu et al 1990). In human cadavers with advanced OA, the trabeculae have higher density, are thicker, smaller in number and are more aligned with the long axis of the bone (Kamibayashi et al 1995).

OA is also characterized by cartilage erosion, even down to subchondral bone in extreme cases. This gives the classic appearance of joint space narrowing, as can be seen in the knee X-rays of OA sufferers. Joint laxity results from this narrowing of cartilage and/or bone as the ligaments on the narrowed side of the joint become lax, or as the ligaments and capsule stretch (Sharma et al 1999). Thus, varus–valgus instability of the knee joint during the stance phase of walking can occur in the later stages of OA (tibiofemoral osteoarthritis (TFOA)). The laxity mentioned above can lead to condylar lift-off during walking, which causes an uneven force distribution at the knee joint. The lateral condyle of the femur lifts off the lateral tibial plateau thus concentrating the entire articular load on the medial condyle (Schipplein and Andriacchi 1991). It is interesting to note that lateral condylar lift might also occur in healthy knees during stance if it was not for the action of the muscles stabilizing the joint (Schipplein and Andriacchi 1991).

Joint loading has been implicated as a major cause of joint OA. In animal models, a number of mechanical factors have been used to induce TFOA; the most important being impact loading (Simon et al 1972) and overloading of the joint (Wu et al 1990). Furthermore, the type of joint loading has been shown to affect the resultant bone changes. Impact loading of the knee (Simon et al 1972) has been shown to produce changes typical of OA in the bone and cartilage. It was hypothesized that impact loading alters the subchondral bone and trabecular bone in the proximal tibia, which stiffens the bone thus reducing its shock-absorbing properties. Consequently, the joint cartilage is required to absorb a greater proportion of the load, which leads to development of TFOA (Radin et al 1991).

A milder form of impact loading occurs when stability of the joint is compromised. For example, an anterior cruciate ligament (ACL) transection (Boyd et al 2000, 2002, Myers et al 1990, O'Connor et al 1989) often leads to joint instability. The unloading of the injured limb causes the trabeculae to become thinner, weakening the support to the subchondral bone and cartilage. Because the trabecular bone is now weaker, the subchondral bone remodels, becoming thicker and denser to increase strength of the bone underlying the cartilage. In turn, this leads to the same outcome as in animal models that have been used in impact loading studies to induce OA. Stiffening of the subchondral bone forces the cartilage to provide greater shock absorption, which leads to fibrillation of this tissue (Radin et al 1991).

Pure overloading of the joint articular surfaces has also been shown to induce OA in animals. Surgically-induced, extreme angulation of the tibia, which concentrates articular forces onto one condyle of the knee, also produced joint degeneration (Wu et al 1990).

Different loading conditions have been shown to cause changes to the cartilage in animal models (Newton et al 1997, Vanwanseele et al 2002). However, the experimental loading conditions employed in these studies make it difficult to delineate the actual cause of the change to the cartilage (i.e. cartilage changes may have been due to alterations to the subchondral bone). Nevertheless, immobilization has a large effect on the joint, causing the cartilage to thin, increasing cartilage calcification, which results in the subchondral bone becoming thicker and encroaching into the cartilage (Vanwanseele et al 2002). Unloading the joint, while maintaining joint mobility, does not elicit the same level of change. Dogs with normal joints, that experience moderate and heavy running programmes do not seem to have compromised cartilage, and moreover have improved cartilage thickness and mechanical properties (Newton et al 1997). Thus exposure of an intact joint to normal physiological loading and ensuring normal joint mobility should not cause knee OA.

Joint loading and OA in humans

Joint overload has been implicated in the development of OA in humans. Obesity in women leads to a faster progression of TFOA (Anderson and Felson 1988, Felson et al 1988), while high levels of physical activity or repetitive and/or high loading during daily work are also risk factors for OA of the hands and knees (Hadler et al 1978). Some people exhibit high impact and articular loading during walking and running, which have been suggested as being an aetiological factor in knee TFOA (Prodromos et al 1985, Radin et al 1991). Based on recent data from 20- to 30-year-old healthy subjects collected from our gait laboratory, approximately 25% displayed high impact loading and about 30% have large external loading of the knee when walking. In addition, people who have knee joint disabilities, such as OA (Kaufman et al 2001), or who have had a recent partial meniscectomy (Sturnieks et al 2001) have larger varus moments (stresses lateral ligament; "bow-legged posture") than normal. These people need gait retraining to reduce impact loading or overloading of the joint.

Greater-than-normal knee varus moments during the stance phase of gait generate large loads on the medial articular surfaces of the tibiofemoral (TF) joint (Prodromos et al 1985, Schipplein and Andriacchi

1991). The varus (adduction) moment tends to adduct the lower leg towards the midline of the body in the frontal plane, pivoting about the medial condyle. In walking this has been shown to be reduced when varus knee alignment was corrected (Kettelkamp et al 1988, Prodromos et al 1985, Weidenhielm et al 1995). Even though subjects had the same varus knee alignment following surgical correction, those with larger varus moments pre-surgery also had larger varus moments post-surgery, poorer clinical outcomes and recurrence of the varus deformity (Prodromos et al 1985). Importantly, static frontal plane alignment of the knee does not predict progression of TFOA (Dougados et al 1992). Therefore, poor knee alignment does not necessarily cause the large varus moments in gait, whereas large varus moments do appear to induce the progression of TFOA.

The varus moments in gait are also related to TF joint bony architecture. In normal young non-OA subjects, larger varus moments are correlated with increased bone density in the medial proximal tibia (Hurwitz et al 1998). Furthermore, higher knee varus moments in gait among TFOA patients are correlated with the more prominent osteophytes and smaller medial joint space width (Sharma et al 1998). These results further suggest that gait patterns, which increase loading of the knee articular surfaces, are critical to the development of TFOA.

Many people exhibit prominent impact forces at heel strike during normal walking (Lloyd et al 1991, Whittle 1999), which generate high impact loads at the knee (Whittle 1999). This is readily seen in the vertical ground reaction (Whittle 1999), where faster walking speed and higher body mass both increase the magnitude of the impact forces (Lloyd et al 1991). Thus the link between obesity and development of OA may in part depend on impact forces during locomotion. Compared with normal, age-matched controls, people with knee pain (but no OA in the joint), exhibit larger heel strike transient forces (Jefferson et al 1990, Radin et al 1991). These people also show reduced quadriceps activity, which is thought to reduce control of eccentric knee flexion, yet concurrently increases leg angular velocity and heel vertical velocity just prior to heel strike. One school of thought suggests that these people are pre-osteoarthritic and the larger heel strike impact loading leads eventually to the development of knee OA (Jefferson et al 1990, Radin et al 1991). This hypothesis has yet to be tested in a pre-osteoarthritic or osteoarthritic population.

Higher levels of muscle activation may cause larger articular loads and this may lead to the development of OA or make the condition worse. For example, people who have larger-than-normal grip strength appear to have greater risk of developing OA in the joints of the hand (Chaisson et al 1999). Whether the same happens at other joints susceptible to OA remains open to question.

Large varus knee moments in gait may lead to condylar lift-off, thereby concentrating the loading on the medial compartment of the knee. This loading has been hypothesized as a possible aetiology for the development or progression of TFOA (Lloyd and Buchanan 1996, 2001, Prodromos et al 1985). As stated earlier, unimpaired people require specific muscle activation patterns to prevent this condylar lift (Schipplein and Andriacchi 1991). Articular forces acting on the medial knee compartment during walking have been estimated to be two to three times body weight with unloading on the lateral condyle during mid-stance and are predictors of the increased bone density in the medial proximal tibia (Hurwitz et al 1998). However, models often used to predict the articular loading of the knee frequently do not include muscle activation patterns as inputs to the model (Prodromos et al 1985, Schipplein and Andriacchi 1991). Preliminary findings suggest that gross underestimates may occur if activation patterns are not included (Besier and Lloyd 2001). Thus, muscular stabilization can be both beneficial and harmful. It is beneficial in that it stabilizes the lax joint and distributes the total joint contact forces between the condyles. It can also be harmful because a more even load distribution may only be achieved by increasing total articular loading. 'Over-stabilization' patterns may also exist in the gait of those who have suffered an injury or have joint laxity, producing higher-than-normal articular forces. Studies conducted in our laboratory have shown a marked increase in the muscular support or 'over-stabilization' of static valgus/varus moments in 20% of unimpaired subjects (Lloyd and Buchanan 2001).

Injury to a joint is one of the primary causes of human OA (Altman 1995). Ligament, cartilage and meniscal injuries occur in sport and traumatic impacts. The loading associated with these injuries, together with altered joint mechanics, may be a cause of the rapid development of OA (Altman 1995, Boyd et al 2002, O'Connor et al 1989, Wu et al 1990). Ligament injuries can compromise the stability of the joint, which increases the impact loading of the articular surfaces. Impact loading may be seen in ACL-deficient subjects where, during stance phase of walking, greater medial–lateral accelerations of the knee joint are indicative of instability (Yoshimura et al 2000). Lateral laxity permits the knee to go into varus postures in normal standing, although this laxity may be stabilized by the muscles surrounding the joint. However, muscular stabilization also increases articular loading during gait (Lloyd and Buchanan 2001).

Neuromuscular factors in OA

Muscle weakness has been strongly linked to the development of OA (Slemenda et al 1997). The quadriceps are reflexively inhibited in a number of knee joint conditions, such as knee pain (Suter et al 1998), joint effusion (Radin et al 1991), ACL deficiency (Snyder-Mackler et al 1994), ACL reconstruction (Urbach et al 2001) and OA (Hurley and Newham 1993). Data on hamstrings inhibition are inconclusive, with studies reporting weaker hamstrings in those with OA (Hurley et al 1994) and an ACL-injured knee (St Clair Gibson et al 2000). In contrast, Slemenda et al (1997) showed no reduction in hamstrings strength for subjects who developed OA. Knee pain (Radin et al 1991) and effusion (Torry et al 2000) have been shown to cause inhibition of quadriceps and facilitation of the hamstrings while walking. Radin et al (1991) showed an increase in impact forces at heel-strike in walking that was related to knee pain via the inhibition of the quadriceps (Jefferson et al 1990). Finally, low knee extension strength has been associated with the development of OA (Slemenda et al 1998). Thus it appears that quadriceps strength is linked to the development of knee OA.

Knee extension strength also plays a role in knee joint stabilization. Quadriceps weakness may create what are called 'quadriceps avoidance gait patterns', whereby a person avoids quadriceps activation during the stance phase of gait, by lowering knee joint extension moments (DeVita et al 1998, Lewek et al 2002). The quadriceps muscles are major stabilizers of the knee in both varus and valgus (Lloyd and Buchanan 2001), and the requirement to generate knee joint extension moments in stance is the main reason for activating this group (Lloyd and Buchanan 2001). In 'avoidance gait', there is less need to generate extension moments leading to lower varus stabilization of the knee. This may increase the loading on the knee ligaments, leading to laxity in these structures. Such an occurrence may be the precursor of a degenerative spiral, where increasing knee instability, damage to other tissues in the joint, and a quadriceps inhibition are linked.

Somatosensation is a general term for all the sensory systems that provide information about the state of the human body and its environment. Such systems include proprioception (joint position and movement sense), pain perception and cutaneous sensation. Feedback from these systems plays a direct role in the lower level reflex pathways and in planning and selection of motor programmes for movement. Somatosensation also enables perception of the state of body systems (e.g. joint position, pain, temperature). Proprioception is poorer after knee injury (Borsa et al 1997, Carter et al 1997) and in those with OA (Sharma and Pai 1997). Balance can also be compromised in people with OA (Hurley 1998, Jones et al 1995). In animal models afferent nerve and ACL transections have been shown to increase the rate of progression to knee OA compared with ACL transection alone. This suggests a neurogenic cause for the progression or development of OA (O'Connor et al 1993). Likewise in people with diabetes, peripheral neuropathies lead to the condition of Charcot arthropathy, a degenerative disease of the knee (O'Connor et al 1993).

In humans, knee pain acts to inhibit the quadriceps muscle group and modify gait patterns that load the knee. As described earlier, those people with knee pain have been shown to inhibit the activity of the quadriceps when walking, which acts to increase the heel-strike impact forces (Radin et al 1991). As knee pain increases there is a corresponding decrease in the varus moments produced during gait. When analgesics reduced pain, increased varus loading was recorded with no increase in the stabilization provided by increased knee extension moments (Hurwitz et al 1999). This is a possible negative consequence of analgesics for OA, where the modified gait pattern may in fact increase the rate of joint degeneration.

Implications for prevention and rehabilitation of OA

Inhibition of the quadriceps can be overcome by strength training (McNair et al 1996). In those who have undergone resistance training, there has been a reduction in the inhibition of the quadriceps and a corresponding increase in knee extension strength. While the effect of this on gait patterns has not been tested, there has been improved knee function in those people who have participated in knee strengthening programmes (Hurley et al 1994). Since it is quadriceps activation and strength and not the hamstrings that is mainly affected by knee trauma and OA, the quadriceps are typically targeted in rehabilitation programmes (Hurley and Newham 1993, Hurley et al 1994).

Poor proprioception has been implicated in the development of OA (Bearne et al 2002), and good sensory input may slow the progression of the disease (O'Connor et al 1993). An intact sensory system is necessary to perceive changes in joint stability brought about through injury or the disease process (Hurley 1999, O'Connor et al 1993). Proprioception has been shown to improve with strength training, balance training (Bearne et al 2002) and through the use of knee braces. One study that investigated balance training and strength training for people with knee OA found improvements in knee extension strength and joint position sense (Bearne et al 2002).

In those people who have sustained a knee injury, early changes in trabecular bone may be the stimulus for initiation of the disease process. This appears to be an unloading response, where rapid changes occur in trabeculae, which become thinner and lose bone quality (Boyd et al 2000, 2002). Even though optimal programmes for treating these people have not been tested, treatment regimes should be characterized, after initial pain and inflammation recede, by a slow return to weight bearing where the joint is stabilized without impact loading. Hydrotherapy appears to be an ideal initial rehabilitation modality, although increased weight bearing is necessary to slowly cause trabecular bone remodelling. Since knee extension strength is most likely inhibited, a gradual increase in knee concentric and eccentric resistance exercises should be included in the training programme.

There has been little research into the effects of various gait patterns and load on the knee. In those people who are overweight, loss of weight is essential as this is directly related to size of the impact loading and magnitude of the varus moments during gait (Hurwitz et al 2000). At least in the early stages of rehabilitation, while body mass is still high, walking at a slow speed could be used to reduce impact loading. In a limited number of studies it has been shown that programmed gait habits are difficult to change. Even when the injury has been fixed by surgery (DeVita et al 1998, Lewek et al 2002), the pre-surgery gait patterns are retained (Prodromos et al 1985). Thus gait retraining may be necessary. Toe-out walking has been shown to reduce the varus moment in the stance phase of gait (Andrews et al 1996, Noyes et al 1996) and this technique may be beneficial in preventing further degeneration. Analgesics are usually used sparingly given that reduced pain in the joint may permit increased varus moments in gait (Hurwitz et al 1999, 2000). For maintenance of cartilage health, it is important to maintain joint motion and avoid high impact loading or repetitive overloading of the joint.

Physical activity pre- and post-surgery

Patients who experience arthritic pain often avoid exercise for fear of exacerbating their symptoms. This inactivity can accelerate the degenerative process. Ettinger and Afable (1994) acknowledged the complex relationship between muscle strength, joint pain and disability. Reduced strength or an imbalance of strength may increase stress on an unstable joint, which may then cause strain on innervated tissues resulting in pain and disability. Avoidance of activity only leads to the disuse of muscles, which may exacerbate muscle weakness, thereby creating a cycle of disuse, muscle weakness, pain and disability (Ettinger and Afable 1994).

Conversely, clinical evidence suggests that fit, strong patients recover faster following surgery in comparison to those who are less fit. Studies have indicated that aerobic and resistance exercise does not exacerbate joint symptoms among patients with OA or rheumatoid arthritis (Gilbey et al 2003, Minor et al 1989). An increasing number of health professionals argue that physical training should be considered to be a part of routine preoperative care in order to increase a patient's general resistance to stress before facing the trauma of surgery (Grimby and Hook 1971, Shilling and Molen 1984).

A recent prospective, randomized controlled study of 68 patients scheduled for total hip arthroplasty (THA), conducted by Gilbey et al (2003), compared the outcome of patients involved in an 8-week presurgery plus 10-week post-surgery exercise programme to a control group. The intervention group attended two 1-hour clinic sessions per week (hydrotherapy plus resistance exercises) and performed a home-based training programme twice per week. Prior to surgery, the intervention group showed improved strength and range of motion in the affected hip, as well as reduced pain, stiffness and difficulty in performing activities of daily living (Figure 5.3) compared with control patients.

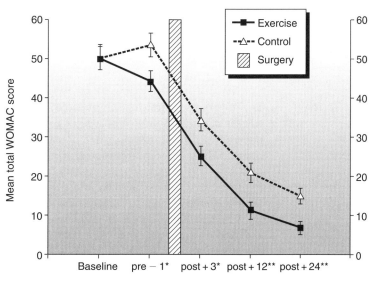

Figure 5.3 The Western Ontario and McMaster Universities Osteoarthritis Index (WOMAC) mean total scores in 57 patients (32 in the exercise group and 25 in the control group) 8 weeks (baseline), and 1 week (pre − 1) before surgery and at 3 (post + 3), 12 (post + 12), and 24 (post + 24) weeks after surgery are shown. *$P < 0.05$; **$P < 0.01$. (Reproduced from Gilbey et al Clinical Orthopaedics and Related Research 2003, 408: 193–200, with permission.)

Both Gilbey et al (2003) and Wang et al (2002) demonstrated that patients with increased levels of hip strength prior to surgery achieved the criteria for early or routine discharge more consistently than other patients.

Improved physical function before surgery also seems to provide a sound base from which to rehabilitate the patient after surgery. Gilbey et al (2003) demonstrated that patients who underwent the pre-surgery exercise programme received a sustained benefit during the subacute, postoperative phase (Figure 5.3). Rapid restoration of muscle strength after THA is an important factor in an individual's ability to return to independent, functional activities.

The post-surgery improvements in strength, range of motion and activities of daily living shown by Gilbey et al (2003) support the findings of Laupacis et al (1993) and Vaz et al (1993), whereby the most rapid improvement in strength of the treated limb occurred within the first 12 weeks. Continued, but less marked improvements are generally observed for up to 12 months among patients who follow the routine course of management, but some relative weakness may persist in comparison to the healthy limb. However, the data of Gilbey et al (2003) demonstrated that exercise group patients exhibited only minimal strength differences between the operated and healthy limb for thigh flexion, thigh extension and isometric thigh abduction (97%, 99% and 98% respectively).

The resultant implications for ambulatory function are striking. Muscle imbalance between limbs may affect gait symmetry and increase the possibility of symptoms developing in other joints. Muscular weakness around the hip will change the hip joint forces and could cause instability which, according to Perrin et al (1985), may lead to accelerated wear or loosening of the prosthesis and the need for early revision surgery. The results of Gilbey et al (2003) suggest that a post-surgery exercise programme may reduce the risk of these sequelae. Furthermore, with respect to patient independence, Wang et al (2002) reported that the exercise group demonstrated significantly greater stride length and gait speed than control subjects at 3-weeks post-surgery. At 12 and 24 weeks post-surgery, both gait speed and 6-minute walking distance among the exercise group were significantly greater than that for the control group.

Protection from falls

The ability to maintain stability following a perturbation (slip, knock or trip) is a fundamental motor skill in the elderly. This ability requires a number of different neuromuscular factors such as muscle strength and coordination to be maintained throughout life.

Muscle strength

Most athletes use strength training as a means of preparing for their sporting life. The same might be said for elderly people, who could include strength training as a means of protecting their quality of life. A number of studies have indicated that the aged exhibit marked increases in muscle strength (40–300%) after 8–12 weeks of training, but less than 10–15% of the increase in strength can be explained by an increase in muscle mass

(Staron et al 1994). Presumably most of the increase in strength, particularly with frail elderly people, is the result of changes to the 'neural drive' (Grabiner and Enoka 1995). It appears that strength training by elderly adults evokes rapid and sustainable increases in the maximum discharge rates of motor units (Patten et al 1995). These neural factors contribute to increases in muscle strength, especially at the beginning of a training programme (Enoka 1997), and to reducing muscle fatigue (Gandevia et al 1995). Strength training is therefore particularly beneficial for elderly people to enable them to perform many of their daily tasks.

There is a paucity of research examining whether benefits from strength training assist in the performance of dynamic actions required for everyday life (e.g. cutting the lawn, general lifting and carrying). However, the important point to be made regarding elderly adults is that activities of daily living do not require high strength levels, so even moderate increases would have a positive effect. It may be that daily activities that load but do not overload the body, while not as beneficial as actual strength training, still provide great benefit to the elderly person.

The result is quite understandable when one considers the biomechanics of walking, particularly among elderly adults. It has been shown (Winter 1991) that with two-thirds of the mass of the body in head, arms and trunk (HAT), balance control of the HAT is very important if upright gait is to be maintained. Muscles controlling hip joint motion balance the HAT (Winter 1991), and the elderly exhibit less hip extension and stay in flexion and forward trunk lean during walking (Kerrigan 1998, 2000). Therefore, increased hip extension strength is generally required to improve the walking gait of elderly persons.

We propose that if strength training programmes are to be beneficial, then specificity of training to function in elderly adults must be examined. However, there has been little research examining the functional deficits of elderly adults to assist in the structure of specific resistance training programmes.

When discussing the role of strength training in falls prevention, it is important to consider the relevant biological changes associated with ageing. Apart from pathological conditions, ageing appears to involve a number of changes in the central nervous system, including a decline in the number of functioning motor units and an increase in the innervation ratio of many of the remaining motor units (Galganski et al 1993). This decline in motor unit numbers is not distributed uniformly across the motor neuron pool, but rather, seems to involve the selective loss of high force-generating, fatigable motor units and an enlargement of the innervation ratio of low force, fatigue-resistant motor units (Faulkner and Brooks 1995). This undoubtedly influences the control strategies and capabilities of the central nervous system to grade muscle force. Strength training may therefore help overcome these reductions in function.

Muscle activation

Muscle co-activation appears to be a default strategy used by the nervous system when there is uncertainty about any task. Older adults often find it difficult to control the rate of change of force and commonly employ a co-activation safety strategy (Spiegel et al 1996). As stated above, strength training is known to affect the neural control used to coordinate movements (Enoka 1997). But one must use caution here since it has been shown that leg flexion/extension strength training leads to a decrease in the co-contraction of the hamstring and quadriceps muscles (Carolan and Cafarrelli 1992). Therefore, greater benefits may be gained with respect to falls prevention by engaging active recreational pursuits and locomotor activities in which both muscle strength and coordination are promoted.

General movement coordination

Variability in patterns of movement has traditionally been considered to be a characteristic of movement in elderly people, whereas skilled athletic performance was linked to precise control. While the outcome of skilled performance is tightly controlled, the notion that this end product may be achieved in a variety of ways is gaining acceptance in a wide variety of disciplines (Hamill et al 1999). The important role of movement variability has been demonstrated in the control of posture and body orientation. Furthermore, Hamill et al (1999) reported greater variability for asymptomatic runners when continuous relative phase plots of lower extremity coupling were compared for individuals with and without patellofemoral pain. Lack of movement variation is indicative of overuse loading on specific cartilage, tendons and ligament structures.

Elderly people often demonstrate a lack of variation in lower extremity movements (Winter 1991), which may impair their ability to handle small perturbations via a slip or bump when walking outdoors or simply about the house. By contrast, a more active person may learn to perform these skills in a variety of different ways and thereby develop strategies to cope with these unanticipated perturbations.

Summary

This chapter has reviewed current literature on biomechanical aspects of activity in elderly people from a functional perspective. It is clear that physical activity plays an important role in protecting a person from many chronic diseases and determining the quality of life. The level of activity should have a positive influence on the body without placing it into an overload situation. Although the type of activity depends on the goal, regular moderate exercise will normally produce health benefits.

References

Ackland T R 1998 Skeletal loading during resistance weight training: ramifications for exercise programs to prevent bone loss. In: Proceedings of the Australasian Society for Human Biology, National Meeting, Perth, Australia, p 31–32

Altman R D 1995 The classification of osteoarthritis. Journal of Rheumatology (Suppl): 43

Anderson J J, Felson D T 1988 Factors associated with osteoarthritis of the knee in the first national Health and Nutrition Examination Survey (HANES I).

Evidence for an association with overweight, race, and physical demands of work. American Journal of Epidemiology 128(1):179–189

Andrews M, Noyes R, et al 1996 Lower limb alignment and foot angle are related to stance phase knee adduction in normal subjects: a critical analysis of the reliability of gait analysis data. Journal of Orthopaedic Research 14(2):289–295

Bailey A J, Mansell J P 1997 Do subchondral bone changes exacerbate or precede articular cartilage destruction in osteoarthritis of the elderly? Gerontology 435:296–304

Bailey A J, Buckland-Wright C, et al 2001 The role of bone in osteoarthritis. Age and Ageing 30(5):374–378

Bearne L M, Scott D L, et al 2002 Exercise can reverse quadriceps sensorimotor dysfunction that is associated with rheumatoid arthritis without exacerbating disease activity. Rheumatology (Oxford) 41(2):157–166

Besier T F, Lloyd D G 2001 Muscle contributions to varus/valgus loads applied to the knee joint during walking. In: Proceedings XVIIIth Congress of the International Society of Biomechanics (CD Rom). Zurich, Switzerland

Borsa P A, Lephart S M, et al 1997 The effects of joint position and direction of joint motion on proprioceptive sensibility in anterior cruciate ligament-deficient athletes. American Journal of Sports Medicine 25(3):336–340

Boyd S K, Muller R, et al 2000 Early morphometric and anisotropic change in periarticular cancellous bone in a model of experimental knee osteoarthritis quantified using microcomputed tomography. Clinical Biomechanics 15(8):624–631

Boyd S K, Muller R, et al 2002 Mechanical and architectural bone adaptation in early stage experimental osteoarthritis. Journal of Bone Mineral Research 17(4):687–694

Carolan B, Cafarrelli E 1992 Adaptations in coactivation after isometric resistance training. Journal of Applied Physiology 73:911–917

Carter N D, Jenkinson T R, et al 1997 Joint position sense and rehabilitation in the anterior cruciate ligament deficient knee. British Journal of Sports Medicine 31(3):209–212

Chaisson C E, Zhang Y, et al 1999 Grip strength and the risk of developing radiographic hand osteoarthritis: Results from the Framingham Study. Arthritis and Rheumatism 42(1):33–38

Cheng Y, Macera C A, et al 2000 Physical activity and self-reported, physician-diagnosed osteoarthritis: is physical activity a risk factor? Journal of Clinical Epidemiology 53:315–322

Chow R, Harrison J, et al 1987 Effect of two randomised exercise programs on bone mass of healthy post menopausal women. British Medical Journal 295:1441–1444

DeVita P, Hortobagyi T, et al 1998 Gait biomechanics are not normal after anterior cruciate ligament reconstruction and accelerated rehabilitation. Medicine and Science in Sports and Exercise 30(10):1481–1488

Dougados M, Gueguen A, et al 1992 Longitudinal radiologic evaluation of osteoarthritis of the knee. Journal of Rheumatology 19(3):378–384

Enoka R 1997 Neural adaptations with chronic physical activity. Journal of Biomechanics 30:447–455

Ettinger W H, Afable R F 1994 Physical disability from knee osteoarthritis: the role of exercise as an intervention. Medicine and Science in Sports and Exercise 26:1435–1440

Farkas T, Boyd R D, et al 1987 Early vascular changes in rabbit subchondral bone after repetitive impulsive loading. Clinical Orthopaedics and Related Research 219:259–267

Faulkner J A, Brooks S A 1995 Muscle fatigue in old animals: unique aspects of fatigue in elderly human beings. In: Gandevia S, Enoka RM, et al (eds) Fatigue: neural and muscular mechanisms. Plenum Press, New York

Felson D T, Anderson J T, et al 1988 Obesity and knee osteoarthritis. The Framingham Study. Annals of Internal Medicine 109(1):18–24

Felson D T, Lawrence R C, et al 2000a Osteoarthritis: new insights. Part 1: the disease and its risk factors. Annals of Internal Medicine 133(8):635–646

Felson D T, Lawrence R C, et al 2000b Osteoarthritis: new insights. Part 2: treatment approaches. Annals of Internal Medicine 133(9):726–737

Forwood M R, Turner C H 1995 Skeletal adaptations to mechanical usage: results from tibial loading studies in rats. Bone 17:1975–2055

Frost H M 1983 A determinant of bone architecture: the minimum effective strain. Clinical Orthopaedics and Related Research 200:198–225

Galganski M E, Fuglevand A J, et al 1993 Reduced control of motor output in a human hand muscle of elderly subjects during submaximal contractions. Journal of Neurophysiology 69:2108–2115

Gallagher J C 1996 Estrogen: prevention and treatment of osteoporosis. In: Marcus R, Feldman D, et al (eds) Osteoporosis. Academic Press, San Diego

Gandevia S C, Enoka R M, et al 1995 Neural and muscular aspects of muscle fatigue. Plenum Press, New York

Gilbey H, Ackland T, et al 2003 Exercise improves early functional recovery after hip arthroplasty. Clinical Orthopaedics and Related Research 408: 193–200

Grabiner M, Enoka R 1995 Change in movement capabilities with aging. Exercise and Sport Science Reviews 23:65–104

Grimby G, Hook O 1971 Physical training of different patient groups: a review. Scandinavian Journal of Rehabilitation Medicine 3:15–25

Hadler N M, Gillings D B, et al 1978 Hand structure and function in an industrial setting. Arthritis and Rheumatism 21(2):210–220

Hamill J, van Emmerick R, et al 1999 A dynamical systems approach to lower extremity running injuries. Clinical Biomechanics 14:297–308

Hurley M V 1998 Quadriceps weakness in osteoarthritis. Current Opinion in Rheumatology 10(3):246–250

Hurley M V 1999 The role of muscle weakness in the pathogenesis of osteoarthritis. Rheumatology Disease Clinics of North America 25(2):283–298

Hurley M V, Newham D J 1993 The influence of arthrogenous muscle inhibition on quadriceps rehabilitation of patients with early, unilateral osteoarthritic knees. British Journal of Rheumatology 32(2):127–131

Hurley M V, Jones D W, et al 1994 Arthrogenic quadriceps inhibition and rehabilitation of patients with extensive traumatic knee injuries. Clinical Science (London) 86(3):305–310

Hurwitz D E, Sumner D R, et al 1998 Dynamic knee loads during gait predict proximal tibial bone distribution. Journal of Biomechanics 31(5):423–430

Hurwitz D E, Sharma L, et al 1999 Effect of knee pain on joint loading in patients with osteoarthritis. Current Opinion in Rheumatology 11(5):422–426

Hurwitz D E, Ryals A R, et al 2000 Knee pain and joint loading in subjects with osteoarthritis of the knee. Journal of Orthopaedic Research 18(4):572–579

Jefferson R J, Collins J J, et al 1990 The role of the quadriceps in controlling impulsive forces around heel strike. Journal of Engineering in Medicine 204(1):21–28

Jones G, Nguyen T, et al 1995 Osteoarthritis, bone density, postural stability, and osteoporotic fractures: a population based study. Journal of Rheumatology 22(5):921–925

Kamibayashi L, Wyss U P, et al 1995 Trabecular microstructure in the medial condyle of the proximal tibia of patients with knee osteoarthritis. Bone 17(1):27–35

Kaufman K R, Hughes C, et al 2001 Gait characteristics of patients with knee osteoarthritis. Journal of Biomechanics 34(7):907–915

Kerr D A, Morton A, et al 1996 Exercise effects on bone mass in postmenopausal women are site specific and strain dependent. Journal of Bone and Mineral Research 11:218–225

Kerr D A, Ackland T R, et al 2001 Resistance training over 2 years increases bone mass in calcium-replete postmenopausal women. Journal of Bone and Mineral Research 16:175–181

Kerrigan D C, Todd M K, et al 1998 Biomechanical gait alterations independent of speed in the healthy elderly: evidence for specific limiting impairments. Archives of Physical and Medical Rehabilitation 79(3):317–322

Kerrigan D C, Lee L W, et al 2000 Kinetic alterations independent of walking speed in elderly fallers. Archives of Physical and Medical Rehabilitation 81(6):730–735

Kettelkamp D B, Hillberry B M, et al 1988 Degenerative arthritis of the knee secondary to fracture malunion. Clinical Orthopaedics and Related Research 234:159–169

Kujala U M, Kaprio J, et al 1994 Osteoarthritis of weight-bearing joints of lower limbs in former elite male athletes. British Medical Journal 308:231–234

Lane N E, Bloch D A, et al 1987 Ageing, long-distance running and the development of musculoskeletal disability. American Journal of Medicine 82:772–780

Lane N E, Micheli B, et al 1993 The risk of osteoarthritis with running and ageing: a 5-year longitudinal study. Journal of Rheumatology 20:461–468

Lanyon L E 1996 Relationship with estrogen of the mechanical adaptation process in bone. Bone 18:375–435

Laupacis A, Bourne R, et al 1993 The effect of elective total hip replacement on health-related quality of life. Journal of Bone and Joint Surgery 75A:1619–1626.

Law M R, Wald N J, et al 1991 Strategies for prevention of osteoporosis and hip fracture. British Medical Journal 303:453–459

Lewek M, Rudolph K, et al 2002 The effect of insufficient quadriceps strength on gait after anterior cruciate ligament reconstruction. Clinical Biomechanics 17(1):56–63

Linsted K D, Tonstad K, et al 1991 Self-report of physical activity and patterns of mortality in Seventh-Day Adventist men. Journal of Clinical Epidemiology 44:355–364

Lloyd D G, Buchanan T S 1996 A model of load sharing between muscles and soft tissues at the human knee during static tasks. Journal of Biomechanical Engineering 118(3):367–376

Lloyd D G, Buchanan T S 2001 Strategies of the muscular contributions to the support of static varus and valgus loads at the human knee. Journal of Biomechanics 34(10):1257–1267

Lloyd D G, Raymond J, et al 1991 The determinants of impulsive forces at heel strike of women walking at a naturally selected walking speed. In: The 13th Conference of International Society of Biomechanics, Perth, Australia, p 233–234

MacRae P G, Feltner M E, et al 1994 A 1-year program for older women: effects on falls, injuries, and physical performance. Journal of Ageing and Physical Activity 2:127–142

McAlindon T E, Wilson P W, et al 1999 Level of physical activity and the risk of radiographic and symptomatic knee osteoarthritis in the elderly: the Framingham study. American Journal of Medicine 106:151–157

McNair P J, Marshall R N, et al 1996 Swelling of the knee joint: effects of exercise on quadriceps muscle strength. Archives of Physical Medicine Rehabilitation 77(9):896–899

McNeal R L 1990 Aquatic therapy for patients with rheumatic disease. Rheumatic Disease Clinics of North America 16(4):915–929

Minor M A, Hewett J E, et al 1989 Efficacy of physical conditioning exercise in patients with rheumatoid arthritis and osteoarthritis. Arthritis and Rheumatism 32:1396–1405

Morris F L, Naughton G A, et al 1997 Prospective ten month exercise intervention on premenarchial girls: positive effects on bone and lean mass. Journal of Bone Mineralisation Research 12:1453–1462

Myers S L, Brandt K D, et al 1990 Synovitis and osteoarthritic changes in canine articular cartilage after anterior cruciate ligament transection. Effect of surgical hemostasis. Arthritis and Rheumatism 33(9):1406–1415

Newton P M, Mow V C, et al 1997 The effect of lifelong exercise on canine articular cartilage. American Journal of Sports Medicine 25(3):282–287

Noyes F R, Dunworth L A, et al 1996 Knee hyperextension gait abnormalities in unstable knees. Recognition and preoperative gait retraining. American Journal of Sports Medicine 24(1):35–45

O'Connor P J, Lanyon L E, et al 1982 The influence of strain rate on adaptive bone remodelling. Journal of Biomechanics 15:767–781

O'Connor B L, Visco D M, et al 1989 Gait alterations in dogs after transection of the anterior cruciate ligament. Arthritis and Rheumatism 32(9):1142–1147

O'Connor B L, Visco D M, et al 1993 Sensory nerves only temporarily protect the unstable canine knee joint from osteoarthritis. Evidence that sensory nerves reprogram the central nervous system after cruciate ligament transection. Arthritis and Rheumatism 36:1154–1163

Panush R S, Brown D G 1987 Exercise and arthritis. Sports Medicine 4:54–64

Patten C, Kamen G, et al 1995 Rapid adaptations of motor unit firing rate during the initial phase of strength development. Medicine and Science in Sport and Exercise 27:S6

Perrin T, Dorr L, et al 1985 Functional evaluation of hip arthroplasty with five-to-ten year follow up evaluation. Clinical Orthopaedics and Related Research 195:252–260

Pollock M L 1988 Exercise prescription for the elderly. In: Spirduso W W, Eckert H M (eds) Physical activity and ageing. Human Kinetics, Champaign, IL

Prodromos C C, Andriacchi T P, et al 1985 A relationship between gait and clinical changes following high tibial osteotomy. Journal of Bone and Joint Surgery 67A(8):1188–1194

Radin E L, Yang H H, et al 1991 Relationship between lower limb dynamics and knee joint pain. Journal of Orthopaedic Research 9:398–405

Rikli R, McManus G G 1990 Effects of exercise on bone mineral content in post menopausal women. Research Quarterly for Exercise and Sport 6:243–249

Rubin C T, Lanyon L E 1984 Regulation of bone formation by applied dynamic loads. Journal of Bone and Joint Surgery 66A:397–402

Rutherford O M 1993 Spine and total body bone mineral density in amenorrhoeic endurance athletes. Journal of Applied Physiology 74(6):2904–2908

Schipplein O D, Andriacchi T P 1991 Interaction between active and passive knee stabilizers during level walking. Journal of Orthopaedic Research 9(1):113–119

Sharma L, Pai Y C 1997 Impaired proprioception and osteoarthritis. Current Opinion in Rheumatology 9(3):253–258

Sharma L, Hurwitz D W, et al 1998 Knee adduction moment, serum hyaluronan level, and disease severity in medial tibiofemoral osteoarthritis. Arthritis and Rheumatism 41(7):1233–1240

Sharma L, Lou C, et al 1999 Laxity in healthy and osteoarthritic knees. Arthritis and Rheumatism 42(5):861–870

Shilling J A, Molen M T 1984 Physical fitness and its relationship to preoperative recovery in abdominal hysterectomy patients. Heart and Lung 13:639–644

Simon S R, Paul I L, et al 1972 The response of joints to impact loading. II. In vivo behaviour of subchondral bone. Journal of Biomechanics 5:267–272

Slemenda C, Brandt D K, et al 1997 Quadriceps weakness and osteoarthritis of the knee. Annals of Internal Medicine 127(2):97–104

Slemenda C D K, Heilman D K, et al 1998 Reduced quadriceps strength relative to body weight: a risk factor for knee osteoarthritis in women? Arthritis and Rheumatism 41(11):1951–1959

Smith E L, Gilligan C, et al 1989 Exercise reduces bone involution in middle aged women. Calcification Tissue International 44:312–321

Snyder-Mackler L, De Luca P F, et al 1994 Reflex inhibition of the quadriceps femoris muscle after injury or reconstruction of the anterior cruciate ligament. Journal of Bone and Joint Surgery 76A(4):555–560

Sohn R S, Micheli L J 1985 The effect of running on the pathogenesis of osteoarthritis of the hips and knees. Clinical Orthopedics 198:106–109

Spiegel K, Stratton J, et al 1996 The influence of age on the assessment of motor unit activation in the human hand muscle. Experimental Physiology 81:805–809

Staron R S, Karapondo D L, et al 1994 Skeletal muscle adaptations during the early phase of heavy resistance training in men and women. Journal of Applied Physiology 76:1247–1255

St Clair Gibson A, Lambert M, et al 2000 Quadriceps and hamstrings peak torque ratio changes in persons with chronic anterior cruciate ligament deficiency. Journal of Orthopaedic and Sports Physical Therapy 30(7):418–427

Sturnieks D L, Lloyd D G, et al 2001 Variations in gait patterns: meniscectomy versus normal group. In: Proceedings of the XVIIIth Congress of the International Society of Biomechanics (CD Rom). Zurich, Switzerland

Suter E, Herzog W, et al 1998 Quadriceps inhibition following arthroscopy in patients with anterior knee pain. Clinical Biomechanics 13(4–5):314–319

Swissa-Sivan A, Simkin I, et al 1989 Effect of swimming on bone growth and development in young rats. Bone Mineralisation 7:91–106

Torry M R, Decker M J, et al 2000 Intra-articular knee joint effusion induces quadriceps avoidance gait patterns. Clinical Biomechanics 15(3):147–159

Urbach D, Nebelung W, et al 2001 Effects of reconstruction of the anterior cruciate ligament on voluntary activation of quadriceps femoris: a prospective twitch interpolation study. Journal of Bone and Joint Surgery 83B(8):1104–1110

US Department of Health and Human Services 1996 Physical activity and health: A report of the Surgeon General. Centers for Disease Control and Prevention, National Center for Chronic Disease Prevention and Health Promotion, Atlanta, GA

Vanwanseele B, Lucchinetti E, et al 2002 The effects of immobilization on the characteristics of articular cartilage: current concepts and future directions. Osteoarthritis and Cartilage 10(5):408–419

Vaz M, Kramer J, et al 1993 Isometric hip abductor strength following total hip replacement and its relationship to functional assessments. Journal of Orthopaedic and Sports Physical Therapy 18:526–531

Vingard E, Alfredsson L, et al 1993 Sports and osteoarthritis of the hip: an epidemiological study. American Journal of Sports Medicine 21:195–200

Wang A, Gilbey H, et al 2002 Perioperative exercise programmes improve early return of ambulatory function after total hip arthroplasty: a randomised controlled trial. American Journal of Physical Medicine and Rehabilitation 81:801–806

Weidenhielm L, Svensson O K, et al 1995 Surgical correction of leg alignment in unilateral knee osteoarthrosis reduces the load on the hip and knee joint bilaterally. Clinical Biomechanics 10:217–221

Whiting W, Zernicke R 1998 Biomechanics of musculoskeletal injury. Human Kinetics, Champaign, IL

Whittle M W 1999 Generation and attenuation of transient impulsive forces beneath the foot: a review. Gait and Posture 10(3):264–275

Winter D 1991 The biomechanics and motor control of human gait: normal, elderly and pathological, 2nd edn. University of Waterloo Press, Waterloo, Canada

World Health Organization 1996 World health report. World Health Organization, Geneva

World Health Organization 1998 World health report. World Health Organization, Geneva

Wu D D, Burr D B, et al 1990 Bone and cartilage changes following experimental varus or valgus tibial angulation. Journal of Orthopedic Research 8(4):572–585

Yoshimura I, Naito M, et al 2000 Analysis of the significance of the measurement of acceleration with respect to lateral laxity of the anterior cruciate ligament insufficient knee. International Orthopedics 24(5):276–278

6

Reducing the risk of osteoporosis: the role of exercise and diet

Shona L Bass, Caryl Nowson and Robin M Daly

CHAPTER CONTENTS

Introduction 99

The role of exercise in osteoporosis prevention 101

The role of diet in osteoporosis prevention 112

References 118

Introduction

Osteoporosis is a disease associated with low bone density and reduced mechanical competence of the skeleton leading to increased bone fragility and susceptibility to fracture. In 2001, nearly two million Australians (approximately 10% of the population) had osteoporosis-related conditions; three-quarters were women. It is estimated that 1 in 4 women and 1 in 6 men will suffer an osteoporotic fracture; this incidence is higher in those over the age of 60 (1 in 2 women and 1 in 3 men) (Osteoporosis Australia 2002). The lifetime risk of a hip fracture from the age of 50 years onwards has been estimated at 17% for white women and 6% for white men in the USA (this risk is lower in individuals from African or Asian heritage) (Cummings 2002, Melton and Cooper 2001). Of the diagnosed fractures, 46% are vertebral, 16% are hip and 16% are radial. In the next two decades, osteoporosis is predicted to reach epidemic proportions due to the demographic trend towards an ageing population. By 2021, it is predicted that three million Australians will be affected by osteoporosis with a fracture occurring every 3½ minutes (Osteoporosis Australia 2002). Thus osteoporosis is a major public health burden because it affects a large proportion of the community and fractures are associated with extensive mortality and morbidity.

Hip fracture is one of the most serious consequences of osteoporosis because of the excessive morbidity and mortality. Hip fracture incidence rates are known to increase exponentially with age in both men and women in most regions of the world. There is, however, considerable variation in hip fracture incidence between populations (Melton and Cooper 2001). In Australia, approximately 20% of those who sustain a hip fracture die within 6 months due to complications; almost 50% will require long-term nursing care, and up to 80% of those who survive will fail to regain their pre-fracture level of function, often suffering prolonged chronic pain, disability and depression (Access Economics 2001). Vertebral fractures are associated with pain, height loss, deformity, diminished quality of life and sometimes death (Access Economics 2001). Furthermore, women who have suffered a vertebral fracture are five times more likely to suffer a subsequent fracture within 12 months (Access Economics 2001).

Low bone mineral density (bone density) is a major risk factor for an osteoporotic fracture. Low bone density can be associated with many factors including advancing age, gender, low body weight, muscle weakness, oestrogen deficiency, smoking, excessive alcohol intake, low calcium intake, and inadequate physical activity. In addition to low bone density, the risk of falling has been identified as a major determinant of fracture. Risk factors associated with falling include impaired gait and balance (mobility impairment), poor vision, recurrent falls, muscle weakness, functional dependency, depression, and use of anti-depressant medications (independent of depression) (Fiatarone 2002).

Exercise and nutrition are two lifestyle factors that have potential to reduce the risk of osteoporosis by increasing and maintaining peak bone mass, reducing the rate of bone loss during adulthood, maintaining bone mass in elderly people and reducing the risk of falling. In this chapter the role of exercise and diet as therapeutic modalities will be discussed in terms of slowing the course of bone fragility in elderly people and the risk of fracture in the frail elderly.

Skeletal metabolism during growth and ageing

The skeleton is an active organ that undergoes change throughout life through the processes of modelling and remodelling. Bone *modelling* refers to the sculpturing of bone (size, shape and spatial location) through the synthesis of new bone on some surfaces and resorption of bone at other surfaces in response to extraneous factors such as mechanical loading. Modelling involves the addition of bone, without prior resorption, and therefore does not depend on any biological coupling between osteoclasts (bone-resorbing cells) and osteoblasts (bone-forming cells) (Baron 1990). It can affect cortical, periosteal, endocortical and trabecular surfaces; it can increase but not decrease the periosteal perimeter, cortical thickness and cortical bone mass; it can only thicken, but not reduce, trabeculae. The majority of bone modelling occurs during the growing years with limited modelling occurring following skeletal maturation (Burr et al 1989). Bone *remodelling* replaces (or 'turns bone over') fatigue-damaged bone in a biologically coupled activation–resorption–formation sequence requiring the coordination of osteoclasts and osteoblasts in a specific 'coupled' sequence. Remodelling acts throughout life on periosteal, Haversian, endocortical and trabecular surfaces.

Figure 6.1 The gain and loss of bone mass over the lifespan. Low bone mass in elderly people may be the result of reduced peak bone mass attained during growth, rapid bone loss during menopause and/or ageing or a combination of both.

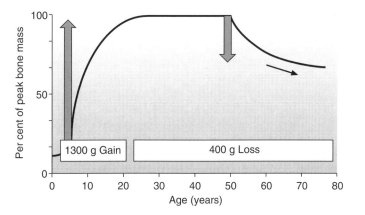

Except on the periosteal surface, remodelling does not usually make more bone than is resorbed – bone is either removed or conserved (Frost 1992).

Non-traumatic osteoporotic fractures occur because of reduced bone strength associated with low bone mass and reduced architectural stability of the skeleton at the site of fracture. Despite fractures typically occurring in elderly people, the pathogenesis of osteoporosis may have its origins early in life. For instance, low bone mass in elderly people may be the result of reduced peak bone mass attained during growth, rapid bone loss during menopause and/or ageing or a combination of both (Figure 6.1). During growth, bone mass increases rapidly with 40% of peak bone mass accrued during the 2 to 4 years of pubertal development (Bailey et al 2000). Peak bone mass is generally maintained until mid-life after which there is rapid bone loss during menopause (up to 4% per year) and a slow gradual bone loss during ageing (~1% per year) (Figure 6.1). The lower risk of fracture in men (compared with women) is thought to be due to gender-related differences in skeletal growth and ageing. Males build a bigger and stronger skeleton during growth and do not experience the rapid bone loss that is associated with menopause, although males and females experience a similar rate of bone loss during ageing (Seeman 2001).

The role of exercise in osteoporosis prevention

Maximizing peak bone mass and preventing age-related bone loss are important approaches to reducing fracture risk in old age. Exercise is one of the most effective lifestyle therapies to contribute to this lifespan approach for osteoporosis prevention. The role of exercise is dependent on the stage of life and the relative risk of fracture. During growth, vigorous exercise leads to large increases in peak bone mass and bone strength (up to 30%). However, in pre- and postmenopausal women moderate to high intensity weight-bearing exercise and high intensity progressive resistance training and impact loading have been shown to increase bone density by more modest amounts (1–4%). In the frail elderly where intense and high impact exercise is not indicated, the benefits of exercise include increased muscle mass and strength, and improved balance and coordination. There may also be psychosocial benefits associated with exercise, such as reduced feelings of depression, anxiety and stress and social isolation that improve well-being and quality of life, which may indirectly contribute to the prevention of falls and lower the risk of fracture.

Precise exercise prescription guidelines in relation to fracture-risk reduction await long term randomized controlled trials (RCTs) that include anti-fracture efficacy as the outcome. However, general exercise recommendations can be made according to the goal of the activity programme and the fracture risk of the individual. In this section, the optimal characteristics of loading and principles of training to maximize bone mass during growth and reduce bone loss during ageing will be presented. Prescription guidelines for the frail elderly will also be discussed.

Characteristics of effective mechanical loading

The skeleton adapts to changes in mechanical loading or strain (*strain* is the deformation that develops in bone in response to an externally applied load) by altering its mass, shape and structure in order to withstand future loads of a similar nature. This unique ability of the skeleton to respond to the different characteristics of loading has been described by Frost's 'mechanostat' theory (Frost 1987). According to this theory, bones have a set-point or threshold level for adaptation called the minimum effective strain (MES) – if strains continually fall within the optimal strain range or MES, no adaptive bone response will occur. In contrast, if strains exceed the upper threshold or set-point of this MES range, bone modelling and/or remodelling will increase (i.e. leading to a change in bone mass) to reduce strains to within the optimal range. However, if strains fall below the set-point of the optimal range (e.g. during periods of disuse, immobilization or detraining), bone tissue will be resorbed resulting in a negative adaptive response. It is thought that MES set-points are genetically controlled and vary depending on the skeletal site, loading history and several hormonal and local agents, including oestrogen (Frost 1987). Furthermore, the MES for bone remodelling is lower than that for bone modelling, and during old age the MES becomes less sensitive and thus greater strains are required to elicit an adaptive bone response (Kohrt 2001).

Extensive research using animal models has shown that the skeleton's response to exercise is regulated by a number of different loading characteristics, including the type, magnitude, rate, distribution (or pattern) and number of loading cycles. While research to confirm these findings has not been conducted in humans, the following are key characteristics of loading associated with an optimal adaptive bone response in animals:

- intermittent dynamic (e.g. jumping), rather than static loads provide greater stimulation for bone formation (Lanyon and Rubin 1984)

- loads which are high in magnitude and applied at a high strain rate (e.g. rapid and high impact activities) are particularly effective for stimulating an osteogenic response (O'Connor et al 1982, Rubin and Lanyon 1985)
- relatively few loading cycles or repetitions are needed to elicit bone formation, and the capacity for bone to respond to a given stimulus is saturated after a few loading cycles (Raab et al 1994, Rubin and Lanyon 1984)
- unusual or diverse loading patterns, differing from that to which the bone is typically accustomed, may be just as important for initiating an adaptive bone response as the magnitude or number of loading cycles (Lanyon et al 1982, Rubin and Lanyon 1984).

The American College of Sports Medicine has also recommended that five basic principles of training be incorporated into exercise programmes designed to augment bone mass and prevent falls (Drinkwater et al 1995):

1. *Principle of specificity*: exercise must be site-specific, e.g. the greatest changes in bone in response to exercise occur at skeletal sites which are directly loaded.
2. *Principle of overload*: exercise must exceed those loads typically encountered during everyday activities, and as the bone responds the stimulus (magnitude, rate, frequency and/or distribution of loading) must be increased progressively.
3. *Principle of reversibility*: any positive effects of exercise on bone will not be maintained if the programme or stimulus is discontinued or removed.
4. *Principle of initial values*: the greatest changes in bone in response to loading occur in those with the lowest initial bone density; those with average or above average bone density do not exhibit marked skeletal changes in response to loading.
5. *Principle of diminished returns*: following an initial adaptation to a given level of exercise, any further gains in bone are likely to be slow and of small magnitude.

The effect of exercise on peak bone strength

For exercise during growth to be effective in the prevention of osteoporosis, the response to loading must be large enough to be considered clinically important and the benefits gained need to be maintained into later life when fractures occur. A 10% increase in bone mass at the femoral neck is associated with halving the risk of fracture (Cumming et al 1993); thus a 5% increase in peak bone mass would be considered to be clinically important. Long-term, intense exercise during growth has been shown to lead to large increases in peak bone mass (5–40%). Large increases in cortical thickness as a result of lifelong exercise were first demonstrated by comparing the playing and non-playing arm of tennis players (Huddleston et al 1980). Higher bone mass of similar magnitudes has also been reported in young elite athletes (Bass et al 1998).

For the benefits of exercise during growth to be considered clinically important, they must be maintained into adulthood. The site-specific higher bone density of gymnasts retired for up to twenty years suggests that this may be the case (Bass et al 1998). Whether these residual benefits are maintained into later life when fractures occur is not known. The study to test this question will never be done because of the long time interval between exposure (exercise during growth) and outcome (fracture in elderly people). However, the limited data in 70- to 80-year-old retired athletes suggest that the effects may be eroded in those who have substantially decreased their training volumes (Karlsson et al 2000).

These data in elite athletes provide us with a model of what is possible rather than probable in normally active children. The results of prospective and retrospective cohort studies, and cross-sectional studies, have shown that children and adolescents who are physically active can accrue between 5% and 15% more bone mass than their sedentary peers (Bailey et al 1999, Cooper et al 1995, Gunnes and Lehman 1996). A limitation of cohort studies is that sampling bias may influence the results. In this case children who are bigger and stronger are likely to be successful in sport. Thus the greater increase in bone mass reported in active children may be a reflection of genetic factors that lead to larger muscles and bones, rather than the result of exercise itself. Despite these limitations, these data do support the notion that long-term physical activity may lead to a higher peak bone mass. However, long-term exercise intervention studies are required to validate these findings.

The few published prospective exercise intervention studies in pre- and peri-pubertal children are all short-term, school-based studies (8 to 11 months) (Bradney et al 1998, Heinonen et al 2000, McKay et al 2000, Morris et al 1997). Not all these studies were randomized, and the interventions included either extra physical education classes or exercise additional to physical education classes. These exercise interventions resulted in a 1.3–5% greater increase in bone density at the legs, while findings were equivocal at the spine. There have been only two studies to date that have quantified loads associated with an osteogenic effect in children. Fuchs reported that bone density at the lumbar spine and femoral neck increased by 4% after children jumped from a 65 cm high bench 100 times three times per week over seven months (Fuchs et al 2001). These jumps loaded the skeleton up to eight times body weight (BW). More recently it has reported that more moderate impact exercise may be sufficient to result in an osteogenic response (Saxon et al 2000). This programme included low (<2 BW), moderate (2–4 BW) and high (>4 BW) impact exercise (74%, 23% and 3% respectively). The increase in bone mineral density (BMD) was comparable to the increases reported by Fuchs et al but the load was less than one half. In this study, however, the loads were progressively increased and were multidirectional. These data are supported by animal studies showing that high impact activities that place unusual strain distributions on the bone elicit a greater osteogenic response than repetitive low impact activities (Chilibeck et al 1995). While the results of these studies are encouraging, more research is required before specific exercise prescription can be developed for improved bone health in children. We know that high impact exercise is important but little is known about the magnitude, duration and frequency of loads required to elicit a clinically important increase in bone density and bone size in children that will be maintained in later life when the fractures occur.

The time period in growth when children exercise may also be important. For instance, up to four times the skeletal benefit appears to be achieved when girls exercise before, rather than after menarche (Kannus et al 1995). In addition, exercise before puberty may have the additional benefit of increasing the external size of the bone (i.e. periosteal expansion) (Bass et al 2002). Apposition of bone on the periosteal (outer) surface of cortical bone is a more effective means of increasing the bending and torsional strength of bone than acquisition of bone on the endocortical (inner) surface (i.e. a greater external bone size increases load-bearing capacity) (Turner and Burr 1993). However, more research is needed before we can understand how the growing skeleton adapts to loading during different stages of growth (Bass 2000, MacKelvie et al 2002).

Summary

Long-term intense training in young athletes leads to increased peak bone mass, with benefits being maintained into adulthood even when training has ceased. The results from short-term, exercise interventions in normally active children provide encouraging evidence for the role of weight-bearing exercises (such as hopping and jumping) in increasing bone strength (due to increased bone density and bone size). It is not known how long or at what intensity young people need to exercise for the benefits to be maintained when the exercise is ceased.

Exercise to maximize bone mass during adulthood

The results from early studies comparing the bone density of athletes to non-athletic controls suggested that exercise had potential to result in large increases (10–15%) in bone density during adulthood. Unfortunately this early enthusiasm was not perpetuated by the results of RCTs. The results of these studies showed that moderate exercise (including weight-bearing exercise and weight training) in normally active adults resulted in much smaller effects on bone density (1–3%). Thus in contrast to childhood, in adulthood the primary benefit of exercise on the skeleton is conservation, not acquisition.

Aerobic training

There is general consensus that walking, jogging and aerobic/endurance activities alone are not particularly beneficial for enhancing skeletal health in healthy, asymptomatic men and women. In pre- and postmenopausal women, brisk walking or jogging over 6 to 24 months resulted in either small increases in bone density (1–3%), no change or bone loss (Brooke-Wavell et al 1997, Cavanaugh and Cann 1988, Dalsky et al 1988, Ebrahim et al 1997, Hatori et al 1993, Humphries et al 2000, Martin and Notelovitz 1993, Snow-Harter et al 1992). There is some evidence, however, that combining walking with more intense bouts of exercise may be more beneficial than walking alone. For instance, a multi-exercise endurance training programme involving walking, jogging, cycling, stair-climbing and graded treadmill exercises at 55–75% of maximum oxygen consumption (VO_{2max}) maintained bone density in older women (Heinonen et al 1998). Others have also reported that moderate to vigorous walking (65–85% of VO_{2max}) combined with stepping exercises, weighted belts, or stair-climbing can be beneficial for skeletal health (Chien et al 2000, Kohrt et al 1995, 1997).

There is little information about the effects of walking/aerobic/endurance training on skeletal health in middle-aged and older men. A recent population-based controlled intervention trial showed that 4 years of low to moderate intensity walking (5 times/week, 60 min at 40–60% of VO_{2max}) had no effect on bone density at the hip or spine (Huuskonen et al 2001). However, 9 months training for a marathon in men aged 38 to 68 years with no previous running experience resulted in increased bone mass at the heel compared with non-exercising controls (Williams et al 1984). In contrast, in a 5-year non-randomized longitudinal study, men aged 55 to 77 years who jogged tended to lose less bone density at the lumbar spine compared with controls (Michel et al 1992).

Resistance training

Resistance or strength training programmes appear to elicit a greater adaptive bone response than walking or jogging. This type of training involves high loads that stimulate the skeleton through the direct action of muscle pulling on bone and/or the increased effect of gravity acting on bone when the skeleton supports heavy weights. In older adults high-intensity resistance programmes undertaken 2–3 times per week have consistently led to modest increases in bone density (1–3%), with the greatest changes occurring at the lumbar spine. For instance, in premenopausal women aged 20 to 40 years, high intensity progressive resistance weight training increased lumbar spine and hip bone density by up to 2% (3 times/week, 8–12 repetitions (reps) $\times$ 3 sets, 12–14 exercises, 70–85% of one repetition maximum strength (1 RM)) (Lohman et al 1995, Snow-Harter et al 1992). In postmenopausal women not on hormone replacement therapy, high-intensity resistance training (2 times/week, 8 reps $\times$ 3 sets, 5 exercises, 80% of 1 RM) has been shown to maintain or increase bone density (Nelson et al 1994). Kerr et al (1996) reported that in postmenopausal women, high-intensity (3 sets $\times$ 8 reps maximum) resistance training was more effective in increasing bone density than low intensity training (3 sets $\times$ 20 reps maximum) despite similar increases in muscle strength in both groups. Similar findings were also reported in elderly women aged 65–79 years (Taaffe et al 1996). In contrast, others have failed to detect a change in bone density following either high- or low-intensity resistance training in postmenopausal women (Pruitt et al 1995). These equivocal findings are likely to be due to differences in the intensity, frequency and duration of the exercise regimens, and/or differences related to the subjects' age, nutritional status, loading history, hormonal status and compliance to the exercise programme.

Few RCTs of resistance training have been conducted in middle-aged and older men, but the results of one short-term trial are encouraging. In men aged 50 to 60 years, 6 months training in a high-intensity free weight exercise programme (8 reps $\times$ 3 sets, 70–90% of 1 RM, 12 exercises, 3 times/week) resulted in a 1.9% gain in lumbar spine bone density (Maddalozzo and Snow 2000). In contrast there was no effect detected from a moderate-intensity machine weight programme (10–13 reps $\times$ 3 sets, 40–60% of 1 RM, 13 exercises, 3 times/week), despite similar increases in muscle strength and lean mass in both groups following training.

Despite the disparate results from RCTs examining the effects of resistance training on bone density in older adults, a common outcome of most resistance training studies is the marked improvements in muscle strength, balance, coordination, mobility and/or reaction time, and the preservation or increase in muscle mass. These factors are particularly important because they have been consistently associated with an increased risk of falling and fractures in elderly people. In addition, resistance training has been shown to be effective in the treatment of depression in elderly people and thus provides an option as a substitute for antidepressant medications, which are known to increase the risk of hip fracture (Fiatarone 2002). However, it is currently unknown whether these benefits translate into fracture-risk reduction.

Impact exercise

Exercise interventions incorporating weight-bearing activities of a moderate to high magnitude and loading rate, such as jumping, appear to provide a better stimulus for promoting bone gain or preventing bone loss in healthy asymptomatic individuals than walking or low-intensity aerobic activities. For instance, in healthy premenopausal women progressive high impact training over 18 months (3 times/week, 60 min jumping, stepping and callisthenics) resulted in 0.7 to 2.4% greater increases in bone density at the weight-bearing sites compared with a non-exercising control group (Heinonen et al 1996). Similar results were reported at the hip following a 5-month non-progressive training programme consisting of 50 vertical jumps (mean height 8.5 cm, 3–4 BW) six days per week in premenopausal women (Bassey et al 1998). However, these results were not replicated in postmenopausal women (regardless of hormone replacement therapy status) after 12 or 18 months training at any skeletal site. But there is some evidence that progressively loaded high impact exercise may have positive skeletal effects in postmenopausal women. Welsh and Rutherford (1996) reported that a 12-month progressive high-impact aerobic exercise programme, which included bench stepping, jumping and skipping, increased hip but not spine bone density in previously sedentary older men and postmenopausal women relative to matched controls. High impact work is contraindicated for individuals with poor balance, strength or stability, osteoporosis, history of fracture, osteoarthritis or artificial joints.

Summary

A combination of decreased hormones (oestrogen, testosterone, growth hormone), the emergence of musculoskeletal and other diseases, retirement and reduced recreational activities can have a negative impact on bone and muscle tissue (Fiatarone 2002). It is for these reasons that exercise is so important in osteoporosis prevention in middle-aged and older adults. It appears resistance-training programmes may be one of the most beneficial forms of exercise in middle-aged and older adults. Magnitude of the load is an important characteristic of the training programmes; one to three sets of 8–12 repetitions at 60–90% of one repetition maximum strength (1 RM) with a 1–2 minute rest period between sets is recommended. A range of upper and lower body and trunk exercises should be selected using a combination of machine weights, free weights and/or rubber tubing. Training should begin at a low intensity (40–50% of 1 RM) until correct technique, form and posture have been learnt. Thereafter, the resistance should be increased gradually (progressive overload) whenever the prescribed number of sets and repetitions can be completed with good technique. In addition, incorporating weight-bearing impact exercises is also beneficial. Programmes involving activities such as single or double legged jumping, skipping, hopping or dancing should be gradually introduced into an exercise programme after an initial skill-specific training period and muscle conditioning to ensure correct techniques have been learnt.

Exercise for individuals with osteopenia, osteoporosis or a history of fracture

Exercise is an essential component for the treatment and management of individuals with osteoporosis. The level of skeletal fragility, functional ability, pain or disability, however, will influence exercise prescription for this group of individuals. Activities that have been shown to increase or maintain bone density in healthy, asymptomatic individuals are often contraindicated for individuals with osteoporosis. Despite limited evidence that exercise in this population can lead to small increases in bone density, the primary focus of any exercise programme in this group should be on improved fitness, muscle strength, posture, flexibility, balance and coordination to prevent falls and their related fractures (Bass et al 2001, Forwood and Larsen 2000).

For relatively pain-free individuals with adequate mobility and muscle strength, a combination of aerobic and resistance exercises is safe and likely to provide the greatest benefits (Forwood and Larsen 2000). For instance, in postmenopausal women with osteopenia, 12 months of exercise (walking, stepping on and off blocks, flexibility exercises and aerobic dance) three times per week for 60 minutes prevented bone loss at the spine, and improved fitness and psychological well-being, and decreased back pain (Bravo et al 1996). In a similar cohort of women, group water-based exercise involving jumping in waist-high water interspersed with muscular exercise maintained hip bone density, improved flexibility, agility, strength and fitness (Bravo et al 1997). Others found that daily outdoor walking and general exercises combined with calcium and vitamin D_3 supplementation increased lumbar spine bone density in postmenopausal osteoporotic women relative to non-exercising controls (Iwamoto et al 2001). Specific exercise programmes aimed at developing muscle strength, balance and coordination can be developed using activities such as walking, tai chi, hydrotherapy or water aerobics, dancing routines, exercise tapes, free weights or rubber tubes attached to a secure object performed 2–3 times per week for 20–30 minutes (Bravo et al 1996, 1997, Carter et al 2001, Chien et al 2000, Forwood and Larsen 2000,

Kronhed and Moller 1998, Malmros et al 1998). A single set of 8–10 resistance exercises performed at least two times per week has been shown to be effective for improving upper and lower body muscle strength in older adults (Forwood and Larsen 2000).

Exercise prescription will be limited for aged or frail individuals suffering osteoporosis-related pain, severe kyphosis, and previous fracture and/or with poor balance and limited movement. Exercise programmes for these high-risk individuals should focus on prevention of falls, maintaining overall health and fitness and where appropriate postural correction and pain management (Bass et al 2001). In these individuals, targeted exercise programmes are likely to be more beneficial that general programmes (Forwood and Larsen 2000). These could include water-based (e.g. hydrotherapy) exercises, mobilization or low intensity home-based exercises which can improve fitness, flexibility, postural stability, coordination and/or muscle strength (Liu-Ambrose et al 2001). Postural exercises to increase back extensor strength, correct forward head postures, maintain and improve shoulder range of motion and trunk stability should be considered on an individual basis (Dilsen et al 1989, Forwood and Larsen 2000, Malmros et al 1998). Exercises that are contraindicated in this high-risk group include dynamic abdominal exercises (e.g. sit-ups), excessive trunk flexion (e.g. toe touching, rowing) and exercises that require twisting (e.g. golf swing), explosive or abrupt movements, or high-impact loading (Forwood and Larsen 2000, Khan et al 2001). Exercises that involve forward flexion of the spine increase the risk of anterior compression fractures of thoracic vertebrae in the presence of ostoepenia.

Exercise and hormone replacement therapy

The rapid decline in bone density during menopause is associated with the reduction in levels of circulating oestrogen. Low levels of circulating oestrogen have also been associated with changes in body composition and in some instances reduced physiological response to training (Shepherd 2001). In terms of skeletal health, low estrogen levels appear also to influence the skeleton's ability to adapt to loading. For instance, oestrogen is thought to be a key regulator of the MES in bone; lower oestrogen levels result in a decrease in the sensitivity of the MES in bone and consequently a greater load is required to elicit an adaptive bone response. Because of this relationship between oestrogen and the MES of bone, it is hypothesized that hormone replacement therapy (HRT) may enhance the effect of exercise in postmenopausal women. For instance, in women aged 60–72 years (10 years past menopause), 9 months of progressive exercise involving walking, jogging and stair climbing (3 times/week, 45 min/day at 65–85% of max heart rate) combined with HRT was more effective in increasing bone density than either exercise alone or HRT alone (Kohrt et al 1995). Furthermore, after 6 months follow-up during which the exercise programme was reduced or discontinued, the benefits of exercise were either preserved or increased in those women continuing to take HRT (Kohrt et al 1997). Prince reported that exercise plus oestrogen-progesterone replacement was more effective than exercise and calcium supplementation in increasing bone mass in post-menopausal women (Prince et al 1991). In contrast, there was no evidence of a combined effect of exercise (3 hours/week, strength training and walking) and HRT in early postmenopausal women (<3 years since menopause), despite HRT and exercise alone preventing bone loss at the lumbar spine and hip (Heikkinen et al 1997). Recently however, it has been reported that high impact exercise combined with HRT had a greater effect on bone strength than exercise or HRT alone (Cheng et al 2002). Given the recent findings of the risks associated with HRT it is recommended that HRT use be short term (<5 years) and primarily for the relief of menopausal symptoms (Baber et al 2003, Rossouw et al 2002).

Does increased dietary calcium enhance the effect of exercise?

Few studies have been specifically designed to examine if increased dietary calcium enhances the adaptive bone response to exercise (French et al 2000). Intervention studies with four groups (exercise and no-exercise combined with calcium and placebo) are required to address this question. The limited data available support the notion that increased dietary calcium may enhance the effect of exercise in individuals on low dietary calcium intakes. For instance, Lau et al (1992) reported an exercise–calcium interaction at the femoral neck resulting in reduced bone loss in postmenopausal Chinese women on low calcium intakes who were supplemented with calcium and participated in an exercise programme (bench stepping four times per week). Greater effects of exercise were also reported at the femoral neck in pre- and postmenopausal women on high calcium intakes (Prince et al 1995). Synergy between exercise and calcium has also been reported at the femur in prepubertal girls who consumed low calcium diets (Iuliano Burns et al 2003). Currently no mechanisms have been identified to explain how exercise and calcium may interact to influence bone metabolism. It has been reported however, that exercise may up-regulate calcium absorption from the gut and small intestine (Yeh and Aloia 1990).

Principles of training for optimal bone health in adults

Recommendations for prescribing exercise that incorporates the different characteristics of loading will vary according to the fracture risk of the individual, the functional ability of the individual and the goal of the exercise programme (Bass et al 2001, Forwood and Larsen 2000) (Figure 6.2). In asymptomatic individuals with normal bone density (i.e. low fracture risk), the goal of the programme should be to maintain or increase bone density while improving muscle strength. Thus, resistance exercises combined with a variety of high impact exercises are appropriate for this group. For individuals with osteopenia (T-score between −1 and −2.5 SD), but with no history of fracture (i.e. moderate risk of fracture) the goal should be to maintain bone density and to reduce the risk of falling as these individuals tend to fracture as a result of falls. Thus moderate to vigorous resistance training is appropriate. For high-risk individuals, which include those with osteoporosis and/or a history of atraumatic fracture, there is no evidence that vigorous

Figure 6.2
Recommendations for exercise prescription for improved bone health and reduced fracture risk in older adults. Recommendations for exercise should consider individual differences and the level of fracture risk as assessed by bone densitometry and associated risk factors or functional status. The algorithm can be used to help guide decisions about exercise prescription or therapy. BMD indicates bone mineral density. SD indicates standard deviation, referring to young normal range. Osteopenia (low bone mass) is −1.0 to −2.5 SD. Osteoporosis is defined as more than −2.5 SD below the young normal mean. (Adapted from Bass et al 2001.)

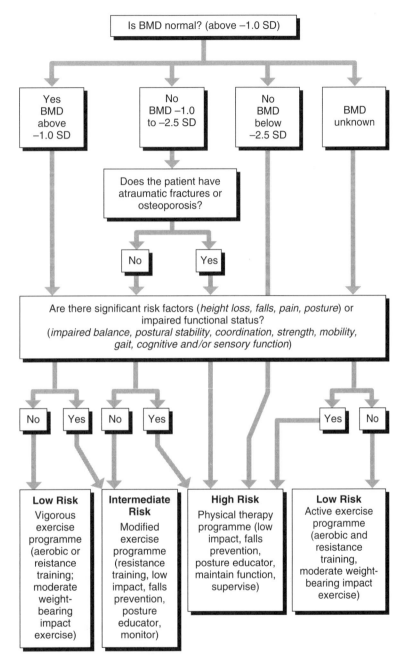

weight-bearing exercise will correct this condition, and it may in fact increase the risk of fracture (Bass et al 2001, Forwood and Larsen 2000). Since fractures in this group are due to a reduction in the mechanical competence of bone, modified exercise programmes are required that primarily focus on preventing falls (improving strength, balance and coordination), and not necessarily building bone mass (Bass et al 2001, Forwood and Larsen 2000).

Summary: the role of exercise across the lifespan for improved bone health	Exercise is important for improved bone health at all stages of life. A generic prescriptive approach is not appropriate for improved bone health because the aims and goals of a programme will vary throughout life and thus are dependent on the health and fragility of the individual. Thus the optimal use of exercise is dependent upon the prescription of an adequate dose of the correct type of exercise appropriate for the age and health of the individual. Furthermore, benefits obtained from any lifestyle or pharmaceutical intervention are only maintained while the treatment is sustained. Thus attention must be given to developing personalized programmes that encourage compliance over long periods of time. Prescription during growth should aim towards increasing peak bone density and strength. Activities should include a wide variety of moderate to high impact weight-bearing activities. During middle and old age, a combination of weight training and moderate impact weight-bearing activities are recommended. In elderly people, weight training and exercises designed to improve balance and coordination are appropriate. In the frail elderly with low bone density and/or fracture, conservative exercise programmes that are designed to increase strength, mobility and improve posture are recommended.

The role of diet in osteoporosis prevention

Nutrition plays an important role in bone health. Calcium and phosphorus are the key building blocks of the skeleton, making up 80–90% of bone mass. Calcium, phosphorus and other dietary components, such as protein, magnesium, zinc, copper, iron, fluoride, and vitamins D, A, C and K, are required for normal bone metabolism. Other ingested compounds not usually categorized as nutrients (e.g. caffeine, alcohol, phyto-oestrogens) may also influence bone metabolism. The relative contributions of nutritional, environmental and genetic factors are not known. Our understanding of the co-dependency of nutrients and the simultaneous interactions with genetic and environmental factors is also limited.

Calcium

Overall variations in calcium intake early in life can account for between 5–10% of the variance in peak bone mass and subsequently influences hip fracture rates in later life (Matkovic et al 1979). Maintaining a high calcium intake into later life appears to reduce the amount of bone loss in women around menopause and there is evidence that long-term high calcium intakes appear to reduce fracture risk (Cumming and Nevitt 1997, Osteoporosis Australia 2002). Although the beneficial effects of dietary calcium have been extensively studied, calcium is not the only nutrient that has an impact on bone development, maintenance and bone loss. Calcium is the main nutrient involved in bone deposition, maintenance and repair, but calcium must be provided together with a range of essential macro- and micronutrients to ensure optimal growth and development, and to minimize bone loss in later years.

The amount of calcium retained in the body is related to dietary intake, intestinal absorption and excretory losses (Weaver 1994). Intestinal calcium absorption and the ability to adapt to low calcium diets decline with ageing and highlight the importance of adequate calcium intakes in elderly people. Dairy foods provide most of the dietary calcium in Australians (60%), but the increasing fortification of other foods with calcium (e.g. cereals and fruit juices) will probably reduce the relative contribution of dietary calcium from dairy products. In addition to providing dietary calcium, dairy products are also good sources of protein, phosphorus and magnesium, which are important in maintaining optimal bone health. Although calcium supplements are useful for increasing dietary calcium intake, supplements do not provide other additional nutrients that may assist with calcium absorption, or facilitate the uptake of calcium into bone. Calcium absorption can vary from about 10 to 60% and can be upregulated through the action of vitamin D, which promotes calcium absorption. Like calcium, vitamin D is important for bone health during both growth and ageing. When calcium intakes are low, vitamin D helps to increase calcium absorption and facilitate the laying down of bone (Jones et al 1998). During menopause when women experience increased bone loss, calcium and/or vitamin D supplementation combined with exercise may help to increase or maintain bone mass.

Vitamin D

Vitamin D deficiency has recently been found to be a major health concern in Australia. The main source of vitamin D for Australians is exposure to sunlight. Recently it has been shown that even young people may be at increased risk of vitamin D deficiency at the end of winter (Pascoe et al 2001). Elderly people, however, are at highest risk where the rate of vitamin D deficiency ranges from 30% to 80% (Nowson and Margerison 2002). Sub-optimal serum vitamin D levels contribute to the development of osteoporosis and have recently been implicated in the propensity to fall. Changes in gait, difficulties in rising from a chair, inability to ascend stairs and diffuse muscle pain are the main clinical symptoms in muscle weakness associated with osteoporosis.

There are several reasons why vitamin D deficiency occurs in elderly people; these include:

- decreased sunlight exposure, because of decreased mobility
- decreased ability of the skin to produce vitamin D (because of less precursor found in the skin and also less activation of the precursor)
- inadequate dietary intake
- decreased intestinal absorption of vitamin D
- decreased hepatic and renal hydroxylation

In general, cutaneous synthesis provides most of the vitamin D to the body (80–100%) and with adequate sunlight exposure, dietary vitamin D can actually be considered unnecessary (Figure 6.3). The majority of the population will obtain most of the vitamin D required by the body through casual exposure to sunlight. Seven-dehydrocholesterol

Figure 6.3 Cutaneous synthesis provides most of the vitamin D to the body and with adequate sunlight exposure, dietary vitamin D can actually be considered unnecessary. Vitamin D assists in maintaining serum ionized calcium levels. When vitamin D status is inadequate parathyroid hormone (PTH) is stimulated to break down bone. The proposed desirable level of 25(OH)D at which PTH is not elevated is 100 nmol/l (Dawson-Hughes 1997, Kinyamu 1998).

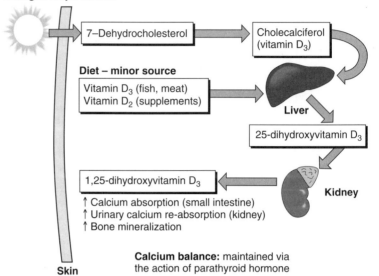

is converted photochemically by solar ultraviolet light into precholecalciferol which is quickly isomerized into the more stable cholecalciferol or vitamin D_3. Once cholecalciferol is formed in the skin it is transported in the bloodstream to the liver where it is converted to 25(OH)D, which although it has some physiological effect in increasing calcium absorption, is not the main active metabolite in the body. Cholecalciferol 1,25(OH)D, which results from the conversion of 25(OH)D to 1,25(OH)D, in the kidney is primarily responsible for upregulating calcium absorption in times of increased requirement (Figure 6.3). The blood levels of 25(OH)D are a direct result of UV irradiation to the skin or, in times of minimal exposure to UV light, can reflect dietary intake. Serum levels of 25(OH)D are measured to assess vitamin status.

An inadequate serum vitamin D status is commonly seen in elderly people as the result of reduced exposure to sunlight, reduced production of 25(OH)D on exposure to sunlight, inadequate diet and reduced renal conversion of 25(OH)D to the active metabolite 1,25(OH)D. Apart from the well-known effects on bone metabolism, this condition is also associated with muscle weakness, predominantly of the proximal muscle groups. Muscle weakness below a certain threshold affects functional ability and mobility, which puts an elderly person at increased risk of falling and fractures. There is some evidence that calcium and vitamin D supplements together might improve neuromuscular function in elderly persons who are deficient in calcium and vitamin D, as supplementation of cholecalciferol in combination with elemental calcium has been shown to reduce hip fractures and other non-vertebral fractures before any effect on bone could have occurred (Chapuy et al 1992).

At present there is no recommended dietary intake (RDI) for vitamin D for the general population but it is recommended that elderly people receive a 5–10 µg vitamin D supplement if they are not directly exposed to sunlight for 1–2 hours per week (National Health and Medical Research Council 1991). This recommendation is based on the premise that at times of low exposure to sunlight (e.g. during winter), dietary intake should be sufficient to maintain serum 25(OH)D at an acceptable level. Recently the US has proposed a daily reference intake (DRI) of 15 µg for those aged 71+ years. This is triple the recommended intake for those less than 50 years of age. Most Australians do not meet an intake of 5 µg vitamin D per day from dietary sources, with the average estimated intake being 2.6–3.0 µg/day for men and 2.0–2.2 µg/day for women (Nowson and Margerison 2002). Few foods contain significant amounts of vitamin D and for elderly people there is a real case for recommending vitamin D supplements to maintain bone health.

Although osteoporosis does not necessarily correlate with vitamin D deficiency, low concentrations of 25(OH)D are often found in older people (usually attributed to lack of sunlight) (Gennari 2001). Distinction between deficiency and insufficiency may no longer be useful since population morbidity associated with insufficiency may be greater than that associated with deficiency (Heaney 2000). It has been suggested that a widespread increase in vitamin D intake will have a far greater effect on osteoporosis and fractures than any other proposed intervention (Utiger 1998).

Vitamin K

Recently it has become evident that vitamin K has a significant role to play in bone health (Meunier 1999). Vitamin K is a unique vitamin in that the major source of vitamin K for humans is actually produced by bacteria that inhabit the large bowel. Dietary intake of foods containing vitamin K (i.e. vegetables, particularly green leafy vegetables such as spinach) makes a small contribution to vitamin status. Human epidemiological and intervention studies have consistently demonstrated that vitamin K can improve bone health (Weber 2001). The benefits of low, non-pharmacological doses of vitamin K on bone health are not known. However, very high pharmacological doses of the vitamin K have been used to prevent bone loss, and in some cases increase bone mass and reduce fracture risk in osteoporotic patients (Iwamoto et al 2000). It appears that vitamins K and D work synergistically on bone density and that vitamin K modulates bone metabolism though the gamma-carboxylation of osteocalcin, a protein believed to be involved in bone mineralization. There is also increasing evidence that vitamin K positively affects calcium balance, a key mineral in bone metabolism. Australia has no stated RDI for vitamin K. However, the Institute of Medicine in the USA has recently increased the dietary reference intakes of vitamin K to 90 µg/day for females and 120 µg/day for males, which is an increase of approximately 50% from previous recommendations.

Phosphorus

As phosphorus is the second most abundant mineral in bone, it would seem reasonable to assume that dietary intake is important for the maintenance of bone health. Phosphorus is widely distributed in foods: meat, poultry, fish, eggs, dairy products, legumes and cereals and cola-based soft drinks. Although phosphorus is an essential dietary mineral there is concern that high intakes may be detrimental to bone. There is no evidence that intakes typically consumed by the general population have detrimental effects on bone. The effect on bone of high phosphorus intakes associated with the consumption of large quantities of carbonated soft drinks is equivocal. The reported adverse effects of carbonated soft drinks may be due to the displacement of milk from the diet (Ilich and Kerstetter 2000).

Zinc, magnesium, sodium

Other dietary minerals also appear to influence bone metabolism, e.g. zinc and magnesium. The majority of evidence supporting the role of these minerals is derived from animal studies; little is known about the impact of low intakes on human bone and risk of fracture. We do know, however, that a high sodium diet causes increased urinary calcium losses, as the excretion of sodium is tied to calcium in the proximal tubule of the kidney. It has been estimated that a sodium excretion of 1 g is associated with a loss of approximately 15 mg of calcium in the urine (Nordin 2000). As more than 90% of the sodium we ingest is processed by the kidneys and passed out of the body in the urine, a high salt (sodium) diet could result in sustained calcium losses from bone. It should be noted, however, that there is no evidence from intervention studies to show that a high intake of sodium has a detrimental effect on bone. As there are other benefits associated with lowering sodium intakes (e.g. on blood pressure), it would be prudent to recommend a reduced sodium intake, whilst maintaining a high calcium intake (Weaver et al 1999).

Antioxidant vitamins and non-nutritive dietary factors

Some vitamins are also associated with bone health: vitamin C acts as an antioxidant and may help to protect bone from the adverse effects of smoking. Other dietary non-nutritive factors appear to have minor effects on bone; high intakes of caffeine have been found in some studies to adversely affect bone, but this is by no means a consistent finding and appears only to have a detrimental effect if calcium intake is low (Massey and Whiting 1993). The effect of alcohol on bone presents a similar story. Chronic alcoholism leads to lower bone mass and higher fracture risk. However, the detrimental effects on bone at lower intakes of alcohol have not been established. Phytochemicals are naturally occurring, plant-derived compounds that may have biological activity. Some of these substances are found in soy products, e.g. phyto-oestrogens. These compounds may act as oestrogen agonists or antagonists. Soy products and phyto-oestrogens have been found to have a positive effect on bone in animal studies, and preliminary studies in humans indicate that there may be some positive effects on bone; an effect on fracture rate, however, has not been demonstrated.

Protein

A number of studies have implicated increased dietary protein with increased calcium losses and increased risk of osteoporosis. Increasing dietary protein does increase urinary calcium excretion and it follows that the higher the protein intake the more calcium is lost from the body. The clinical and epidemiological data addressing this hypothesis are controversial. On one hand many epidemiological studies have found a positive association between protein intake and bone density; conversely many studies report a higher fracture rate in those consuming a high protein diet (Abelow et al 1992). More recent studies, however, indicate that increased dietary protein intake may have a favourable effect on bone density when combined with calcium and vitamin D supplements in older people (Dawson-Hughes and Harris 2002). This again indicates some interactive component and highlights the difficulty in making recommendations for single nutrients across all age groups (Dawson-Hughes and Harris 2002).

Older people

Preventive strategies implemented early in life will result in the greatest reductions in risk of osteoporosis; however, the importance of adequate nutrition being maintained into old age should not be dismissed. This presents a challenge. Older people have distinct metabolic characteristics that alter the requirements for specific nutrients. The variability in requirements for nutrients increases in the older population, making it difficult to make general recommendations on nutrient needs. A range of physical and environmental factors impact on eating habits and nutritional status. Eating is not just a physiological response; it has social, cultural and symbolic meaning. Social isolation and lack of social support places older people at greater risk of developing depression, which results in reduction in food intake. The reduction in food intake, particularly low intakes of vitamin B_{12} and folate, may also exacerbate depression, leading to the development of frank malnutrition. Physical activity is also important as this assists in maintaining appetite. Energy expenditure, in relation to physical activity is the most variable component of total energy expenditure. Many older people lead very sedentary lives, with greatly reduced energy expenditure. Balancing energy intake with energy expenditure is fundamental in maintaining a relatively constant body weight. A high-energy intake relative to energy expenditure will result in overweight and obesity, which is associated with increased morbidity and mortality in those less than 70 years old. On the other hand, a low energy intake will result in undernutrition and low body weight, which is also associated with increased morbidity and mortality particularly in those over the age of 80 years. Low body weight is also a risk factor for fracture.

It is recognized that energy expenditure and consequently energy intake and therefore nutrient intake reduces with ageing. This occurs at a time where there are likely to be increased requirements for some nutrients, making it more difficult to meet these nutrient requirements through dietary sources. There is some evidence that dietary protein requirements are increased with ageing (Kurpad and Vaz 2000). Increased dietary recommendations for calcium and magnesium have been proposed for older people (e.g. calcium, vitamin D, riboflavin, vitamin B_6, and vitamin B_{12}).

There are not sufficient data on vitamin K, phosphorus, iodine, manganese, fluoride and molybdenum to make a critical judgement about the appropriateness of the dietary recommendations for elderly people (Wood et al 1995).

It is difficult to meet the increased requirement for more nutrients in older people because of the decline in energy expenditure, energy intake and reduced food intake. Providing older people with nutrient fortified drinks and/or food does not necessarily improve nutritional status, as total dietary intake appears to remain low if physical activity is low. One study found that when elderly residents were provided with supplemental drinks, they took the special drink but subsequently reduced their intake of food from meals, so their overall energy intake was not greater (Fiatarone et al 1994). A recent study conducted in frail elderly persons for 17 weeks combined an exercise regime with nutrient-dense foods containing a range of vitamins and minerals including 25% of the recommended daily allowance for calcium. They demonstrated a preservation of lean mass and a slight increase in bone density (de Jong et al 2000). This demonstrates the possible synergy between physical activity and dietary intake.

Dietary recommendations

Everyone loses bone as they age, and the emphasis should be to build maximum bone during growth by ensuring adequate intakes of all nutrients, particularly calcium, especially during times of peak growth (800–1500 mg/day), vitamin D, and protein (at least 0.75 g/kg body weight) in conjunction with regular physical activity. The aim in old age is to minimize the age-related loss of bone by ensuring an adequate intake of energy (dependent on a reasonable level of physical activity) and at least 1000 mg calcium/day and 10 μg/day of vitamin D plus some regular exposure to sunshine, and including protein-containing foods at least twice per day, e.g. meat, fish, legumes and dairy products. The diet should also include a variety of fruit and vegetables everyday as these contain a number of antioxidants as well as folate. From the best evidence available this will maintain quality of life in the older years, assist in reducing age-related bone loss and reduce the risk of hip and other fractures in later life.

References

Access Economics 2001: The burden of brittle bones: costing osteoporosis in Australia. Osteoporosis International Canberra

Abelow B, Holford T, Insogna K 1992 Cross-cultural association between dietary animal protein and hip fracture: a hypothesis. Calcified Tissue International 50(1):14–18

Baber R J, O'Hora J L, Boyle F M 2003 Hormone replacement therapy: to use or not to use? Medical Journal of Australia 178:630–633

Bailey D, McKay H, Mirwald R L, Crocker P R E, Faulkner R A 1999 A six year longitudinal study of the relationship of physical activity to bone mineral accrual in growing children: the University of Saskatchewan Bone Mineral Accrual Study. Journal of Bone and Mineral Research 14(10):1672–1679

Bailey D A, Martin A D, McKay H A, Whiting S, Mirwald R 2000 Calcium accretion in girls and boys during puberty: a longitudinal analysis. Journal of Bone and Mineral Research 15(11):2245–2250

Baron R 1990 Anatomy and ultrastructure of bone. In: Favus M J (ed) Primer on metabolic bone diseases and disorders of mineral metabolism, 3rd edn. American Society for Bone and Mineral Research, California, p 3–7.

Bass S L 2000 The prepubertal years: a uniquely opportune stage of growth when the skeleton is most responsive to exercise? Sports Medicine 30(2):73–78

Bass S, Pearce G, Bradney M, et al 1998 Exercise before puberty may confer residual benefits in bone density in adulthood: studies in active prepubertal and retired female gymnasts. Journal of Bone and Mineral Research 13(3):500–507

Bass S, Forwood M, Larsen J, Saxon L 2001 Prescribing exercise for osteoporosis. International Journal of Sports Medicine 5:1–13

Bass S, Saxon L, Daly R, et al 2002 The effect of mechanical loading on the size and shape of cortical bone in pre- peri- and postpubertal tennis players. Journal of Bone and Mineral Research 17:2274–2280

Bassey E J, Rothwell M C, Littlewood J J, Pye D W 1998 Pre- and postmenopausal women have different bone mineral density responses to the same high-impact exercise. [See Comment in: Journal of Bone and Mineral Research 1998 Dec;13(12).] Journal of Bone and Mineral Research 13(12):1792–1796

Bradney M, Pearce G, Naughton G, et al 1998 Moderate exercise during growth in prepubertal boys: changes in bone mass, size, volumetric density, and bone strength: a controlled prospective study. Journal of Bone and Mineral Research 13(12):1814–1821

Bravo G, Gauthier P, Roy P M, et al 1996 Impact of a 12-month exercise program on the physical and psychological health of osteopenic women. Journal of the American Geriatrics Society 44(7):756–762

Bravo G, Gauthier P, Roy P M, Payette H, Gaulin P 1997 A weight-bearing, water-based exercise program for osteopenic women: its impact on bone, functional fitness, and well-being. Archives of Physical Medicine and Rehabilitation 78(12):1375–1380

Brooke-Wavell K, Jones P R M, Hardman A E 1997 Brisk walking reduces calcaneal bone loss in post-menopausal women. Clinical Science 92:75–80

Burr D, Schaffler M, Yang K H, et al 1989 Skeletal change in response to altered strain environments: is woven bone a response to elevated strain? Bone 10:223–233

Carter N D, Khan K M, Petit M A, et al 2001 Results of a 10 week community based strength and balance training programme to reduce fall risk factors: a randomised controlled trial in 65–75 year old women with osteoporosis. British Journal of Sports Medicine 35(5):348–351

Cavanaugh D J, Cann C E 1988 Brisk walking does not stop bone loss in post-menopausal women. Bone 9(4):201–204

Chapuy M C, Arlot M E, Duboeuf F D, et al 1992 Vitamin D3 and calcium to prevent hip fractures in elderly women. New England Journal of Medicine 327:1637–1642

Cheng S, Sipla S, Taffe D, Puolakka J, Suominen H 2002 Change in bone mass distribution induced by hormone replacement therapy and high impact physical exercise in post-menopausal women. Bone 31(1):126–135

Chien M Y, Wu Y T, Hsu A T, Yang R S, Lai J S 2000 Efficacy of a 24-week aerobic exercise program for osteopenic postmenopausal women. Calcified Tissue International 67(6):443–448

Chilibeck P, Sale D, Webber C 1995 Exercise and bone mineral density. Sports Medicine 19(2):103–122

Cooper C, Cawley M, Bhalla A, et al 1995 Childhood growth, physical activity, and peak bone mass in women. Journal of Bone and Mineral Research 10(6):940–947

Cumming R, Nevitt M 1997 Calcium for prevention of osteoporotic fractures in postmenopausal women. Journal of Bone and Mineral Research 12:1321–1329

Cummings S R 2002 Epidemiology and outcomes of osteoporotic fractures. Lancet 359:1761–1767

Cumming S R, Black D M, Nevitt M C, et al 1993 Bone density at various sites for prediction of hip fracture. The study of osteoporotic fracture research group. Lancet 341:962–963

Dalsky G P, Stocke K S, Ehsani A A, et al 1988 Weight-bearing exercise training and lumbar bone mineral content in postmenopausal women. Annals of Internal Medicine 108(6):824–828

Dawson-Hughes B, Harris S S, Krall E A, Dallal G E 1997 Effect of calcium D supplementation on bone density in men and women 65 years of age or older. New England Journal of Medicine 337(10):670–676

Dawson-Hughes B, Harris S 2002 Calcium intake influences the association of protein intake with rates of bone loss in elderly men and women. American Journal of Clinical Nutrition 75(4):773–779

de Jong N, Paw M, de Groot L, Hiddink G, van Staveren A 2000 Dietary supplements and physical exercise affecting bone and body composition in frail elderly persons. American Journal of Public Health 90:947–954

Dilsen G, Berker C, Oral A, Varan G 1989 The role of physical exercise in prevention and management of osteoporosis. Clinical Rheumatology 8 (Suppl 2):70–75

Drinkwater B L, Grimston S K, Raab-Cullen D M, Snow-Harter C M 1995 ACSM position stand on osteoporosis and exercise. Medicine and Science in Sports and Exercise 27(4):i–vii

Ebrahim S, Thompson P W, Baskaran V, Evans K 1997 Randomized placebo-controlled trial of brisk walking in the prevention of postmenopausal osteoporosis. Age and Ageing 26(4):253–260

Fiatarone M 2002 Exercise comes of age: rationale and recommendations for a geriatric exercise prescription. Journal of Gerontology 57A(1):M262–282

Fiatarone M, O'Neill E, Ryan N, et al 1994 Exercise training and nutritional supplementation for physical frailty in very elderly people. New England Journal of Medicine 330:1769–1775

Forwood M, Larsen J 2000 Exercise recommendations for osteoporosis. Australian Family Physician 29(8):761–764

French S A, Fulkerson J A, Story M 2000 Increasing weight-bearing physical activity and calcium intake for bone mass growth in children and adolescents: a review of intervention trials. Preventive Medicine 31(6):722–731

Frost H M 1987 Bone 'mass' and the 'mechanostat': a proposal. Anatomical Record 219:1–9

Frost H M 1992 Perspectives: the role of changes in mechanical usage set points in the pathogenesis of osteoporosis. Journal of Bone and Mineral Research 7:253–262

Fuchs R K, Bauer J J, Snow C M 2001 Jumping improves hip and lumbar spine bone mass in prepubescent children: A randomized controlled trial. Journal of Bone and Mineral Research 16(1):148–156

Gennari C 2001 Calcium and vitamin D nutrition and bone disease of the elderly. Public Health and Nutrition 4(2B):547–559

Gunnes M, Lehman E H 1996 Physical activity and dietary constituents as predictors of forearm cortical and trabecular bone gain in healthy children and adolescents: a prospective study. Acta Paediatrica 85:19–25

Hatori M, Hasegawa A, Adachi H, et al 1993 The effects of walking at the anaerobic threshold level on vertebral bone loss in postmenopausal women. Calcified Tissue International 52(6):411–414

Heaney R P 2000 Vitamin D: how much do we need, how much is too much? Osteoporosis International 11:553–555

Heikkinen J, Kyllonen E, Kurttila-Matero E, et al 1997 HRT and exercise: effects on bone density, muscle strength and lipid metabolism. A placebo controlled 2-year prospective trial on two estrogen-progestin regimes in healthy premenopausal women. Maturitas 26:139–149

Heinonen A, Kannus P, Sievanen H, et al 1996 Randomised controlled trial of effect of high-impact exercise on selected risk factors for osteoporotic fractures. Lancet 348:1343–1347

Heinonen A, Oja P, Sievanen H, Pasanen M, Vuori I 1998 Effect of two training regimens on bone mineral density in healthy perimenopausal women: a randomized controlled trial. Journal of Bone and Mineral Research 13(3):483–490

Heinonen A, Sievanen H, Kannus P, et al 2000 High-impact exercise and bones of growing girls: a 9-month controlled trial. Osteoporosis International 11(12):1010–1017

Huddleston A L, Rockwell D, Kulund D N, Harrison R B 1980 Bone mass in lifetime tennis athletes. JAMA 244(10):1107–1109

Humphries B, Newton R, Bronks R, et al 2000 Effect of exercise intensity on bone density, strength, and calcium turnover in older women. Medicine and Science in Sports and Exercise 32(6):1043–1050

Huuskonen J, Vaisanen S B, Kroger H, et al 2001 Regular physical exercise and bone mineral density: a four-year controlled randomized trial in middle-aged men. The DNASCO study. Osteoporosis International 12(5):349–355

Ilich J, Kerstetter J 2000 Nutrition in Bone Health Revisited: a story beyond calcium. Journal of the American College of Nutrition 19:715–735

Iuliano Burns S, Saxon L, Naughton G, Gibbons K, Bass S 2003 Regional specificity of exercise and calcium during growth in girls: a randomised controlled trial. Journal of Bone and Mineral Research 18:156–162

Iwamoto J, Takeda T, Ichimura S 2000 Effect of combined administration of vitamin D3 and vitamin K2 on bone mineral density of the lumbar spine in postmenopausal women with osteoporosis. Journal of Orthopaedic Research 5(6):546–551

Iwamoto J, Takeda T, Ichimura S 2001 Effect of exercise training and detraining on bone mineral density in postmenopausal women with osteoporosis. Journal of Orthopaedic Science 6(2):128–132

Jones G, Strugnell S, DeLuca H 1998 Current understanding of the molecular actions of vitamin D. Physiology Review 78(4):1193–1231

Kannus P, Haapasalo H, Sankelo M, et al 1995 Effect of starting age of physical activity on bone mass in the dominant arm of tennis and squash players. Annals of Internal Medicine 123:27–31

Karlsson M, Linden C, Karlsson C, et al 2000 Exercise during growth and bone mineral density and fractures in old age. Lancet 355:469–470

Kerr D, Morton A, Dick I, Prince R 1996 Exercise effects on bone mass in postmenopausal women are site-specific and load-dependent. Journal of Bone and Mineral Research 11(2):218–225

Khan K M, Liu-Ambrose T, Donaldson M G, McKay H A 2001 Physical activity to prevent falls in older people: time to intervene in high risk groups using falls as an outcome. British Journal of Sports Medicine 35(3):144–145

Kinyamu H K, Gallagher J C, Rafferty K A, Balhorn K E 1998 Dietary calcium and vitamin D intake in elderly women: effect on serum parathyroid hormone and vitamin D metabolites. American Journal of Clinical Nutrition 67:342–348

Kohrt W M 2001 Aging and the osteogenic response to mechanical loading. International Journal of Sports Nutrition and Exercise Metabolism 11:S137–142

Kohrt W M, Snead D B, Slatopolsky E, Birge S J 1995 Additive effects of weight-bearing exercise and estrogen on mineral density in older women. Journal of Bone and Mineral Research 10(9):1303–1311

Kohrt W M, Ehsani A A, Birge S J 1997 Effects of exercise involving predominately either joint-reaction or ground-reaction forces on bone mineral density in older women. Journal of Bone and Mineral Research 12(8):1253–1261

Kronhed A C, Moller M 1998 Effects of physical exercise on bone mass, balance skill and aerobic capacity in women and men with low bone mineral density, after one year of training – a prospective study. Scandinavian Journal of Medicine and Science in Sports 8(5 Pt 1):290–298

Kurpad A, Vaz M 2000 Protein and amino acid requirements in the elderly. European Journal of Clinical Nutrition 54 (Suppl 3):131–142

Lanyon L E, Rubin C T 1984 Static vs dynamic loads as an influence of bone remodelling. Journal of Biomechanics 17(12):897–905

Lanyon L E, Goodship A E, Pye C J, MacFie J H 1982 Mechanically adaptive bone remodelling. Journal of Biomechanics 15(3):141–154

Lau E M, Woo J, Leung P C, Swaminathan R, Leung D 1992 The effects of calcium supplementation and exercise on bone density in elderly Chinese women. Osteoporosis International 2(4):168–173

Liu-Ambrose T, Khan K M, McKay H A 2001 The role of exercise in preventing and treating osteoporosis. International Sports Medicine Journal 2(4):1–14

Lohman T, Going S, Pamenter R, et al 1995 Effects of resistance training on regional and total bone mineral density in premenopausal women: a randomized prospective study. Journal of Bone and Mineral Research 10(7):1015–1024

MacKelvie K, Khan K, McKay H 2002 Is there a critical period for bone response to weight-bearing exercise in children and adolescents? A systematic review. British Journal of Sports Medicine 36:250–257

Maddalozzo G F, Snow C M 2000 High intensity resistance training: effects on bone in older men and women. Calcified Tissue International 66(6):399–404

Malmros B, Mortensen L, Jensen M B, Charles P 1998 Positive effects of physiotherapy on chronic pain and performance in osteoporosis. Osteoporosis International 8:215–221

Martin D, Notelovitz M 1993 Effects of aerobic training on bone mineral density of postmenopausal women. Journal of Bone and Mineral Research 8(3):931–936

Massey L, Whiting S 1993 Caffeine, urinary calcium, calcium metabolism and bone. Journal of Nutrition 123:1611–1614

Matkovic V, Kostial K, Simonovic I, et al 1979 Bone status and fracture rates in two regions of Yugoslavia. American Journal of Clinical Nutrition 32:540–549

McKay H, Petit M A, Schutz R W, et al 2000 Augmented trochanteric bone mineral density after modified physical education classes: a randomised school-based exercise intervention study in prepubescent and early pubescent children. Journal of Pediatrics 136(2):156–162

Melton J I, Cooper C 2001 Magnitude and impact of osteoporosis and fractures. In: Kelsey J (ed) Osteoporosis, 2nd edn. Academic Press, San Diego, p 557–567

Meunier P 1999 Calcium, vitamin D and vitamin K in the prevention of fractures due to Osteoporosis. Osteoporosis International 9 (Suppl 2):48–52

Michel B A, Lane N E, Bjorkengren A, Bloch D A, Fries J F 1992 Impact of running on lumbar bone density: a 5-year longitudinal study. Journal of Rheumatology 19(11):1759–1763

Morris F L, Naughton G A, Gibbs J L, Carlson J S, Wark J D 1997 Prospective ten-month exercise intervention in premenarcheal girls: positive effects on bone and lean mass. Journal of Bone and Mineral Research 12(9):1453–1462

National Health and Medical Research Council 1991 Recommended dietary intakes for use in Australia. Australian Government Publishing Service, Canberra.

Nelson M E, Fiatarone M A, Morganti C M, et al 1994 Effects of high-intensity strength training on multiple risk factors for osteoporotic fractures – a randomized controlled trial. JAMA 272(24):1909–1914

Nordin B C 2000 Calcium requirement is a sliding scale. American Journal of Clinical Nutrition 71(6):1381–1383

Nowson C, Margerison C 2002 Vitamin D intake and vitamin D status of Australians. Medical Journal of Australia 177(3):149–152

O'Connor J A, Lanyon L E, MacFie H 1982 The influence of strain rate on adaptive bone remodelling. Journal of Biomechanics 15(10):767–781

Osteoporosis Australia 2002 Preventing osteoporosis: outcomes of the Australian Fracture Prevention Summit. Medical Journal of Australia 176(Suppl):S1–16

Pascoe J, Henry M, Nicholson G, et al 2001 Vitamin D status of women in the Geelong Osteoporosis Study: association with diet and casual exposure to sunlight. Medical Journal of Australia 175:401–405

Prince R, Smith M, Dick I M, et al 1991 Prevention of postmenopausal osteoporosis. A comparative study of exercise, calcium supplementation, and hormone-replacement therapy. New England Journal of Medicine 325(17):1189–1195

Prince R, Devine A, Dick I, et al 1995 The effects of calcium supplementation (milk powder or tablets) and exercise on bone density in postmenopausal women. Journal of Bone and Mineral Research 10(7):1068–1075

Pruitt L A, Taaffe D R, Marcus R 1995 Effects of a one-year high-intensity versus low-intensity resistance training program on bone mineral density in older women. Journal of Bone and Mineral Research 10(11):1788–1795

Raab Cullen D M, Akhter M P, Kimmel D B, Recker R R 1994 Bone response to alternate-day mechanical loading of the rat tibia. Journal of Bone and Mineral Research 9(2):203–211

Rossouw S E, Anderson G L, Prentice R L, et al 2002 Risks and benefits of estrogen plus progestin in healthy postmenopausal women: principle results from the Women's Health Initiative randomized controlled trial writing group for Women's Health Initiative. JAMA 288:321–333

Rubin C T, Lanyon L E 1984 Regulation of bone formation by applied dynamic loads. Journal of Bone and Joint Surgery 66A(3):397–402

Rubin C T, Lanyon L E 1985 Regulation of bone mass by mechanical strain magnitude. Calcified Tissue International 37(4):411–417

Saxon L, Iuliano-Burns S, Naughton G, Bass S 2000 The osteotrophic response to different mechanical loading regimes in pre- and early pubertal girls. International Bone and Hormone Meeting. Elsevier Science, Australia, p 47S

Seeman E 2001 Clinical review 137: sexual dimorphism in skeletal size, density, and strength. Journal of Clinical Endocrinology and Metabolism 86(10):4576–4584

Shepherd R (ed) 2001 Gender, physical activity and aging. Chapman & Hall, London

Snow-Harter C, Bouxsein J L, Lewis B T, Carter D R, Marcus R 1992 Effects of resistance and endurance exercise on bone mineral status of young women: A randomized exercise intervention trial. Journal of Bone and Mineral Research 7(7):761–769

Taaffe D R, Pruitt L, Pyka G, Guido D, Marcus R 1996 Comparative effects of high- and low-intensity resistance training on thigh muscle strength, fibre area, and tissue composition in elderly women. Clinical Physiology 16(4):381–392

Turner C H, Burr D B 1993 Basic biomechanical measurements of bone: a tutorial. Bone 14(4):595–608

Utiger R 1998 The need for more vitamin D [editorial comment]. New England Journal of Medicine 338:828–829

Weaver C 1994 Age related calcium requirements due to changes in absorption and utilization. Journal of Nutrition 124(8 Suppl):1418–1425

Weaver C, Proulx W, Heaney R 1999 Choices for achieving adequate dietary calcium with a vegetarian diet. American Journal of Clinical Nutrition 70(3 Suppl):543–548

Weber P 2001 Vitamin K and bone health. Nutrition 17(10):880–887

Welsh L, Rutherford O M 1996 Hip bone mineral density is improved by high-impact aerobic exercise in postmenopausal women and men over 50 years. European Journal of Applied Physiology 74(6):511–517

Williams J A, Wagner J, Wasnich R, Heibrun L 1984 The Effect of Long Distance Running upon Appendicular Bone Mineral Content

Wood R, Suter P, Russell R 1995 Mineral requirements of elderly people. American Journal of Clinical Nutrition 62:493–505

Yeh J K, Aloia J F 1990 Effect of physical activity on calciotropic hormones and calcium balance in rats. American Journal of Physiology 258(2 Pt 1):263–268

7

Strength training for older people

Karen J Dodd, Nicholas F Taylor
and Scott Bradley

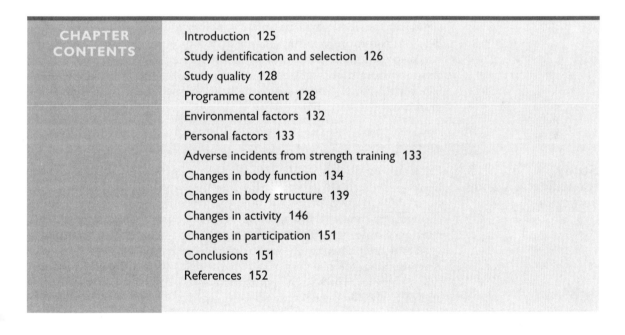

CHAPTER CONTENTS

Introduction 125

Study identification and selection 126

Study quality 128

Programme content 128

Environmental factors 132

Personal factors 133

Adverse incidents from strength training 133

Changes in body function 134

Changes in body structure 139

Changes in activity 146

Changes in participation 151

Conclusions 151

References 152

Introduction

Muscle weakness can be a major health problem for older people. After the age of 50 years, muscle mass decreases by more than 6% each decade and muscle strength decreases by more than 10% each decade (Lynch et al 1999). Weakness is associated with decreased bone mineral density (Bevier et al 1989) and increased risk of falls (Campbell et al 1989, Whipple et al 1987), fractures (Aniansson et al 1984), and contributes to disability.

For these reasons, a means of preventing or even reversing muscle weakness may be an important health intervention for older people.

Recently there has been interest in the role of exercise in preventing or reversing age-related muscle mass and strength losses in older people. Based on the premise that strength training increases muscle strength and leads to improved functional capacity, community-based strength training programmes for older people have flourished. There has also been substantial research into whether strength training in community-dwelling older people increases muscle strength and physiological function.

This chapter reports the results of a systematic review on the effects of strength training for healthy, community-dwelling people over 50 years of age. To evaluate the effects of strength training, we examined outcomes using the International Classification of Functioning, Disability and Health (ICF) framework for classifying health status (WHO 2001). According to this framework, response to an intervention can be considered in terms of changes to body function (e.g. muscle strength, flexibility, endurance) and structure (e.g. skeletal muscle morphology, bone mineral density), functional activity (e.g. walking, stair-climbing, sit-to-stand) and societal participation (e.g. ability to take part in social activities, join community groups, make decisions about finances). Evidence was also evaluated about the effect of personal and environmental contextual factors that might have an impact on the feasibility and success of strengthening programmes, such as the setting in which the programme was conducted.

Study identification and selection

Electronic databases (MEDLINE, PubMed, EMBASE, CINAHL, Sports Discus, PsychInfo, AusportMed, Cochrane) were searched to find trials from 1966 to 2002 using the following search terms: strengthening, strength training, weight training, resistance training and progressive resistance training combined with aging, ageing, elderly, older, middle-aged and aged. This search was supplemented by citation tracking, which is where the reference lists of relevant articles were scanned to identify further articles. The search was limited to full articles written in English and published in peer-reviewed journals.

The titles and abstracts of papers identified by the initial search strategy were assessed independently by two researchers for the following inclusion criteria:

1. Population: independent community-living older people (>50 years of age). Trials that focused on populations with specific pathology, for example people with diabetes or osteoarthritis, were excluded.
2. Intervention: progressive resistance exercise programme.
3. Outcome: quantitative data measuring change in (i) body systems and functions, (ii) functional activities and/or (iii) societal participation.
4. Study design: randomized controlled trials.

When it was not clear from the title or abstract whether a paper should be included, the full paper was obtained and read for the inclusion criteria.

Papers were required to fulfil all four inclusion criteria. Differences were resolved by discussion until consensus was reached.

Trials that met inclusion criteria were rated for quality using the PEDro scale (PEDro 1999). With the PEDro scale, the following indicators of methodological rigour were scored independently by two researchers (two of KD, NT, SB) as either present or absent:

1. Specification of eligibility criteria.
2. Random allocation.
3. Concealed allocation.
4. Prognostic similarity at baseline.
5. Subject blinding.
6. Therapist blinding.
7. Assessor blinding.
8. Greater than 85% follow-up for at least one key outcome.
9. Intention-to-treat analysis.
10. Between group statistical analysis for at least one key outcome.
11. Point estimates of variability provided for at least one key outcome.

The PEDro guidelines specify that criteria 2–11 are used for scoring purposes so that a score out of 10 is obtained (PEDro 1999). For the review in this chapter we predicted that participants and therapists administering the programme would not be blind to the intervention, so a maximum score of eight was expected. The PEDro scale has high content validity, being developed from the Delphi list described by Verhagen et al (1998) and has demonstrated high inter-observer reliability (kappa = 0.88) (Dodd et al 2002). To further improve reliability, any disagreements between the two reviewers were resolved by discussion until consensus was reached.

Data were summarized on a standardized form that included the following headings: study objective, study design, subject details (including inclusion/exclusion criteria, subject demographics and recruitment procedures), description of intervention, outcome measures used (including evidence of reliability and validity of the outcome measurement tools used), results, conclusions and other comments (including details of programme adherence and adverse events). From these forms, data were extracted about changes in body structure and function, functional activities, societal participation, as well as environmental and personal contextual factors.

For the data analysis, effect sizes with 95% confidence intervals were calculated to enable comparison between the outcome measurements of the selected studies. These were calculated on web-based software (Schwarzer 1989) according to the method described by Hedges and Olkin (1985). The mean of the control group post-intervention was subtracted from the mean of the experimental group post-intervention, and divided by the pooled standard deviation of both groups. This approach assumes that no baseline differences exist between groups. When there were significant baseline differences between the experimental and control groups the data were excluded from the analysis. Therefore, to calculate effect sizes, the paper had to report post-intervention means and standard deviations for both groups, or the absolute change and standard deviations for both groups. Although it is recognized that other methods are available for transforming data, such as F values (Hedges and Olkin 1985), for the purposes of this review data were only included that reported post-intervention means or absolute change and standard deviations. Results were grouped according to whether upper body strength or lower limb strength was measured when calculating the effect sizes for strength. When multiple measures of strength were reported those relating to knee extensor strength or leg press strength were calculated.

To calculate an overall effect, a random effects model was used for the meta-analysis programmes (Schwarzer 1989). The random effects model assumes a different effect for each study and has been recommended for use when data are heterogeneous (Egger et al 1997, Lau et al 1998). Some data were found to be heterogeneous, for example data for upper body strength ($Q(14) = 46.5$, $P = 0.00002$), where only 19.1% of the variance was explained by sampling error. Therefore, for consistency overall effects were all assessed with random effects models.

Some studies investigated the effects of more than one strength training programme. For example, a number of studies had both high-intensity and low-intensity training groups (Pruitt et al 1995, Taaffe et al 1995, 1996, Willoughby and Pelsue 1998), while programmes of different frequency (either one, two or three days per week) were also investigated (Taaffe et al 1999). Under these circumstances, the training group subjected to the greatest stimulus (i.e. high-intensity strength training groups, or three days per week training groups) was used for study analysis.

Study quality

The initial search strategy yielded 2132 articles. After applying the inclusion criteria, 50 randomized controlled trials remained for detailed review. Study quality as assessed by the PEDro ranged from a score of three to a score of seven (Chandler et al 1998, Judge et al 1994) with a median score of five. Most studies ($n = 40$) obtained a PEDro score of four, five or six (Table 7.1). None of the 50 randomized controlled trials reported that the allocation process concealed the treatment allocation (PEDro criterion 3). Only three papers reported that measurements were taken by assessors who were blind to group allocation (PEDro criterion 7) (Buchner et al 1997, Chandler et al 1998, Westhoff et al 2000). Juni et al (1999) reported that effect sizes were, on average, exaggerated by 35% when assessment of outcomes was not blinded (Juniet al 1999). Since all except three of the papers included in this review did not blind assessors, the effect sizes reported in the following sections may slightly overestimate the true effects of strength training in older people.

Programme content

There was consistency in the content of the strength training programmes reported in the 50 randomized controlled trials studied. The typical training programme for older people comprised 8–10 exercises

Table 7.1 Description of included papers on strength training for older people

Author/year	PEDro score	Sample size	Sex	Age (mean)	Muscle group	Type of weights	Load	Sets and repetitions	Frequency and duration
Adams et al 2001	6	19	F = 19	50.7	Arms and legs	Machine and free weights	70–80% 1 RM	3 sets 8–10 reps	2/wk for 8 wks
Ades et al 1996	6	24	F = 13 M = 11	70.4	Arms and legs	Machine weights	50–80% 1 RM	3 sets 8 reps	3/wk for 12 wks
Balagopal et al 2001	4	39	Not stated	Range: 46–79	Arms and legs	Machine weights	50–80% 1 RM	3 sets 8 reps	3/wk for 12 wks
Bermon et al 1999a, b	6	32	F = 16 M = 16	70.1	Arms and legs	Machine weights	80% 1 RM	3 sets 8 reps	3/wk for 8 wks
Brandon et al 2000	6	85	F = 60 M = 25	72.3	Legs	Machine weights	50–70% 1 RM	3 sets 8–12 reps	3/wk for 16 wks
Buchner et al 1997	6	55	F = 28 M = 27	74.5	Arms, trunk and legs	Machine weights	1st set 50–60% 1 RM; 2nd set 75% 1 RM	2 sets 10 reps	3/wk for 24–26 wks
Chandler et al 1998	7	100	F = 50 M = 50	77.6	Legs	Theraband and body weight	10 RM	2 sets 10 reps	3/wk for 10 wks
Charette et al 1991	4	19	F = 19	69	Legs	Machine weights	65–75% 1 RM	3–6 sets 6 reps	3/wk for 12 wks
Damush and Damush 1999	6	62	F = 62	68	Arms, trunk and legs	Theraband and body weight	Reach exertion rating of 'somewhat hard or strong exertion' on Borg scale	1 set of as many reps as necessary to reach target exertion level	2/wk for 8 wks
Flynn et al 1999	5	29	F = 29	72	Legs	Not stated	70–80% 1 RM	3 sets 8 reps	3/wk for 10 wks
Hagberg et al 1989	5	31	M and F	72	Arms and Legs	Machine weights	12 RM	1 set 8–12 reps	3/wk for 26 wks
Hagerman et al 2000	5	18	M = 18	63.7	Legs (quadriceps)	Machine weights	85–90% 1 RM	3 sets 6–8 reps	2/wk for 16 wks
Haykowsky et al 2000	4	20	M = 20	68	Arms and legs	Machine weights	60–80% 1 RM	3–10 reps Sets not stated	3/wk for 16 wks
*Hortobagyi et al 2001	5	27	Not stated	72	Legs (extensors)	Machine weights	80% 1 RM or 40% 1 RM	5 sets 4–6 or 8–12 reps	3/wk for 10 wks
Jette et al 1996	4	83	M = 52 F = 31	71	Trunk and proximal extremities	Theraband	10 RM	10 reps Sets not stated	3/wk for 12–15 wks
Jette et al 1999	6	215	M = 48 F = 167	75.4	Not stated	Theraband	10 RM	10 reps	3/wk for 26 wks

(continued)

Table 7.1 (continued)

Author/year	PEDro score	Sample size	Sex	Age (mean)	Muscle group	Type of weights	Load	Sets and repetitions	Frequency and duration
Jubrias et al 2001	6	26	M and F	69.2	Legs (quadriceps)	Machine weights	60–85% 1 RM	3–5 sets 4–15 reps	3/wk for 24 wks
Judge et al 1994	7	54	F = 21 M = 33	80.5	Legs	Sandbag, body and machine weights	Sandbag: 13 RM Machine: up to 75% 1RM	2–3 sets up to 13 reps	3/wk for 13 wks
Macaluso et al 2000	5	16	F = 16	75	Elbow flexion	Kin-Com dynamometer	20–80% MVC	15 sets 10 reps	3/wk for 6 wks
McCartney et al 1995	4	119	M and F	Range: 60–80	Arms, trunk and legs	Machine weights	50–80% 1 RM	2–3 sets 10–12 reps	2/wk for 10 months
McCartney et al 1996	5	113	F = 63 M = 50	Range: 60–80	Arms, trunk and legs	Machine weights	50–80% 1 RM	2–3 sets 10–12 reps	2/wk for 10 months in each of 2 yrs
Mikesky et al 1994	5	55	F = 34 M = 21	69.2	Arms and legs	Theraband	12 RM	1–3 sets 10–12 reps	3/wk for 12 wks
Nelson et al 1994, 1996	4	39	F = 39	59.2	Legs and trunk	Machine weights	80% 1 RM	3 sets 8 reps	2/wk for 52 wks
Nichols et al 1993	5	36	F = 36	67.1	Arms, trunk and legs	Machine weights	80% 1 RM	1–3 sets 8–10 reps	3/wk for 24 wks
Nicholson et al 2000	4	14	F = 12 M = 2	72.5	Legs	Elastic tubing and body weight	Reach exertion rating of 'somewhat hard'	3 sets 12 reps	3/wk for 12 wks
Panton et al 1990	5	32	F = 17 M = 15	72.2	Arms, trunk and legs	Machine weights	12 RM	1 set 8–12 reps	3/wk for 26 wks
Parkhouse et al 2000	4	22	F = 22	68	Legs	Not stated	75–80% 1 RM	3 sets 8–10 reps	3/wk for 32 wks
Perrig Chiello et al 1998	6	46	F = 18 M = 28	73.2	Arms, trunk and legs	Machine weights	Not stated	Not stated	1/wk for 8 wks
Pollock et al 1991	5	32	F = 17 M = 15	72.2	Arms, trunk and legs	Machine weights	12 RM	1 set 10–12 reps	3/wk for 26 wks
*Pruitt et al 1995	4	26	F = 26	68.3	Arms, trunk and legs	Machine weights	80% 1 RM or 40% 1 RM	3 sets 7 or 14 reps	3/wk for 52 wks
Pyka et al 1994	4	14	F = 9 M = 5	67.2	Arms, trunk and legs	Machine weights	65–75% 1 RM	3 sets 8 reps	3/wk for 50 wks
Rhodes et al 2000	6	38	F = 38	68.8	Arms and legs	Machine weights	75% 1 RM	3 sets 8 reps	3/wk for 52 wks
Rooks et al 1997	5	81	F = 58 M = 23	73.9	Arms and legs	Weighted belt, body weight,	Variable, dependent on	3 sets 8 reps	3/wk for 42 wks

Study					muscle group	machine and free weights			
Schlicht et al 2001	5	22	F = 14 M = 8	72	Legs	Machine weights	77.8% 1 RM	2 sets 10 reps	3/wk for 8 wks
Sforzo et al 1995	3	35	F = 22 M = 13	69	Legs	Not stated	12 RM	Not stated	Times/wk not stated 32 of 42 wks
Sipila et al 1995, 1996	4	21	F = 21	Range: 76–78	Legs	Machine weights	60–75% 1 RM	3–4 sets 8–10 reps	3/wk for 18 wks
Skelton et al 1995	5	40	F = 40	79.5	Arms and legs	Body weight, rice bags and Theraband	8 RM	3 sets 4–8 reps	3/wk for 12 wks
Skelton and McLaughlin 1996	3	18	F = 18	Range: 74–89	Arms and legs	Body weight, Theraband, tin cans and sponge balls	8 RM	1–3 sets 4–8 reps	3/wk for 8 wks
*Taaffe et al 1995	5	32	F = 32	Range: 65–79	Arms, trunk and legs	Machine weights	80% 1 RM or 40% 1 RM	3 sets 7 or 14 reps	3/wk for 52 wks
*Taaffe et al 1996	4	32	F = 32	Range: 65–79	Thigh	Machine weights	80% 1 RM or 40% 1 RM	3 sets 7 or 14 reps	3/wk for 52 wks
*Taaffe et al 1999	5	46	F = 17 M = 29	Range: 65–79	Arms and legs	Machine weights	80% 1 RM	3 sets 10 reps	1, 2, or 3/wk for 24 wks
Topp et al 1993	4	55	Not stated	71	Arms and legs	Elastic tubing	12 RM	Upper body: 2 sets 10 reps; lower body: 3 sets 10 reps	3/wk for 12 wks
Topp et al 1996	3	42	F = 23 M = 19	71.5	Arms, trunk and legs	Theraband	10 RM	Upper body: 2 sets 10 reps; lower body: 3 sets 10 reps	3/wk for 14 wks
*Tsutsumi et al 1997	5	41	F = 8 M = 33	68.8	Arms, trunk and legs	Machine weights	75–85% 1 RM or 55–65% 1 RM	2 sets 8–10 or 14–16 reps	3/wk for 12 wks
Tsutsumi et al 1998	6	36	F = 36	68.5	Arms, trunk and legs	Machine weights	75–85% 1 RM	2 sets 8–10 reps	3/wk for 12 wks
Westhoff et al 2000	5	21	Not stated	75.9	Knee extensors	Elastic bands and body weight	8 RM	1–3 sets 4–8 reps	3/wk for 10 wks
*Willoughby and Pelsue 1998	6	18	M = 18	69.3	Arms, trunk and legs	Machine weights	75–80% 1 RM or 60–65% 1 RM	3 sets 8–10 or 15–20 reps	3/wk for 12 wks

* Indicates the studies that investigated the effects of more than one intensity of strength training programme.

using weight machines aimed at strengthening the arms, lower limbs and trunk. Participants typically completed 2–3 sets of 6–12 repetitions of each exercise with a training intensity of 70–80% of the one repetition maximum (1 RM). The term 1 RM refers to the amount of weight that can be lifted only once through full range with good form. Participants typically trained 2–3 times per week for periods ranging from 6 weeks to 2 years. Seventeen papers investigated programmes that lasted for 26 weeks or more (Table 7.1).

The programme content was similar to guidelines for strength training recommended by the American College of Sports Medicine (ACSM) for healthy young adults (Kraemer et al 2002). However, the amount of training in the studies reviewed in this chapter was generally greater than recommended by ACSM for older adults. The ACSM recommends that older adults complete one set of each exercise for 10–15 repetitions to fatigue (ACSM 1998a, 1998b, Kraemer et al 2002). In contrast, most of the studies in the systematic review completed 2–3 sets of 6–12 RM.

A few investigations with less training also reported strength benefits from their programmes. Training was specifically investigated at a lower intensity of 40–65% 1 RM for 14 repetitions (Pruitt et al 1995, Taaffe et al 1995, Tsutsumi et al 1997), training with only one set of each exercise (e.g. Damush and Damush 1999, Hagberg et al 1989) or training only one session per week (Perrig Chiello et al 1998, Taaffe et al 1999). These investigations found that strength benefits in older people can also be achieved with moderate strength training programmes. A distinction could also be made between novice and previously trained older people. The ACSM (2002) recommends that while strength gains can be made by the novice strength trainer (as was typical of the participants in the included studies) with a lesser training load, ongoing strength gains might require intensities of closer to 80% 1 RM with the use of multiple sets.

Although most studies evaluated training programmes that used weight machines, nine successfully used graduated elastic tubing to provide the progressive resistance. The practical advantage of using elastic tubing was that it allowed participants to complete their exercises at home, compared to weight machines located in a facility such as a gymnasium, hospital or laboratory.

Environmental factors

The setting in which the exercise programme was performed was not specified in many cases. Since most programmes completed training on weight machines, it might be assumed that training was typically conducted in a facility with gymnasium equipment. Examples of specified facilities included a hospital (Sforzo et al 1995, Skelton et al 1995), community centre (Rooks et al 1997) and research laboratory (Macaluso et al 2000). Several papers ($n = 24$) specified that training sessions were supervised by qualified staff.

Nine of the papers specified that strength training occurred in the home setting (Chandler et al 1998, Jette et al 1996, 1999, Mikesky et al 1994, Skelton et al 1995, Skelton and McLaughlin 1996, Topp et al 1993, 1996,

Westhoff et al 2000), and typically used simple equipment such as graduated elastic tubing to provide resistance. These papers are of particular interest to clinicians because they provide information about the practicality of prescribing strengthening programmes for older people in routine clinical practice. A number of these programmes also included one or two weekly supervised sessions in addition to the home programme (Skelton et al 1995, Skelton and McLaughlin 1996, Topp et al 1993, 1996, Westhoff et al 2000).

Personal factors

The effects of strength training have been investigated more in older women than in men. Thirty studies included both males and females, while 17 studies investigated females exclusively, and only three studies were restricted to males (Hagerman et al 2000, Haykowsky et al 2000, Willoughby and Pelsue 1998). The emphasis on older women may reflect the concern for the bone health and subsequent risk of fracture in this population (Sambrook et al 2002).

Participants in the strength training programmes were typically healthy older people with few health problems. All studies investigated independent community-dwelling adults over the age of 50 years, and the health status of the participants was often verified by thorough physical screening.

The efficacy of any intervention is dependent upon both the effectiveness of the programme and programme adherence. Most studies reported high levels of programme completion and adherence. Drop-out rates of less than 20% were typical, and compared favourably to drop-out rates for general exercise programmes of 20–50% in the first 5–6 months (Dishman et al 1985, Pollock 1988). Of those who completed the programmes, there was a consistently high rate of adherence, as measured by the percentage of scheduled sessions attended. Many of the papers reported attendance rates of greater than 90%. Of the studies reporting higher drop-outs (e.g. Westhoff et al (2000): 28.6%) or lower levels of adherence (e.g. Jette et al (1996): 58%), most were home-based programmes. Jette et al (1999) implemented a number of strategies in his home-based programme to improve adherence to 89% (Jette et al 1999). These included periodic telephone monitoring and incentives such as sending a new dollar bill to each participant on return of each exercise log book.

The ability to have time off from training and largely maintain the benefits may make strength training a feasible long-term exercise option for older people. McCartney et al (1996) found that a rest period of 3 weeks after 1 year of training led to little strength loss when training resumed. Sforzo et al (1995) also found that a rest of up to five weeks did not produce significant loss of strength.

Adverse incidents from strength training

Relatively few injuries or adverse effects as a result of strength training have been reported in older people. The injuries that were reported were typically of a minor nature that allowed participants to continue with their training. Pollock et al (1991) reported a 19.3% injury rate, defined as missing or modifying training for at least 1 week. It was noted that almost all musculoskeletal injuries occurred during 1 RM testing, and that there were minimal problems during strength training. Similarly, Judge et al (1994) reported that 18% of participants had musculoskeletal complaints such as back and knee pain, yet all continued in the programme with exercise modification. These injury rates for strength training compare favourably to the injury rate of 42% for older participants undertaking aerobic training with treadmill jogging (Pollock et al 1991).

There was little evidence that strength training led to any cardiovascular events in older people. Jette et al (1996) reported that one participant dropped out of the programme due to shortness of breath, and Skelton and McLaughlin (1996) reported one fainting episode. However, it is difficult to conclude that strength training does not increase cardiovascular risk to older people as many of the studies heavily screened their participants for cardiovascular risk factors. This screening is consistent with recommendations that the major contraindications for exercise are recent ECG changes or myocardial infarction, unstable angina, uncontrolled arrhythmias, third degree heart block, and acute congestive heart failure (ACSM 1998a).

Changes in body function

Upper body strength

Fifteen studies reported sufficient post-intervention data to calculate effect sizes for upper body strength after a strength training programme (Figure 7.1). As can be seen, there was a positive outcome for strength training on upper body strength, with the meta-analysis indicating there was a large effect ($d = 1.32$, $z = 3.45$, $P = 0.0003$). According to Cohen's (1988) conventions, effect sizes greater than $d = 0.80$ are considered to be large. The duration of the programmes that led to this treatment effect ranged from 8 to 52 weeks (mean = 26.9 weeks, SD = 16.9). Percentage strength gains ranged from 5.8% (Pruitt et al 1995) to 57.7% (Pyka et al 1994). The weighted average strength gain was 26.9%. There was no significant correlation between the effect size and the duration of the strengthening programme (Pearson's $r = -0.19$, $P = 0.50$).

Lower limb strength

The results of the studies that reported sufficient data to calculate effect sizes for increasing strength in the knee extensors and for the leg press can be viewed in Figures 7.2 and 7.3. Overall, meta-analysis revealed a significant effect for strength training in increasing the strength of the knee extensors ($d = 1.20$, $z = 3.54$, $P = 0.0004$) and increasing strength of the leg press ($d = 1.43$, $z = 8.89$, $P < 0.000\,01$).

The groups undertaking strength training had a net weighted average strength gain of 43.1% in their knee extensors and a net average

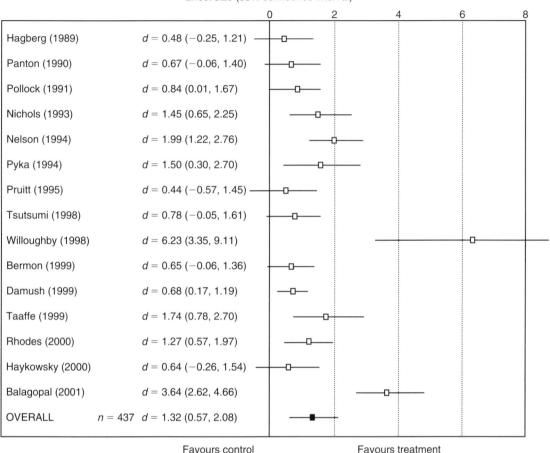

Upper body strength
Effect size (95% confidence interval)

Hagberg (1989)	$d = 0.48 (-0.25, 1.21)$
Panton (1990)	$d = 0.67 (-0.06, 1.40)$
Pollock (1991)	$d = 0.84 (0.01, 1.67)$
Nichols (1993)	$d = 1.45 (0.65, 2.25)$
Nelson (1994)	$d = 1.99 (1.22, 2.76)$
Pyka (1994)	$d = 1.50 (0.30, 2.70)$
Pruitt (1995)	$d = 0.44 (-0.57, 1.45)$
Tsutsumi (1998)	$d = 0.78 (-0.05, 1.61)$
Willoughby (1998)	$d = 6.23 (3.35, 9.11)$
Bermon (1999)	$d = 0.65 (-0.06, 1.36)$
Damush (1999)	$d = 0.68 (0.17, 1.19)$
Taaffe (1999)	$d = 1.74 (0.78, 2.70)$
Rhodes (2000)	$d = 1.27 (0.57, 1.97)$
Haykowsky (2000)	$d = 0.64 (-0.26, 1.54)$
Balagopal (2001)	$d = 3.64 (2.62, 4.66)$
OVERALL $n = 437$	$d = 1.32 (0.57, 2.08)$

Favours control   Favours treatment

Figure 7.1 Effect sizes for upper body strength changes after progressive resistance exercise programmes for independent older adults.

weighted strength gain of 28.1% for the leg press. Strength gains reported by individual studies ranged from 5.1% (Nichols et al 1993) to 101.4% (Pyka et al 1994). The duration of the programmes that led to knee extensor strengthening ranged from 8 to 52 weeks (mean 23.4 weeks, SD 15.1). There was no significant correlation between the effect size and the duration of the strengthening programme (Pearson's $r = 0.16$, $P = 0.59$).

To synthesize, older adults can achieve significant strength increases in their arms and lower limbs with a progressive strength training programme. This is despite early opinions in the literature that, 'the gift however to increase strength by training is lost in the course of ageing' (Muller 1957). The capacity of older people to adapt to training and increase strength appears at least equal to that of younger adults. The average strength gains in this review were 26.9%, 28.1% and 43.1% for upper body, leg press and knee extension, respectively, compared with the average improvement in young and middle-aged adults of 25–30% for up to 6 months of training (Fleck and Kraemer 1997).

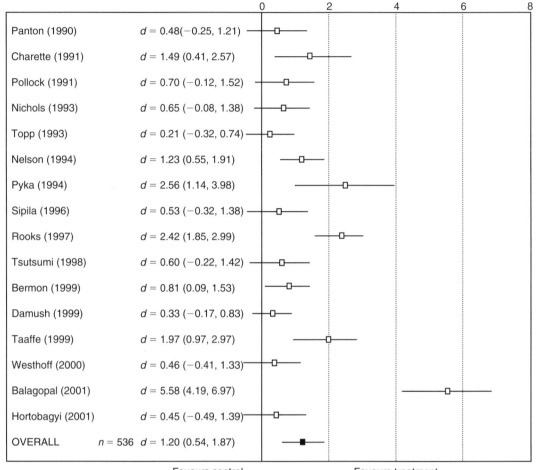

Figure 7.2 Effect sizes for strength changes in knee extensors after progressive resistance exercise programmes for independent older adults.

It is possible that older participants in a home-based strength training programme may not gain strength to the same extent as when the programme is closely supervised and uses gymnasium equipment. Only two of the studies included in the knee extension meta-analysis were home-based programmes (Topp et al 1996, Westhoff et al 2000). These two studies reported effect sizes less than the overall effect. In addition, the home-based programme evaluated by Jette et al (1999) reported only moderate strength increases (6–12%) in lower limb strength. In a home-based programme, participants may not train at the same intensity as when closely supervised in a clinical or research laboratory setting. Also, it is more difficult to quantify the progression of resistance with the use of graduated elastic tubing, as used in the home-based programmes. Strength in the home-based programmes was not measured on the equipment the participants used during training. Consistent with the principle of specificity of training, it has been demonstrated that

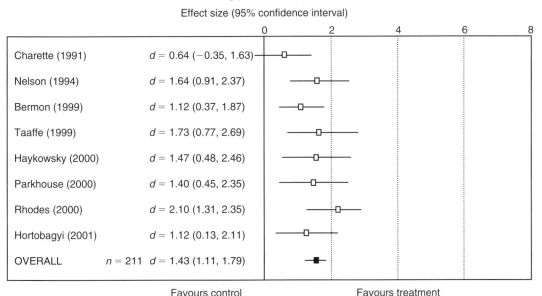

Leg press strength

Effect size (95% confidence interval)

Charette (1991)	$d = 0.64 \, (-0.35, 1.63)$	
Nelson (1994)	$d = 1.64 \, (0.91, 2.37)$	
Bermon (1999)	$d = 1.12 \, (0.37, 1.87)$	
Taaffe (1999)	$d = 1.73 \, (0.77, 2.69)$	
Haykowsky (2000)	$d = 1.47 \, (0.48, 2.46)$	
Parkhouse (2000)	$d = 1.40 \, (0.45, 2.35)$	
Rhodes (2000)	$d = 2.10 \, (1.31, 2.35)$	
Hortobagyi (2001)	$d = 1.12 \, (0.13, 2.11)$	
OVERALL	$n = 211 \quad d = 1.43 \, (1.11, 1.79)$	

Favours control   Favours treatment

Figure 7.3 Effect sizes for strength changes in the leg press after progressive resistance exercise programmes for independent older adults.

strength increases are lower when not measured on the equipment used for training (Fleck and Kraemer 1997).

Aerobic capacity

This review did not find strong evidence for increased aerobic capacity after strength training. The three studies that reported sufficient data to calculate effect sizes of aerobic capacity (VO_{2max}) are displayed in Figure 7.4. Each of these had 95% confidence intervals that crossed zero. However, Hagerman et al (2000) reported a statistically significant interaction effect in favour of strength training. When the results of these three studies were aggregated with a random effects model the total sample of 65 subjects confirmed the impression of no significant effect ($d = 0.32, z = 1.26, P = 0.10$). The weighted average improvement in aerobic capacity (VO_{2max}) across training programmes of duration of 16 to 26 weeks was 4.1%. This calculation included the results of Buchner et al (1997), who provided sufficient information for calculation of percentage change in aerobic capacity yet insufficient data to calculate effect sizes.

The American College of Sports Medicine (1998b) recommends training should be at least 55–65% of maximum heart rate for 20–60 minutes for 3–5 days per week to increase cardiorespiratory fitness. When followed, these guidelines generally show a minimum increase in aerobic capacity of 10–15% (ACSM 1998b). Therefore, strength training programmes, in isolation, may not provide sufficient stimulus and intensity to train cardiorespiratory fitness (Fleck and Kraemer 1997).

Endurance

Strength training in older people led to significant increases in muscular endurance as assessed by walking endurance (Ades et al 1996,

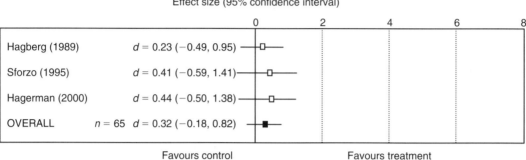

Figure 7.4 Effect sizes for strength changes in aerobic capacity (VO_{2max}) after progressive resistance exercise programmes for independent older adults.

McCartney et al 1995, McCartney et al 1996) and the number of bench and leg presses performed at sub-maximal load (50–70% 1 RM) (Adams et al 2001). Calculated effect sizes for these studies were d (walking endurance) = 1.52 (95% CI: 0.61, 2.43) (Ades et al 1996), d (bench press) = 1.60 (0.54, 2.66) and d (leg press) = 1.59 (0.53, 2.65) (Adams et al 2001). There were insufficient data to calculate the effect sizes from the 1995 and 1996 studies of McCartney et al. From a total of 204 subjects, the weighted average gain in endurance was 44.6%.

This is consistent with findings that strength training can increase muscular endurance in younger adults (Anderson and Kearney 1982, Huczel and Clarke 1992). The clinical significance of these findings is that the ability to perform repeated daily activities, such as walking, might be particularly affected by the level of muscle endurance older people have. Improvements in endurance in this review were not just muscle specific (e.g. number of bench presses), but also demonstrated in the functional activity of walking endurance.

Flexibility

Strength training appeared to have no effect on the flexibility of older people. The effect of strength training on flexibility was documented in four papers (Adams et al 2001, Mikesky et al 1994, Rhodes et al 2000, Westhoff et al 2000). Flexibility was measured using the sit and reach test (Adams et al 2001, Rhodes et al 2000) and by measurement of knee flexion range (Mikesky et al 1994, Westhoff et al 2000). None of these studies reported changes in flexibility. This was confirmed with effect sizes calculated at $d = 0.00$ (95% CI: −0.53, 0.53) (Mikesky et al 1994), $d = 0.22$ (−0.42, 0.86) (Rhodes et al 2000) and $d = -0.20$ (−1.06, 0.66) (Westhoff et al 2000). There were insufficient data to calculate the effect size for the Adams et al (2001) study.

The percentage change in flexibility across 112 subjects was 1.2%, ranging from a reduction in flexibility of 2% in the Westhoff et al (2000) study to a reported increase in 6.1% in the Adams et al (2001) study. Overall no reduction in flexibility was detected. This finding should allow the clinician to counter the anecdotal claims that strength training can result in loss of flexibility.

Changes in psycho-logical functioning

The effects of strength training on the psychological function of older people remains unclear. A total of seven articles evaluated the effect of strength training on psychological functioning (Damush and Damush 1999, Jette et al 1996, 1999, Perrig Chiello et al 1998, Skelton and McLaughlin 1996, Tsutsumi et al 1997, Tsutsumi et al 1998). A range of psychological factors were measured. However, the most common were changes in negative symptoms known to be associated with ageing such as anxiety, fatigue, confusion, vigour and depression. Figure 7.5 summarizes the results of the studies that reported sufficient data to calculate effect sizes for changes in psychological function. Visual inspection of the effect sizes suggests that most psychological factors remained unchanged after a strength training programme. It is difficult, however, to draw firm conclusions about the effects of strength training on the psychological functioning of older people because few randomized controlled trials have measured change in psychological function after strength training.

Personal factors such as the degree of improvement in muscle strength, whether the participants had psychological impairments, as well as the age and sex of the participants in the experimental group may have an impact on the psychological benefits of strength training (Jette et al 1999). The effect of these factors has yet to be systematically investigated. For this reason it remains unknown whether certain subsections of the older population benefit more than others.

The psychological benefits from strength training might be due to programme factors such as the duration, intensity and setting of the exercise programme, as well as the physiological changes that occur with training. This issue is illustrated by comparing the effect sizes for vigour calculated from data collected in a study by Tsutsumi (1998) compared with that from a study by Jette (1999) (Figure 7.5). Tsutsumi's participants trained for 12 weeks on machine weights in a gymnasium setting under close individual supervision. In contrast, Jette's participants trained for 24 weeks using resistance elastic tubing in their own home with minimal supervision. As Figure 7.5 shows, Tsutsumi's programme appeared to have a large positive effect on vigour while Jette's programme did not. The effects of programme factors on psychological function in older people remain unknown.

Changes in body structure

Skeletal muscle

Ageing is associated with decreases in skeletal muscle mass and muscle strength (Lindle et al 1997, Lynch et al 1999). There is considerable interest in whether strength training can induce skeletal muscle hypertrophy in older people. The following sections deal firstly with the effect of training on total body muscle mass, and then secondly with changes in muscle morphology such as whole muscle cross-sectional area and individual muscle fibre cross-sectional area.

Muscle mass

Seven papers measured the effect of strength training on skeletal muscle mass (Ades et al 1996, Hagberg et al 1989, Hagerman et al 2000, Nelson et al 1996, Nichols et al 1993, Sipila and Suominen 1995, Taaffe et al 1999). All studies reported sufficient data to calculate effect sizes (Figure 7.6). The calculated effect sizes ranged from $d = 0.17$ (Nelson et al 1996) to $d = 0.69$ (Hagberg et al 1989). Absolute changes in lean body mass ranged from $-0.1\,kg$ (Nelson et al 1996) to $1.8\,kg$ (Hagerman et al 2000). Meta-analysis demonstrated a significant increase in lean body mass and lean tissue mass ($d = 0.38$, $z = 2.52$, $P = 0.01$), and by implication total muscle mass after strength training. This finding supports the notion that training leads to an increase in strength, at least in part, by inducing muscle hypertrophy.

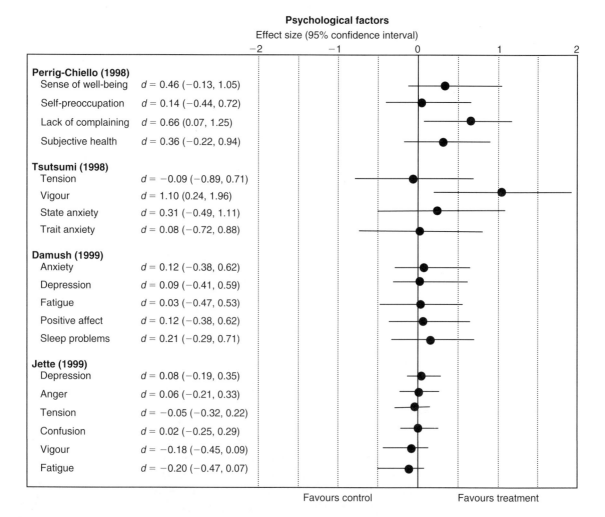

Figure 7.5 Effect sizes for changes in psychological variables after progressive resistance exercise programmes for independent older adults.

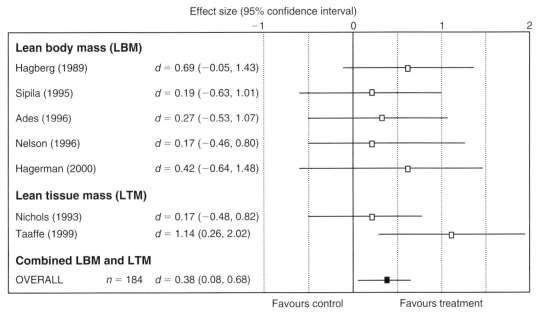

Figure 7.6 Effect sizes for changes in lean body mass and lean tissue mass after progressive resistance exercise programmes for independent older adults.

Skeletal muscle morphology

Skeletal muscle cross-sectional area

Five studies examined the effects of strength training on muscle cross-sectional area (Jubrias et al 2001, McCartney et al 1995, 1996, Nelson et al 1996, Sipila and Suominen 1995). Four of these measured cross-sectional area of the quadriceps muscle group. Compared with the control group, quadriceps cross-sectional area increased from 4.8% (Sipila and Suominen 1995), to 11.5% (Jubrias et al 2001) after strength training. Because only two of these studies provided sufficient data to calculate effect sizes (Jubrias et al 2001, Sipila and Suominen 1995) (Figure 7.7) an overall effect size of strength training on quadriceps muscle cross-sectional area was not calculated. However, these studies provide some evidence that strength training can cause skeletal muscle hypertrophy that could contribute to the increase in strength.

Skeletal muscle fibre cross-sectional area

Three studies investigated the effects of strength training on type I (slow-twitch) and type II (fast-twitch) muscle fibre cross-sectional area in the quadriceps muscle (Charette et al 1991, Pyka et al 1994, Taaffe et al 1996). The percentage increase in type I muscle fibre cross-sectional area ranged from 13.4% (Charette et al 1991) to 29.7% (Taaffe et al 1996), and the percentage increase in type II muscle fibre cross-sectional area ranged from 9.6% (Pyka et al 1994) to 38.4% (Charette et al 1991). Meta-analysis revealed that both type I ($d = 1.23$, $z = 2.90$, $P = 0.004$) and type II ($d = 1.16$, $z = 3.21$, $P = 0.001$) muscle fibre cross-sectional area significantly increased after strength training (Figure 7.7). The large effect

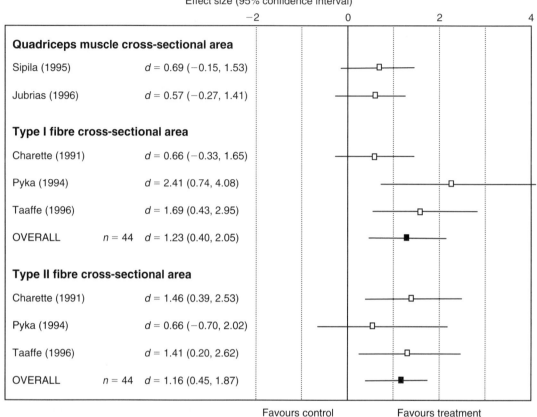

Figure 7.7 Effect sizes for changes in quadriceps muscle cross sectional area, and vastus lateralis type I and type II muscle fibre cross-sectional area after progressive resistance exercise programmes for independent older adults.

sizes suggest that significant hypertrophy of individual skeletal muscle fibres (both type I and type II fibres) occurs in response to strength training. These changes account for the increase in total muscle mass and cross-sectional area, and would ultimately contribute to an increase in muscle strength. It is apparent that ageing skeletal muscle retains the ability to hypertrophy in response to resistance training.

Bone mineral density

The effect of strength training on bone mineral density (BMD) in older people remains equivocal. Six studies evaluated the effects of strength training on lumbar spine or femoral neck BMD. Three of these examined the effects of strength training on BMD in an exclusively female population (Nelson et al 1994, Pruitt et al 1995, Rhodes et al 2000) (Figure 7.8). One study reported significant increases in both lumbar spine and femoral neck BMD after strength training (Nelson et al 1994). The other two studies found no effect of strength training on either lumbar spine or femoral neck BMD (Pruitt et al 1995, Rhodes et al 2000).

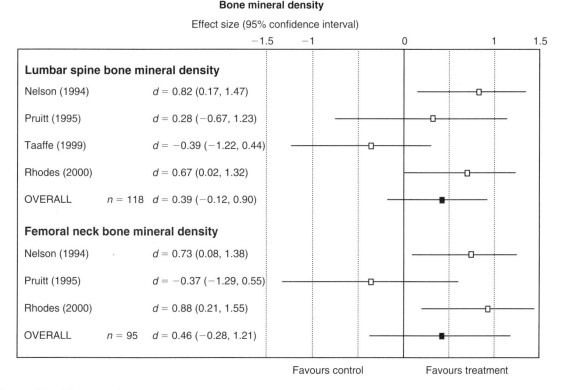

Bone mineral density

Effect size (95% confidence interval)

Lumbar spine bone mineral density

Nelson (1994) $d = 0.82$ (0.17, 1.47)

Pruitt (1995) $d = 0.28$ (-0.67, 1.23)

Taaffe (1999) $d = -0.39$ (-1.22, 0.44)

Rhodes (2000) $d = 0.67$ (0.02, 1.32)

OVERALL $n = 118$ $d = 0.39$ (-0.12, 0.90)

Femoral neck bone mineral density

Nelson (1994) $d = 0.73$ (0.08, 1.38)

Pruitt (1995) $d = -0.37$ (-1.29, 0.55)

Rhodes (2000) $d = 0.88$ (0.21, 1.55)

OVERALL $n = 95$ $d = 0.46$ (-0.28, 1.21)

Favours control   Favours treatment

Figure 7.8 Effect sizes for changes in bone mineral density (BMD) of the lumbar spine and femoral neck after progressive resistance exercise programmes for independent older adults.

The remaining three studies examined the effects of strength training on lumbar spine BMD in a mixed sex cohort. None of these studies found a positive effect of strength training (McCartney et al 1995, 1996, Taaffe et al 1999). Two of these studies provided insufficient post-intervention data to calculate effect sizes (McCartney et al 1995, 1996); the effect size for the Taaffe et al (1999) study is shown in Figure 7.8, and was included in the meta-analysis.

Meta-analysis showed a positive trend for both lumbar spine BMD ($d = 0.39$, $z = 1.51$, $P = 0.14$) and femoral neck BMD ($d = 0.46$, $z = 1.22$, $P = 0.09$) to increase slightly in the training group compared with the control group.

Two previous meta-analyses have evaluated the effects of resistance exercise training on BMD in women. Similar to the findings of our review, Wolff et al (1999) showed a non-significant trend for strength training to increase both lumbar spine BMD and femoral neck BMD in four randomized controlled trials in postmenopausal women. Kelley et al (2001) found a small yet significant effect of resistance training for maintaining lumbar spine BMD in strength-trained women compared with a 1.45% decrease in control groups (Kelley et al 2001). Similarly they found that training increased femoral BMD by 0.40%, whereas it decreased in the control group by 0.21%.

Despite some positive trends, the effect of strength training on BMD remains uncertain in older people. With effect sizes maintained in larger randomized controlled trials strength training may yet prove to have some beneficial effects on BMD in older people. However, the results suggest that compared to weight-bearing aerobic/endurance training, strength training may have a relatively small effect on bone health (Kelley 1998a, 1998b).

Body fat

Strength training appears to have little effect on reducing body fat in older people. The effect of strength training on body fat was evaluated in 13 studies. The effect was reported as sum of skinfolds, percentage body fat, and/or total body fat mass. One study did not provide sufficient post-intervention data to calculate effects sizes (Adams et al 2001), whilst two further studies were excluded because baseline percentage body fat (Hagerman et al 2000) or baseline total fat mass (Taaffe et al 1999) was significantly different between the strength training group and the control group. Calculated effect sizes for the remaining studies are shown in Figure 7.9. Each study individually reported no significant

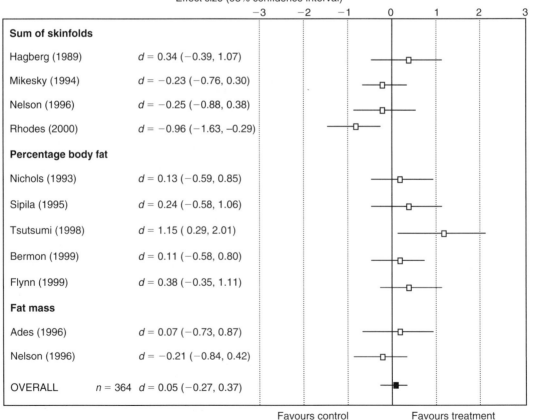

Figure 7.9 Effect sizes for changes in body fat after progressive resistance exercise programmes for independent older adults.

effect of strength training on body fat. Meta-analysis confirmed no overall effect of strength training on body fat ($d = 0.05, z = 0.31, P = 0.75$).

Haematology

Six studies investigated the effects of strength training on haematological parameters in older people. These parameters included plasma hormone levels, immune markers and plasma lipids. A summary of these studies is provided in Table 7.2.

Bone formation may be increased in older people after strength training. One study found that parathyroid hormone and plasma osteocalcin levels were increased after 1 year of strength training in older women (Nelson et al 1994). Parathyroid hormone directly increases bone resorption, whilst osteocalcin is a protein produced by osteoblasts, the cells which generate new bone tissue. Considered together these changes in bone generation and resorption suggest that bone formation may be increased in older people.

Two studies examined the effects of strength training on insulin-like growth factor one (IGF-1). IGF-1 is thought to promote increases in muscle and bone mass (Benbassat et al 1997, Cohick and Clemmons 1993, Langlois et al 1998, Ravn et al 1995). Bermon et al (1999a) found no significant effect of 8 weeks of strength training on IGF-1. By contrast, Parkhouse et al (2000) reported a 67% increase in IGF-1 concentration ($P < 0.05$) following 8 months of strength training in older women with initially low IGF-1 levels and low bone mineral density (Parkhouse et al 2000). These contrasting results may be due to the effects of strength training on IGF-1 levels in individuals that have initially low IGF-1 levels, such as the women in the Parkhouse et al (2000) study.

Table 7.2   The effects of strength training in older people on haematological parameters

	Indication	Studies	Result
Hormones			
Parathyroid hormone and osteocalcin	Bone formation	Nelson et al 1994	Parathyroid hormone: ↑18% Osteocalcin: ↑19% Both significant ($P < 0.05$)
IGF-1	Promotes increased muscle and bone mass	Bermon et al 1999a Parkhouse et al 2000	NS ↑67% ($P < 0.05$)
Catecholamines (adrenaline, noradrenaline)	Reflect sympathetic nervous system activity	Bermon et al 1999b	NS
Cortisol	Reflects physical or psychological stress	Bermon et al 1999b Flynn et al 1999	NS NS
Immune markers		Bermon et al 1999b Flynn et al 1999	NS NS
Plasma lipids (e.g. cholesterol)		Hagerman et al 2000	NS

NS: non-significant.

The remaining studies failed to detect any significant effects of strength training on hormones (Bermon et al 1999b), immune markers (Bermon et al 1999b, Flynn et al 1999) or plasma lipid profile (Hagerman et al 2000) in older people (Table 7.2).

Changes in activity

Nineteen articles examined the effects of strength training on at least one activity-related outcome. The most common activities measured were walking (maximum or self-selected speed, endurance), sit-to-stand (speed, endurance, kinetics), stair-climbing (speed or endurance) and balance (static or dynamic standing).

Walking

Thirteen studies reported the effects of strength training on walking (Ades et al 1996, Brandon et al 2000, Buchner et al 1997, Judge et al 1994, McCartney et al 1995, 1996, Schlicht et al 2001, Skelton et al 1995, Sipila et al 1996, Skelton and McLaughlin 1996, Topp et al 1993, 1996, Westhoff et al 2000). Ten of these measured change in walking speed and three measured change in walking endurance. Figure 7.10 shows the results of the studies that reported sufficient data to calculate effect sizes for increasing walking speed. Overall, meta-analysis demonstrated that strength training increased the maximum walking speed of older people ($d = 0.31$, $z = 2.06$, $P = 0.04$) but appeared to have no effect on their self-selected walking speed ($d = -0.03$, $z = -0.25$, $P = 0.80$). It has been postulated that stronger lower limb muscles would be able to generate larger propulsion forces that could in turn increase walking speed. Several studies have demonstrated a strong positive relationship between muscle strength and walking speed in frail older people (Bassey et al 1988, 1992, Fiatarone et al 1990). However, the results of this review reveal that only maximum walking speed and not habitual walking speed increased. This differential effect of strength training on maximum versus self-selected walking speed may be explained by the activity limitation the person experiences. Most of the studies in this review included healthy older people with sufficient strength to walk at speeds adequate for normal everyday functioning. Because habitual walking speed produced no activity limitation, strengthening would be unlikely to lead to changes in self-selected walking speed. Only when the demands of the activity are increased such as when asked to walk at maximum speed would limitations be evident. In this case muscle strengthening would be expected to lead to increased maximal walking speed.

A separate longitudinal study examining the effect of progressive resistance training on walking endurance detected significant improvements after both 1 year (McCartney et al 1995) and 2 years (McCartney et al 1996) of training. These findings were replicated in a separate study of 24 men and women aged 65–79 years of age who exercised for only 12 weeks (Ades et al 1996). Although the mechanism responsible for improved endurance after strength training has not been identified, it

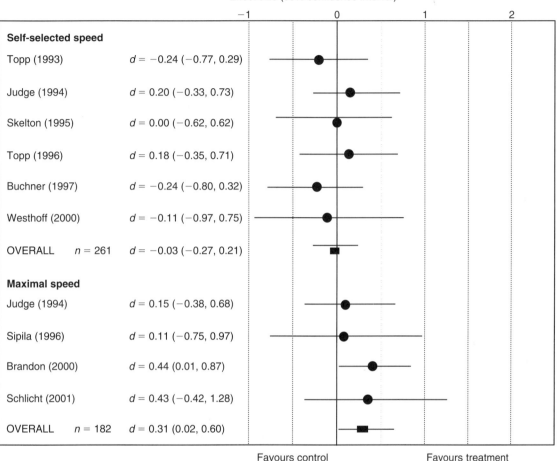

Figure 7.10 Effect sizes for changes in self-selected and maximum walking speed after progressive resistance exercise programmes for independent older adults.

has been proposed that stronger muscles are able to generate force more efficiently. This is likely to result in a reduced perception of effort, which in turn enables physical activities to be performed for longer before symptoms of fatigue occur (McCartney et al 1996).

Sit-to-stand

The effects of strength training on an older person's ability to move from sitting to standing remains unclear. Six papers measured changes in the performance of sit to stand (Judge et al 1994, Nicholson and Emes 2000, Schlicht et al 2001, Skelton et al 1995, Skelton and McLaughlin 1996, Taaffe et al 1999). All of these trials measured change in self-selected and/or maximum speed of sit-to-stand, with one trial also measuring change in the power generated during sit-to-stand (Nicholson and Emes

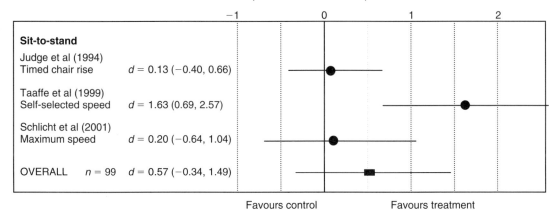

Timed sit-to-stand

Effect size (95% confidence interval)

Sit-to-stand

Judge et al (1994)
Timed chair rise $\quad d = 0.13\ (-0.40, 0.66)$

Taaffe et al (1999)
Self-selected speed $\quad d = 1.63\ (0.69, 2.57)$

Schlicht et al (2001)
Maximum speed $\quad d = 0.20\ (-0.64, 1.04)$

OVERALL $\quad n = 99 \quad d = 0.57\ (-0.34, 1.49)$

Favours control $\qquad\qquad$ Favours treatment

Figure 7.11 Effect sizes for changes in speed of sit-to-stand after progressive resistance exercise programmes for independent older adults.

2000). Figure 7.11 summarizes the results of the three studies that reported sufficient data to calculate effect sizes. Only one trial reported a significantly increased speed of sit-to-stand and this was for self-selected speed (Taaffe et al 1999). Speed of sit-to-stand was generally unchanged after participation in a strength training programme ($d = 0.57$, $z = 1.23$, $P = 0.20$). With respect to the three trials that did not report sufficient data to calculate effect sizes, one reported a significant increase in maximum speed (Nicholson and Emes 2000), another reported a significant increase in self-selected speed (Skelton and McLaughlin 1996), and the last reported no change in either self-selected or maximum speed of sit-to-stand (Skelton et al 1995). Overall, half of the studies that examined the effects of training on chair rise reported improvements, while the other half did not. In addition to finding a significant effect for speed of sit-to-stand, Nicholson and Emes (2000) found that strength training increased the maximum power generated during sit-to-stand.

Stair-climbing

Seven papers measured the effects of strength training on the speed or endurance of stair-climbing in older people (Brandon et al 2000, Buchner et al 1997, McCartney et al 1995, 1996, Rooks et al 1997, Skelton et al 1995, Skelton and McLaughlin 1996). Figure 7.12 shows the results of the four studies that reported sufficient data to calculate effect sizes for increasing stair-climbing speed. Overall, meta-analysis demonstrated that strength training increased the speed of stair-climbing in older people ($d = 0.39$, $z = 2.09$, $P = 0.04$). This result is primarily based on self-selected speed, rather than maximum speed. The only other study to examine the effect of training on speed of stair-climbing also detected a significant increase in the self-selected speed of stair-climbing (Skelton and McLaughlin 1996). McCartney et al's longitudinal study examined the effect of progressive resistance training on the endurance of stair-climbing. This study detected significant improvements in endurance

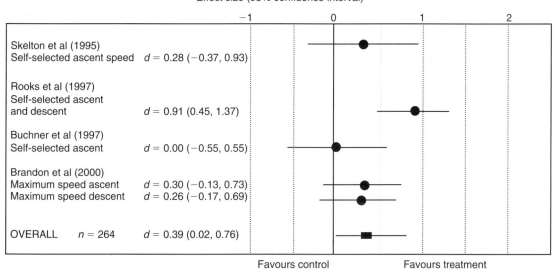

Timed stair-climbing

Effect size (95% confidence interval)

Skelton et al (1995)
Self-selected ascent speed $d = 0.28$ (−0.37, 0.93)

Rooks et al (1997)
Self-selected ascent
and descent $d = 0.91$ (0.45, 1.37)

Buchner et al (1997)
Self-selected ascent $d = 0.00$ (−0.55, 0.55)

Brandon et al (2000)
Maximum speed ascent $d = 0.30$ (−0.13, 0.73)
Maximum speed descent $d = 0.26$ (−0.17, 0.69)

OVERALL $n = 264$ $d = 0.39$ (0.02, 0.76)

Favours control   Favours treatment

Figure 7.12 Effect sizes for changes in speed of climbing stairs after progressive resistance exercise programmes for independent older adults.

after both 1 year (McCartney et al 1995) and 2 years (McCartney et al 1996) of training.

Balance

Muscle weakness has been associated with an increased risk of falls and fractures (Aniansson et al 1984, Campbell et al 1989, Whipple et al 1987) in older people and therefore the effects of strength training on preventing these debilitating health problems has received great interest. Eleven articles measured the effects of strength training on balance in standing. Three of these measured change in static balance (Buchner et al 1997, Schlicht et al 2001, Westhoff et al 2000), three in dynamic standing balance (Nelson et al 1994, Skelton et al 1995, Taaffe et al 1999), and five in both static and dynamic balance (Jette et al 1999, Rooks et al 1997, Skelton and McLaughlin 1996, Topp et al 1993, 1996). Static balance is defined as the ability to maintain balance when there is no self-generated or external perturbation. This includes the ability to maintain single limb stance or tandem stance. Dynamic balance is defined as the ability to maintain balance when there is either self-generated or external perturbation. This includes the ability to maintain balanced when reaching as far as possible out of the base of support (i.e. the functional reach test) or when performing either forward or backward tandem walking. Figure 7.13 summarizes the results of studies that reported sufficient data to calculate effect sizes. Overall, meta-analysis demonstrated a highly significant effect for strength training in increasing dynamic standing balance ($d = 0.23$, $z = 2.39$, $P = 0.02$), but did not detect a significant effect on static standing balance ($d = 0.18$, $z = 1.43$, $P = 0.15$). The mechanism(s) responsible for improving dynamic balance in standing is not

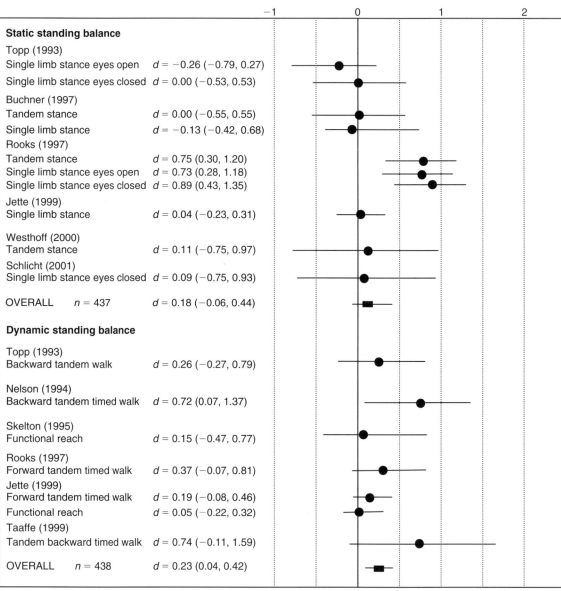

Standing balance

Effect size (95% confidence interval)

Static standing balance

Topp (1993)
Single limb stance eyes open $d = -0.26 (-0.79, 0.27)$
Single limb stance eyes closed $d = 0.00 (-0.53, 0.53)$

Buchner (1997)
Tandem stance $d = 0.00 (-0.55, 0.55)$
Single limb stance $d = -0.13 (-0.42, 0.68)$
Rooks (1997)
Tandem stance $d = 0.75 (0.30, 1.20)$
Single limb stance eyes open $d = 0.73 (0.28, 1.18)$
Single limb stance eyes closed $d = 0.89 (0.43, 1.35)$

Jette (1999)
Single limb stance $d = 0.04 (-0.23, 0.31)$

Westhoff (2000)
Tandem stance $d = 0.11 (-0.75, 0.97)$

Schlicht (2001)
Single limb stance eyes closed $d = 0.09 (-0.75, 0.93)$

OVERALL $n = 437$ $d = 0.18 (-0.06, 0.44)$

Dynamic standing balance

Topp (1993)
Backward tandem walk $d = 0.26 (-0.27, 0.79)$

Nelson (1994)
Backward tandem timed walk $d = 0.72 (0.07, 1.37)$

Skelton (1995)
Functional reach $d = 0.15 (-0.47, 0.77)$

Rooks (1997)
Forward tandem timed walk $d = 0.37 (-0.07, 0.81)$
Jette (1999)
Forward tandem timed walk $d = 0.19 (-0.08, 0.46)$
Functional reach $d = 0.05 (-0.22, 0.32)$
Taaffe (1999)
Tandem backward timed walk $d = 0.74 (-0.11, 1.59)$

OVERALL $n = 438$ $d = 0.23 (0.04, 0.42)$

Favours control   Favours treatment

Figure 7.13 Effect sizes for changes in static and dynamic standing balance after progressive resistance exercise programmes for independent older adults.

known. However, in 7 of the 11 trials, the exercises closely mimicked balance tasks and functional activities rather than more isolated strengthening exercises using machine weights. It is possible, therefore, that in clinical practice the specificity of the strength training programme is important if the aim is to improve balance.

Changes in participation

Participation restrictions are defined in the ICF framework as the inability or restriction of individuals to perform roles and everyday tasks expected of individuals within their society. Only four papers evaluated the effect of strength training on the societal participation of older people (Buchner et al 1997, Damush and Damush 1999, Jette et al 1996, 1999). The findings of these studies were inconsistent. Two studies reported significant improvements in the social activity and role limitation domains of the Short Form (SF-36) health survey following strength training (Buchner et al 1997, Jette et al 1996). By contrast, the other two studies reported no change in the participation domain of the Sickness Impact Profile-68 (Jette et al 1999) or the Health Related Quality of Life measure (Damush and Damush 1999).

Clients and health service providers are often interested in the effect of interventions that reflect meaningful improvements to an older person's ability to function within society. However, little information is currently available about the effects of strength training on the participation dimension of functioning and disability of older people. There remains a need to demonstrate that health-related programmes are effective from the client's perspective. To achieve this, researchers must first incorporate distinct measures of participation restriction when assessing the effects of interventions; and second, demonstrate that these outcome measures improve with training.

Conclusions

There is strong evidence that strength training programmes in older adults living independently in the community lead to large muscle strength gains for lower limbs and arms. A smaller number of studies has also shown that strength training programmes in older adults can result in significant improvements in muscle endurance. Strength training in older adults did not have significant positive or negative effects on other components of body function: aerobic capacity, flexibility and psychological impairment.

Muscle strength increases are attributable, at least in part, to increases in muscle size and lean body mass after strength training. The increase in muscle size is due to hypertrophy of both type I and type II skeletal muscle fibres. Despite positive trends, it remains uncertain whether strength training leads to beneficial effects on bone mineral density in older people.

There is evidence that strength training programmes in older adults living independently in the community can lead to improvements in the performance of everyday activities such as walking and stair-climbing. Strength training in older adults can also enhance dynamic standing balance, which in turn may lead to a decreased risk of falls. Training that strengthens muscles in a way that is similar to their use when performing physical activities is likely to have a greater impact on functional performance than training that increases muscle strength in isolation. The degree of activity limitation experienced by subjects may have an effect on whether changes are detected in activity performance.

The content of programmes leading to improvements in muscle strength and activity are consistent with the ACSM guidelines for strength training in young healthy adults, and are generally more intense than programmes advocated for older people. Programmes typically consist of 2–3 sets of 6–12 repetitions of each exercise, with a training intensity of 70–80% 1 RM performed 2–3 times per week. These programmes report a low risk of injury, demonstrating that programmes of such intensity can safely and effectively be undertaken by community-dwelling older people.

In conclusion, this review has shown that muscle weakness in older people can be reversed with strength training. Furthermore, gains in muscle strength can positively impact on the health of older people by improving functional capacity.

Acknowledgement

The authors acknowledge the valuable advice provided by the Council on the Ageing (COTA) for this review.

References

ACSM 1998a American College of Sports Medicine Position Stand. Exercise and physical activity for older adults. Medicine and Science in Sports and Exercise 30(6):992–1008

ACSM 1998b American College of Sports Medicine Position Stand. The recommended quantity and quality of exercise for developing and maintaining cardiorespiratory and muscular fitness, and flexibility in healthy adults. Medicine and Science in Sports and Exercise 30(6):975–991

ACSM 2002 American College of Sports Medicine Position Stand. Progression models in resistance training for healthy adults. Medicine and Science in Sport and Exercise 34(2):364–380

Adams K J, Swank A M, et al 2001 Progressive strength training in sedentary, older African American women. Medicine and Science in Sports and Exercise 33(9):1567–1576

Ades P A, Ballor D L, et al 1996 Weight training improves walking endurance in healthy elderly persons. Annals of Internal Medicine 124(6):568–572

Anderson T, Kearney J T 1982 Effects of three resistance training programs on muscular strength and absolute and relative endurance. Research Quarterly 53:1–7

Aniansson A, Zetterberg C, et al 1984 Impaired muscle function with aging. A background factor in the incidence of fractures of the proximal end of the femur. Clinical Orthopaedics and Related Research 191:193–201

Balagopal P, Schimke J C, Ades P, Adey D, Nair K S 2001 Age effect on transcript levels and synthesis rate of muscle MHC and response to resistance exercise. American Journal of Physiology, Endocrinology and Metabolism 280:E203–E208

Bassey E, Bendall M, et al 1988 Muscle strength in the triceps surae and objectively measured customary walking activity in men and women over 65 years of age. Clinical Science 74:85–89

Bassey E J, Fiatarone M A, et al 1992 Leg extensor power and functional performance in very old men and women. Clinical Science 82:321–327

Benbassat C A, Maki K C, et al 1997 Circulating levels of insulin-like growth factor (IGF) binding protein-1 and -3 in aging men: relationships to insulin, glucose, IGF, and dehydroepiandrosterone sulfate levels and anthropometric measures. Journal of Clinical Endocrinology and Metabolism 82(5):1484–1491

Bermon S, Ferrari P, et al 1999a Responses of total and free insulin-like growth factor-I and insulin-like growth factor binding protein-3 after resistance exercise and training in elderly subjects. Acta Physiologica Scandinavica 165(1):51–56

Bermon S, Philip P, et al 1999b Effects of a short-term strength training programme on lymphocyte subsets at rest in elderly humans. European Journal of Applied Physiology and Occupational Physiology 79(4):336–340

Bevier W C, Wiswell R A, et al 1989 Relationship of body composition, muscle strength, and aerobic capacity to bone mineral density in older men and women. Journal of Bone and Mineral Research 4(3):421–432

Brandon L J, Boyette L W, et al 2000 Effects of lower extremity strength training an functional mobility in older adults. Journal of Aging and Physical Activity 8(3):214–227

Buchner D M, Cress M E, et al 1997 The effect of strength and endurance training on gait, balance, fall risk, and health services use in community-living older adults. Biological Sciences and Medical Sciences 52(4):218–224

Campbell A J, Borrie M J, et al 1989 Risk factors for falls in a community-based prospective study of people 70 years and older. Journal of Gerontology 44(4):M112–117

Chandler J M, Duncan P W, et al 1998 Is lower extremity strength gain associated with improvement in physical performance and disability in frail, community-dwelling elders? Archives of Physical Medicine and Rehabilitation 79(1):24–30

Charette S L, McEvoy L, et al 1991 Muscle hypertrophy response to resistance training in older women. Journal of Applied Physiology 70(5):1912–1916

Cohen J 1988 Statistical power analysis for behavioral sciences. Academic Press, New York

Cohick W S, Clemmons D R 1993 The insulin-like growth factors. Annual Review of Physiology 55:131–153

Damush T M, Damush J G Jr 1999 The effects of strength training on strength and health-related quality of life in older adult women. Gerontologist 39(6):705–710

Dishman R K, Sallis J, et al 1985 The determinants of physical activity and exercise. Public Health Report 100:158–180.

Dodd K J, Taylor N F, et al 2002 A systematic review on effectiveness of strength training programs for people with cerebral palsy. Archives of Physical Medicine and Rehabilitation 83(8):1157–1164

Egger M, Davey Smith G, et al 1997 Meta-analysis: principles and procedures. British Medical Journal 315:1533–1537

Fiatarone M A, Marks E C, et al 1990 High-intensity strength training in nonagenarians: effects on skeletal muscle. JAMA 263:3029–3034

Fleck S J, Kraemer W J 1997 Designing resistance training programs. Human Kinetics, Champaign, IL

Flynn M G, Fahlman M, et al 1999 Effects of resistance training on selected indexes of immune function in elderly women. Journal of Applied Physiology 86(6):1905–1913

Hagberg J M, Graves J E, et al 1989 Cardiovascular responses of 70- to 79-yr-old men and women to exercise training. Journal of Applied Physiology 66(6):2589–2594

Hagerman F C, Walsh S J, et al 2000 Effects of high-intensity resistance training on untrained older men. I. Strength, cardiovascular, and metabolic responses. Journals of Gerontology Series A Biological Sciences and Medical Sciences 55(7):B336–346

Haykowsky M, Humen D, et al 2000 Effects of 16 weeks of resistance training on left ventricular morphology and systolic function in healthy men >60 years of age. American Journal of Cardiology 85(8):1002–1006

Hedges L V, Olkin I 1985 Statistical methods for meta-analysis. Academic Press, Orlando

Hortobagyi T, Tunnel D, Moody J, De Vita P 2001 Low- or high-intensity strength training partially restores impaired quadriceps force accuracy and steadiness in aged adults. Journal of Gerontology: Biological Sciences 56A(1):B38–B47

Huczel H A, Clarke D H 1992 A comparison of strength and muscle endurance in strength-trained and untrained women. Journal of Applied Physiology 64:467–470

Jette A M, Harris B A, et al 1996 A home-based exercise program for nondisabled older adults. Journal of the American Geriatrics Society 44(6):644–649

Jette A M, Lachman M, et al 1999 Exercise – it's never too late: the Strong-for-Life program. American Journal of Public Health 89(1):66–72

Jubrias S A, Esselman P C, et al 2001 Large energetic adaptations of elderly muscle to resistance and endurance training. Journal of Applied Physiology 90(5):1663–1670

Judge J O, Whipple R H, et al 1994 Effects of resistive and balance exercises on isokinetic strength in older persons. Journal of the American Geriatrics Society 42(9):937–946

Juni P, Witschi A, et al 1999 The hazards of scoring the quality of clinical trials for meta-analysis. JAMA 282(11):1054–1060

Kelley G A 1998a Aerobic exercise and bone density at the hip in post-menopausal women: a meta-analysis. Preventive Medicine 27(6):798–807

Kelley G A 1998b Exercise and regional bone mineral density in postmenopausal women: a meta-analytic review of randomized trials. American Journal of Physical Medicine and Rehabilitation 77(1):76–87

Kelley G A, Kelley K S, et al 2001 Resistance training and bone mineral density in women: a meta-analysis of controlled trials. American Journal of Physical Medicine and Rehabilitation 80(1):65–77

Kraemer W J, et al 2002 American College of Sports Medicine position stand. Progression models in resistance training for healthy adults. Medicine and Science in Sports and Exercise 34(2):364–380

Langlois J A, Rosen C J, et al 1998 Association between insulin-like growth factor I and bone mineral density in older women and men: the Framingham Heart Study. Journal of Clinical Endocrinology and Metabolism 83(12):4257–4262

Lau J, Ioannides J P A, et al 1998 Quantitative synthesis in systematic reviews. In: Mulrow C, Cook D (eds) Systematic reviews: synthesis of best evidence for health care decisions. American College of Physicians, Philadelphia, p 91–101

Lindle R S, Metter E J, et al 1997 Age and gender comparisons of muscle strength in 654 women and men aged 20–93 yr. Journal of Applied Physiology 83(5):1581–1587

Lynch N A, Metter E J, et al 1999 Muscle quality. I. Age-associated differences between arm and leg muscle groups. Journal of Applied Physiology 86(1):188–194

Macaluso A, De Vito G, et al 2000 Electromyogram changes during sustained contraction after resistance training in women in their 3rd and 8th decades. European Journal of Applied Physiology 82(5–6):418–424

McCartney N, Hicks A L, et al 1995 Long-term resistance training in the elderly: effects on dynamic strength, exercise capacity, muscle, and bone. Biological Sciences and Medical Sciences 50(2):97–104

McCartney N, Hicks A L, et al 1996 A longitudinal trial of weight training in the elderly: continued improvements in year 2. Biological Sciences and Medical Sciences 51(6):425–433

Mikesky A E, Topp R, et al 1994 Efficacy of a home-based training program for older adults using elastic tubing. European Journal of Applied Physiology and Occupational Physiology 69(4):316–320

Muller E A 1957 The regulation of muscular strength. Journal of the Association for Physical and Mental Rehabilitation 11:41–47

Nelson M E, Fiatarone M A, et al 1994 Effects of high-intensity strength training on multiple risk factors for osteoporotic fractures: a randomized controlled trial. JAMA 272(24):1909–1914

Nelson M E, Fiatarone M A, et al 1996 Analysis of body-composition techniques and models for detecting change in soft tissue with strength training. American Journal of Clinical Nutrition 63(5):678–686

Nichols J F, Omizo D K, et al 1993 Efficacy of heavy-resistance training for active women over sixty: muscular strength, body composition, and program adherence. Journal of the American Geriatrics Society 41(3):205–210

Nicholson J M, Emes C G 2000 From the field. Effect of strength training on the vertical force of a chair rise in the elderly. Clinical Kinesiology. Journal of the American Kinesiotherapy Association 54(2):36–42

Panton L B, Graves J E, Pollock M L, Hagberg J M, Chen W 1990 Effect of aerobic and resistance training on fractionated reaction time and speed of movement. Journal of Gerontology: Medical Sciences 45(1):M26–M31

Parkhouse W S, Coupland D C, et al 2000 IGF-1 bioavailability is increased by resistance training in older women with low bone mineral density. Mechanisms of Ageing and Development 113(2):75–83

PEDro 1999 The Physiotherapy evidence database (PEDro) frequently asked questions: how are trials rated? Available at: http://www.cchs.usyd.edu.au/pedro. Accessed February 2002

Perrig Chiello P, Perrig W J, et al 1998 The effects of resistance training on well-being and memory in elderly volunteers. Age and Ageing 27(4):469–475

Pollock M L 1988 Prescribing exercise for fitness and adherence. In: Dishman R K (ed) Exercise adherence: its impact on public health. Human Kinetics, Champaign, IL

Pollock M L, Carroll J F, et al 1991 Injuries and adherence to walk/jog and resistance training programs in the elderly. Medicine and Science in Sports and Exercise 23(10):1194–1200

Pruitt L A, Taaffe D R, et al 1995 Effects of a one-year high-intensity versus low-intensity resistance training program on bone mineral density in older women. Journal of Bone and Mineral Research 10(11):1788–1795

Pyka G, Lindenberger E, et al 1994 Muscle strength and fiber adaptations to a year-long resistance training program in elderly men and women. Journal of Gerontology 49(1):22–27

Ravn P, Overgaard K, et al 1995 Insulin-like growth factors I and II in healthy women with and without established osteoporosis. European Journal of Endocrinology 132(3):313–319

Rhodes E C, Martin A D, et al 2000 Effects of one year of resistance training on the relation between muscular strength and bone density in elderly women. British Journal of Sports Medicine 34(1):18–22

Rooks D S, Kiel D P, et al 1997 Self-paced resistance training and walking exercise in community-dwelling older adults: effects on neuromotor performance. Biological Sciences and Medical Sciences 52(3):M161–168

Sambrook P N, Seeman E, et al 2002 Preventing osteoporosis: outcomes of the Australian fracture prevention summit. Medical Journal of Australia 176(Suppl):S1–S16

Schlicht J, Camaione D N, et al 2001 Effect of intense strength training on standing balance, walking speed, and sit-to-stand performance in older adults. Journals of Gerontology Series A Biological Sciences and Medical Sciences 56(5):M281–286

Schwarzer R 1989 Meta-analysis programs. Version 5.1. Free University of Berlin

Sforzo G A, McManis B G, et al 1995 Resilience to exercise detraining in healthy older adults. Journal of American Geriatrics Society 43(3):209–215

Sipila S, Suominen H 1995 Effects of strength and endurance training on thigh and leg muscle mass and composition in elderly women. Journal of Applied Physiology 78(1):334–340

Sipila S, Multanen J, et al 1996 Effects of strength and endurance training on isometric muscle strength and walking speed in elderly women. Acta Physiologica Scandinavica 156(4):457–464

Skelton D A, McLaughlin A W 1996 Training functional ability in old age. Physiotherapy 82(3):159–167

Skelton D A, Young A, et al 1995 Effects of resistance training on strength, power, and selected functional abilities of women aged 75 and older. Journal of the American Geriatrics Society 43(10):1081–1087

Taaffe D R, Pruitt L, et al 1995 Effect of sustained resistance training on basal metabolic rate in older women. Journal of the American Geriatrics Society 43(5):465–471

Taaffe D R, Pruitt L, et al 1996 Comparative effects of high- and low-intensity resistance training on thigh muscle strength, fiber area, and tissue composition in elderly women. Clinical Physiology 16(4):381–392

Taaffe D R, Duret C, et al 1999 Once-weekly resistance exercise improves muscle strength and neuromuscular performance in older adults. Journal of the American Geriatrics Society 47(10):1208–1214

Topp R, Mikesky A, et al 1993 The effect of a 12-week dynamic resistance strength training program on gait velocity and balance of older adults. Gerontologist 33(4):501–506

Topp R, Mikesky A, et al 1996 Effect of resistance training on strength, postural control, and gait velocity among older adults. Clinical Nursing Research 5(4):407–427

Tsutsumi T, Don B M, et al 1997 Physical fitness and psychological benefits of strength training in community dwelling older adults. Applied Human Science 16(6):257–266

Tsutsumi T, Don B M, et al 1998 Comparison of high and moderate intensity of strength training on mood and anxiety in older adults. Perceptual and Motor Skills 87(3 Pt 1):1003–1011

Verhagen A, de Vet H, et al 1998 The Delphi list: a criteria list for quality assessment of randomized clinical trials for conducting systematic reviews developed by Delphi consensus. Journal of Clinical Epidemiology 51:1235–1241

Westhoff M H, Stemmerik L, et al 2000 Effects of a low-intensity strength-training program on knee-extensor strength and functional ability of frail older people. Journal of Aging and Physical Activity 8(4):325–342

Whipple R H, Wolfson L I, et al 1987 The relationship of knee and ankle weakness to falls in nursing home residents: an isokinetic study. Journal of American Geriatrics Society 35(1):13–20

WHO 2001 ICF: International Classification of Functioning, Disability and Health (Short Version). World Health Organization, Geneva

Willoughby D S, Pelsue S C 1998 Muscle strength and qualitative myosin heavy chain isoform mRNA expression in the elderly after moderate- and high-intensity weight training. Journal of Aging and Physical Activity 6(4):327–339

Wolff I, van Croonenborg J J, et al 1999 The effect of exercise training programs on bone mass: a meta-analysis of published controlled trials in pre- and postmenopausal women. Osteoporosis International 9(1):1–12

8

Declining muscle function in older people – repairing the deficits with exercise

Dennis R Taaffe

CHAPTER
CONTENTS

Alterations in muscle mass, muscle function and physical performance 159

Factors responsible for the age-related changes in muscle mass
and function 163

Role of exercise in restoring muscle function 166

Exercise prescription 175

Conclusion 179

References 179

Normal ageing is characterized by a decline in muscle mass, termed sarcopenia, which largely contributes to the loss in muscle strength. These alterations in skeletal muscle have a dramatic effect on functional performance, quality of life and maintenance of independent living for older people, as well as contributing to frailty and fracture risk. The decline in muscle mass is approximately 40% from age 20 to 70 years (Rogers and Evans 1993), with similar declines reported for muscle strength (Brooks and Faulkner 1994, Ringsberg 1993). Data from the Framingham study in the USA revealed that the number of women unable to lift 4.5 kg increased from 40% in 55–64-year-olds to 65% in those aged 75–84 (Jette and Branch 1981). Unfortunately, the decrease in muscle mass and strength accelerates with advancing age, severely compromising the functioning of the oldest old (Evans 1995).

Alterations in muscle mass and strength can be viewed as stages in the disablement process (Figure 8.1) that lead to musculoskeletal disability (Schroll 1994, Verbrugge and Jette 1994). In this conceptual model for the pathway to disability, the pathology is a loss in muscle mass (muscle fibre atrophy and decreased fibre number) that results in impaired muscle strength. The reduction in strength results in restrictions in basic

Figure 8.1 The disablement process according to Verbrugge and Jette (1994), the Institute of Medicine (1991) and Nagi (1965, 1979), showing the pathway leading to disability

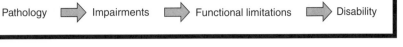

Pathology ⟹ Impairments ⟹ Functional limitations ⟹ Disability

physical activities, such as being able to rise from a chair, step certain heights, walk at the required speed to successfully negotiate a traffic intersection or cross a street, shop for groceries or even lift groceries onto shelves. These limitations result in disability, and assistance may then be required or activities will need to be altered.

Although the age-related loss in muscle mass and strength is due to normal biological ageing as well as lifestyle patterns, effective counter-measures have been developed. Exercise, specifically resistance training, has been repeatedly shown over the past decade to repair these age-related deficits in the muscular system, which may improve the ability to undertake daily activities and maintain independence. Apart from the personal, social and community benefits, maintaining independence and physical functioning has significant implications for containing healthcare expenditure, especially those associated with disability and extended nursing home care. This chapter will address: (1) the alterations in muscle mass, muscle function and physical performance that occur with age, (2) the factors responsible for the age-related decline in muscle mass and muscle function, (3) the role of exercise in restoring these deficits and the associated benefits to physical performance, and (4) exercise prescription for improving muscle function.

Alterations in muscle mass, muscle function and physical performance

Muscle mass

The reduction in skeletal muscle size with age is due to a decrease in the total number of muscle fibres and a reduction in the size of individual fibres, especially for type II or fast-twitch fibres. The reduction in fibre number and size was demonstrated in an elaborate study undertaken by Lexell and colleagues (1988) on whole human autopsied thigh muscles. Fibre loss commenced at 25 years of age with an average reduction in fibre size of 26% between age 20 and 80. The net effect is a significant decrease in muscle area, as shown in Figure 8.2. For type II fibres, it has been reported that by age 85 individual fibre cross-sectional area (CSA) may be less than 50% of that for type I fibres (Tomonaga 1977). However, there is some controversy regarding preferential loss of the major fibre types with age, with some researchers reporting a preferential loss of type II fibres (Larsson et al 1978) while others report no change (Grimby et al 1984). Although Lexell and colleagues (1988) did not find a preferential loss of type II fibres in their investigation, due to the preferential atrophy of this fibre type, the proportion of the muscle area occupied by type II fibres is nevertheless reduced. Apart from a reduction in fibre

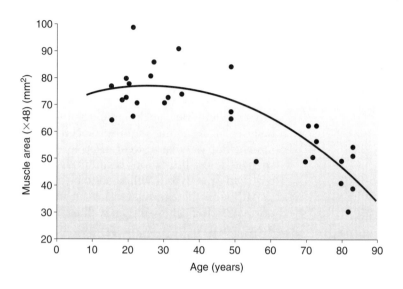

Figure 8.2 Age-related change in area of the vastus lateralis muscle ($P < 0.001$). Muscle area peaks in the third decade and declines thereafter, the rate accelerating with advancing age with an average reduction of 40% between age 20 and 80 years. (Reprinted from Lexell J, Taylor C C, Sjöström M (1988) What is the cause of the aging atrophy? Total number, size, and proportion of fiber types studied in whole vastus lateralis muscle from 15- to 83-year-old men. Journal of the Neurological Sciences, 84, 275–294, with permission from Elsevier Science.)

number and area, the amount of muscle area composed of muscle fibres is also reduced with age (Lexell et al 1988).

Recently, in studying individuals aged 72–98 years, Fiatarone Singh and co-workers (1999) noted severe selective atrophy of type II fibres and ultrastructural damage with evidence of Z band and myofibrillar disruption that may also negatively impact muscle function. It has been reported by Larsson et al (1997) that the specific force of muscle fibres (force per CSA) is lower in older than in younger adults, and this contributes to the decline in force at the whole muscle level. Indeed, Jubrias and co-workers (1997) reported that although quadriceps CSA was reduced by 20% between age 65 and 80 years, force production decreased by 40%. Ultrastructural alterations as well as changes in calcium release by the sarcoplasmic reticulum (Delbono et al 1995), which permits the contractile filaments to interact, may be responsible for the decline in specific force.

Muscle function

Information on age-related changes in muscle strength is derived from cross-sectional and longitudinal data. Cross-sectional data on 847 subjects from the Baltimore Longitudinal Study of Aging, a cohort of healthy volunteers, indicated that summed grip strength increases into the thirties and then declines, such that by the ninth decade strength is 37% lower (Kallman et al 1990). However, with advancing years the rate of decline accelerates. These results concur with those found for muscles of the arms, legs and back in adults aged 30–80 years (Grimby and Saltin 1983). This pattern of an accelerating decline with age was also evident when longitudinal data from a subset of the Baltimore cohort with an average follow-up of 9 years were examined. Interestingly, not all subjects lost grip strength as they aged. During the follow-up period, 48% of subjects less than 40 years old, 29% aged 40–59 years, and 15% of subjects older than 60 years showed no decline. In the same study, muscle mass was estimated by urinary creatinine excretion and by forearm circumference. There was a reasonably strong correlation between grip strength and muscle mass ($r = 0.60$). However, in multiple regression analysis, grip strength was more strongly correlated with age than muscle mass. Therefore, other factors apart from muscle mass alone account for the decline in muscle force.

The rate of decline in muscle strength with age generally varies between 1 and 2% per year, depending on the age group studied. Rantanen and colleagues (1998) assessed grip strength of 3741 men participating in the Honolulu Heart Program 27 years after initial measurements were performed (age range at follow-up was 71–96 years). The annualized strength change was 1.0% per year with a steeper decline of >1.5% in those with older age at baseline. Similarly, Bassey and Harries (1993) examined grip strength in a cohort of men and women over the age of 65 years. The cross-sectional decline in strength was 2% per year; however, follow-up evaluation 4 years later showed a decline in men and women of 12% and 19%, respectively. In a similar fashion, Aniansson and colleagues (1986) examined 23 men aged 73–83 years for muscle strength of the knee extensors 7 years after an initial examination. Isometric and isokinetic strength at several movement velocities decreased by 10–22% while body cell mass, calculated from total body potassium, declined by 6%, again indicating that changes apart from muscle mass contribute to decrements in strength.

Apart from muscle strength, muscle power (the product of force and velocity of contraction) is also severely comprised with age. An early study examining muscle power in older adults was performed by Bosco and Komi (1980) with power assessed using a vertical jump test. Whereas average force was about 50% lower in men and women in their 70s compared to those in their 20s, muscle power was 70–75% less. Similarly, Skelton and associates (1994) assessed strength and power in healthy independent living men and women aged 65–89 years. The decline in strength for several muscle groups was 1–2% per year while for knee extensor power the rate was ~3.5% per year. As previously mentioned, the type II or fast-twitch muscle fibres exhibit the greatest degree of degeneration with age (Izquierdo et al 1999). A result of this is a dramatic loss in the ability to generate muscle force rapidly (De Vito et al 1998), so that muscle power decreases at a faster rate than muscle strength. The decline in muscle power may be particularly important in the performance of daily tasks, as many activities require rapid force production.

Muscle endurance is a less researched and reported area than muscle strength, primarily due to the ease of assessing maximal voluntary strength and its relation to physical performance tasks. When normalized to maximal voluntary force, there appears to be little change in fatiguability of ageing muscle. Larsson and Karlsson (1978) examined 50 men aged 22–65 years for isometric and dynamic endurance in relation to muscle strength and found that while maximum isometric and dynamic strength decreased in the older groups, there was no significant change in muscle endurance. Age-related changes in muscle remodelling (see below) may partially account for the maintenance of endurance with advancing age. However, when absolute loads are involved then endurance is reduced in older persons due to their decreased maximal force; consequently, they have to work at a higher percentage of their maximum strength compared with their younger counterparts.

Physical performance

Numerous studies have reported significant relationships between muscle strength and walking speed (Bassey et al 1988, Fiatarone et al 1990), balance and fall risk (Whipple et al 1987, Wolfson et al 1995), self-reported mobility difficulties (Rantanen et al 1994) and disability (Giampoli et al 1999, Van Heuvelen et al 2000). In a cohort of 705 community-dwelling women participating in the Hawaii Osteoporosis Study, hand grip and knee extensor muscle strength were positively associated with several performance measures that included usual and rapid walking speed, chair stands and the Get Up and Go test (Davis et al 1998). Notably, those with greater grip performance on strength had less difficulty with most activities of daily living (ADL). A one standard deviation difference in grip strength was associated with a 20–30% decrease in the odds ratio for ADL difficulty. These results are comparable to several other studies that report an association between strength and ADL (Avlund et al 1994, Ensrud et al 1994, Hyatt et al 1990, Posner et al 1995).

However, muscle power may be more important for functional performance than muscle strength. Bassey and colleagues (1992) reported that leg extensor muscle power accounted for 86% of the variance in walking speed in frail elderly people and those requiring assistance with ambulation had less than half the muscle power than those people who could walk freely. Recently, Foldavi et al (2000) found that leg press power, rather than muscle strength, was an independent predictor of functional status in community-dwelling elderly women with pre-existing impairments. Similarly, in an elderly cohort of mobility-limited people, leg muscle power, although strongly correlated to muscle strength, exerted a greater influence on physical performance than strength (Bean et al 2002).

An important consequence of the decline in muscle function is a diminished reserve capacity for the performance of many daily tasks, such as walking at a sufficient speed, rising from a chair or seated position, climbing stairs, or lifting groceries. As can be seen in Figure 8.3, a young adult woman may only require approximately half of her quadriceps strength to rise from an armless chair, whereas an 80-year-old woman may be close to her muscle strength threshold when performing this activity (Young 1986). An acute illness or injury resulting in temporary bedrest or immobilization can have a negative effect on muscle strength and may result in the individual being no longer able to perform the activity. In turn, the individual might have to employ alternative strategies to rise from a chair, compromising their independence and quality of life. Moreover, a downward spiral in physical functioning could result, where the reduced movement from poor muscle performance negatively impacts upon the remaining muscle strength, leading to a diminished ability to perform other tasks.

Figure 8.3 The effect of age on the ability to rise from a chair. A woman aged 80 years may be close to her muscle strength threshold for performing this activity. MVC stands for maximal voluntary contraction of the quadriceps. (Reprinted with permission of Blackwell Publishing, from Young A (1986) Exercise physiology in geriatric practice. Acta Medica Scandinavica Supplementum, 711, 227–232.)

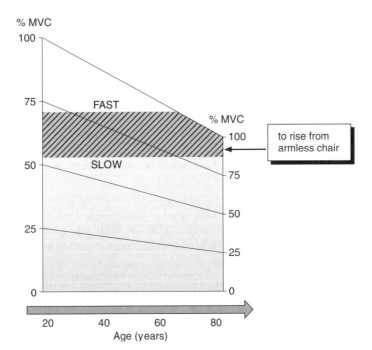

Apart from gross motor skills, fine motor skills are also compromised with advancing age. A reduced ability to control or regulate submaximal contractile forces, referred to as steadiness, occurs with advancing age (Patten 2000). This manifests in slowness of movement, loss of accuracy, and increased force variability. Denervation–reinnervation cycles that lead to larger but fewer motor units within the muscle (see below), an increase in fibrous tissue and increased tissue stiffness may contribute to the reduced ability to modulate force with advanced age. Decreases in the motor unit discharge rate at moderate-to-high force levels may also be a contributing factor (Roos et al 1997).

Factors responsible for the age-related changes in muscle mass and function

The underlying cause of diminished muscle mass and muscle function with age is multifactorial, and it is unlikely that all contributing mechanisms have yet been identified. Moreover, the contribution of various factors may vary among individuals. Several contributing factors are described below, the two principal ones being motor unit loss and remodelling, and reduced physical activity.

Neuropathic change: motor unit loss and remodelling

With age there is a reduction in the total number of motor units, although the size of the remaining units are increased through collateral reinnervation. Doherty et al (1993b) reported a 47% decrease in estimated numbers of motor units between the ages of 22–38 years and 60–81 years, with a 23% increase in unit size. These findings are comparable to the estimated neuronal loss found in the lumbospinal segments by Tomlinson and Irving (1977) in individuals aged between 13 and 95 years. These alterations in size of motor units are evidenced histochemically by fibre type grouping, where muscle cross-sections display a greater degree of homogeneity with age compared with the mosaic appearance observed in young adult muscle (Lexell et al 1988). Apart from reductions in the total number of motor units, there are age-related reductions in motor axon conduction velocity, such that there is a general slowing of all nerve fibres (Doherty et al 1994). These findings are consistent for proximal and distal limb muscles across numerous studies employing anatomical and electrophysiological methods (Doherty et al 1993a). Motor unit remodelling and reduction in conduction velocity negatively impacts on the ability to generate force and to generate force rapidly, which are critical for maintaining balance and preventing falls.

Reduced physical activity

It has long been recognized that the characteristics associated with ageing are similar to those of enforced physical inactivity. Unfortunately, with advancing age there is a decline in recreational and occupational physical activity (Bortz 1982). Due to reduced functional demands with inactivity and immobilization, there is a selective reduction in the size and relative area of type II muscle fibres (Lexell 1993) and an accompanying decrease in muscle strength and physical performance. As such, these biological alterations are subject to correction with physical exercise (Bortz 1982).

A number of studies indicate that individuals who have higher levels of physical activity as they age preserve their muscle performance. Sipilä and colleagues (1991) compared male strength-trained, speed-trained, and endurance-trained athletes aged 70–81 years with an age-matched control group for isometric strength of the knee flexors and extensors, elbow flexors and extensors, trunk extension and flexion, and hand grip, as well as vertical jump for muscle power. Most of the athletes had trained throughout their lives and continued to compete in sports events. Absolute isometric strength and vertical jump performance were greater in athletes than controls, with the values for strength-trained athletes generally higher than those for the endurance-trained individuals. When strength was adjusted for lean body mass, differences between athletes and controls still existed, albeit at a reduced level. Moreover, in a subgroup of these men, ultrasound imaging of the quadriceps revealed that people with a history of long-term training had maintained their muscle architecture whereas the untrained men had an increased proportion of connective tissue and fat within the muscle (Sipilä and Suominen 1991). These findings were reproduced when female athletes and controls aged 66–85 years were compared (Sipilä and Suominen 1993). Similarly, Klitgaard et al (1990) observed a decrease in maximal isometric force, speed of movement and muscle CSA of the knee extensors and elbow flexors in sedentary older men compared with younger men. When they examined older runners, swimmers and strength-trained subjects with 12–17 years training prior to measurement, muscle strength and size were well maintained in the strength-trained men and were identical to those of the young men.

Dietary insufficiency	A factor seldom considered as contributing to loss of muscle mass is protein and energy undernutrition. Although more prevalent in hospitalized and institutionalized elders, community-dwelling older adults may also succumb to the negative consequences of an inadequate intake of protein and energy (Vellas et al 2001). A number of factors may contribute to the loss in appetite and decreased food intake including a reduction in taste and olfactory sensitivity, reliance on dentures and difficulty chewing, acute and chronic diseases, psychiatric disorders, lack of finances, social isolation, reduced mobility and functional disabilities (Fischer and Johnson 1990). Low protein diets have been shown to lead to a loss in muscle mass and function in older people (Castaneda et al 1995). Moreover, the requirement of protein may be greater than that recommended for nitrogen equilibrium of 0.8 g/kg body weight/day. In a 14-week controlled diet study, Campbell and colleagues (2001) reported a loss in mid-thigh muscle area (determined by computed tomography scanning) in older men and women on eucaloric diets (weight-maintaining) that contained 0.8 g/kg body weight/day. Consequently, protein intakes of at least 1 g/kg body weight/day may be more appropriate to prevent gradual losses in muscle with age (Campbell et al 2001, Evans 1995, Kurpad and Vaz 2000).
Hormonal decline	Ageing is associated with a decline in the growth hormone (GH)-insulin-like growth factor-1 (IGF-1) axis and the sex hormones, testosterone and oestrogen. The somatic changes that occur with ageing are associated temporally with a reduction in GH, the effects of which are mediated by IGF-1 (Rudman et al 1981). This decline in hormone secretion, termed the somatopause, has led researchers to speculate that GH replacement may restore muscle mass and muscle strength. Although alterations in body composition with GH deficiency are similar to those that occur with ageing, and these changes in GH-deficient adults are reversed with GH replacement therapy (Salomon et al 1989), studies to date in healthy elders lend little support for replacement GH to improve muscle mass and function (Marcus 1996). In randomized placebo-controlled trials in healthy older (Taaffe et al 1994) and younger men (Yarasheski et al 1992), strength was not shown to be augmented when recombinant human GH was combined with resistance training. Although there was a slight rise in lean body mass and decrease in adiposity, GH was associated with a non-trivial risk for adverse effects, including polyarthralgias and oedema.

With normal ageing, plasma total and free testosterone levels slowly decline in men, which may contribute to age-related changes in muscle, fat and bone mass, and muscle strength (Tenover 1999). Evidence suggests that testosterone replacement in older men may improve body composition and strength. However, as with GH replacement therapy, there are a number of potential adverse consequences including unknown long-term effects on the prostate (Tenover 1999). In women, there is evidence that oestrogen withdrawal at the time of menopause leads to reduced muscle mass (Aloia et al 1991) and muscle function. A cross-sectional investigation by Phillips and colleagues (1993) generated considerable interest in this area when they reported that the decline in specific force of the adductor pollicis muscle at the time of menopause was halted in those taking hormone replacement therapy (HRT). Subsequently, in a prospective 39-week HRT trial in early postmenopausal women, Greeves et al (1999) found that hormone replacement preserved quadriceps and hand-grip strength. However, cross-sectional data from a national (England) survey reported by Bassey and co-workers (1996) and from the Study of Osteoporotic Fractures in the United States (Seeley et al 1995) lend no support for the ergogenic effect of HRT on muscle performance. Therefore, the role of long-term hormone replacement in the elderly remains unclear.

Low-level systemic inflammation

A chronic state of low-level systemic inflammation in older persons may also underlie sarcopenia and loss in muscle strength. Ageing is associated with an elevation in pro-inflammatory cytokines such as interleukin-6 (IL-6), which play a central role in the production of C-reactive protein (CRP) and other acute-phase proteins involved in the inflammatory response (Gabay and Kushner 1999). Inflammatory markers such as IL-6 and CRP are associated with a myriad of chronic diseases that afflict the elderly such as cardiovascular disease, osteoporosis, arthritis, type 2 diabetes, and periodontal disease (Taaffe et al 2000). Several lines of evidence indicate that multiple cytokines disrupt muscle homeostasis leading to muscle wasting (Mitch and Goldberg 1997). In community-dwelling elderly people, Cohen and colleagues (1997) demonstrated a gradient of increasing IL-6 levels with poorer functional ability. In addition, catabolic cytokines may minimize the anabolic response to diet and exercise (Roubenoff and Castaneda 2001). Apart from the potential use of anti-cytokine agents, minimizing increases in body fat with age, especially intra-abdominal fat (Kuller 1999), and engaging in regular physical activity (Taaffe et al 2000) may stem the increase in inflammatory cytokines.

Role of exercise in restoring muscle function

It is critical that treatment strategies for declining muscle mass and function be developed and incorporated into programmes for older persons to maximize their functional lifespan, postpone requirement for assisted care and maintain/enhance their quality of life. To this end, resistance training or strength/weight training has been repeatedly shown over the past decade to be an effective countermeasure to these alterations in muscle function, even in the very old. Importantly, this form of training is well tolerated in the older adult and dramatic improvements rapidly accrue. The ability of resistance training to preserve existing muscle function as well as restore lost function illustrates the high degree of residual plasticity that remains in the ageing neuromuscular system. Although this mode of training typically involves the use of free weights or machine weights, body weight can also be used, as can elastic tubing or other devices. In contrast, aerobic exercise, such as walking and jogging, although providing benefit for the cardiovascular system, enhancing energy expenditure and possibly preventing mobility disability, has little effect on restoring muscle strength or mass. More importantly, unless an individual has the muscle strength to rise from a chair, they are not able to walk or jog.

Muscle strength and hypertrophy	Over two decades ago, Moritani and deVries (1980) published the findings of their 8-week progressive resistance-training programme of the elbow flexors in young and older men. The results showed a similar improvement in muscle strength, although the mechanisms underlying the strength change differed. In young men, strength improvement was attributed to neural factors during the initial stage with hypertrophy becoming dominant during the last 4 weeks. In contrast, there was no evidence of hypertrophy in older men as determined by anthropometric techniques. The technique used to assess hypertrophy may not have been sensitive enough to detect subtle changes in muscle size in older men. A subsequent study by Aniansson and Gustafsson (1981) also reported improvements in muscle strength with training with little change in hypertrophy as determined by histochemical techniques.

A landmark study published in 1988 by Frontera and colleagues (1988) clearly demonstrated that older adults have the potential for gross muscle hypertrophy in addition to obtaining dramatic gains in muscle strength with an appropriate regimen of resistance training. Twelve men aged 60–72 years underwent 12 weeks of training for the knee extensors and flexors three times per week at 80% of their one repetition maximum (1 RM, the maximal amount of weight lifted one time with acceptable form). At the conclusion of the training period, knee extensor strength increased by 107% and knee flexor strength by 227% (Figure 8.4). These substantial improvements in strength were accompanied by an 11.4% increase in thigh muscle CSA as determined by computed tomography (CT) scanning (Figure 8.5). In addition to CT scanning, muscle biopsies of the vastus lateralis muscle were taken and subjected to histochemical analysis. An increase in CSA of both type I (33.5%) and type II (27.6%) fibres was evident, with the increase progressive as training continued.

The study by Frontera and colleagues (1988) generated considerable interest in the beneficial effects of resistance training for older adults, and many studies have since been undertaken. A sample of these studies is shown in Table 8.1. In these studies, muscle function is consistently assessed by voluntary maximal muscle strength. As can be seen, substantial improvements in 1 RM strength (with measurements generally performed on the apparatus used for training) were obtained in all

Figure 8.4 Muscle strength change for the knee extensors (triangles) and knee flexors (squares) during 12 weeks of high-intensity resistance training in older men. (Reprinted with permission of the American Physiological Society, from Frontera W R, Meredith C N, O'Reilly K P, Knuttgen H G, Evans W J (1988) Strength conditioning in older men: skeletal muscle hypertrophy and improved function. Journal of Applied Physiology, 64, 1038–1044.)

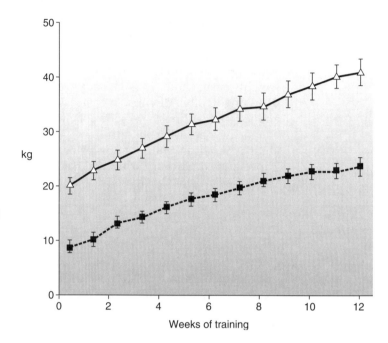

Figure 8.5 Right and left mid-thigh muscle cross-sectional area as determined by computed tomography scanning in response to a 12-week programme of high-intensity resistance training in older men. (Reprinted with permission of the American Physiological Society, from Frontera W R, Meredith C N, O'Reilly K P, Knuttgen H G, Evans W J (1988) Strength conditioning in older men: skeletal muscle hypertrophy and improved function. Journal of Applied Physiology, 64, 1038–1044.)

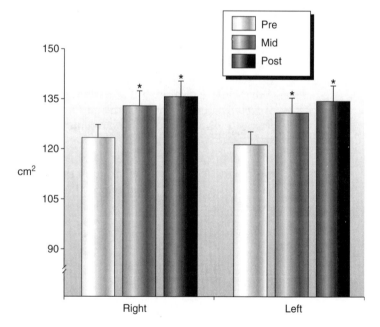

studies, regardless of exercise duration, which ranged from 8 weeks to 2 years. Moreover, strength changes were accompanied by muscle hypertrophy as evidenced by increases in fibre CSA determined by muscle biopsy specimens or by increases in whole muscle CSA obtained by CT and magnetic resonance imaging (MRI).

Table 8.1 Muscle strength and hypertrophy responses to resistance training in frail and healthy older people

Study	Subject age (years)	Gender	Duration (weeks)	Muscles	Strength change (% 1 RM)	Fibre CSA (% change)	Muscle CSA* (% change)
Fiatarone et al (1990)	86–96	M, F	8	Knee extensors	174		8.4–10.9
Charette et al (1991)	64–86	F	12	Lower body	28–115	Type I, 7.3 (NS) Type II, 20.1	
Nichols et al (1993)	>60	F	24	Whole body	5–65		
Pyka et al (1994)	61–78	M, F	52	Whole body	30–97	Type I, 58.5 Type II, 66.6	
Fiatarone et al (1994)	72–98	M, F	10	Lower body	113		2.7
Nelson et al (1994)	50–70	F	52	Whole body	35–76		
Hunter et al (1995)	60–77	F	16	Whole body	52		
Lexell et al (1995)	70–77	M, F	11+	Elbow flexors Knee extensors	49 163	Type I, 13 (EF) Type II, 17 (EF)	
McCartney et al (1996)	60–80	M, F	84	Whole body	32–90		8.7
Sipilä et al (1996; 1997)	76–78	F	18	Knee extensors Knee flexors	60 40	Type I, 34 Type II, 20 (NS)	4.5
Taaffe et al (1999)	65–79	M, F	24	Whole body	40		
Hagerman et al (2000) and Hikida et al (2000)	60–75	M	16	Lower body	50–84	Type I, 46 Type IIA, 34 Type IIB, 52	
Jubrias et al (2001)	69	M, F	24	Knee extensors	64		9.8[†]

M = male; F = female; NS = not significant; EF = elbow flexors; 1 RM = 1 repetition maximum; *muscle cross-sectional area (CSA) by computed tomography (CT) and magnetic resonance imaging (MRI); [†] MRI.

Several of the studies listed in Table 8.1 are worthy of comment. Following the findings by Frontera et al (1988) in men, Charette and colleagues (1991) reported the results of a similar study in healthy community-dwelling women aged 64–86 years. For several muscle groups of the lower body including the knee extensors/flexors and hip extensors/flexors, 12 weeks of moderate- to high-intensity training resulted in improvements in muscle strength ranging from 28 to 115%, depending on muscle group, with a 20% increase in type II fibre CSA. These relatively short-term exercise trials were followed by training studies of 1 year and longer in duration. Pyka et al (1994) found continual increases in strength over the course of their year-long study in men and women, although the gains were greatest in the first 3 months. Type I fibre CSA increased by 15 weeks with further gains evident by 30 weeks, along with hypertrophy of type II fibres. This study showed that strength gains were progressive, as was fibre hypertrophy with prolonged training. In addition, this study demonstrated that older adults could safely undertake high-intensity training with reasonable compliance for an extended period of time. The longest intervention to date was subsequently reported by McCartney and co-workers (1996) from McMaster University in Canada. They undertook a 2-year progressive resistance training study in men and women aged 60–80 years and found continual increases in strength with an increase in muscle hypertrophy in each year.

Although these studies in community-dwelling older adults are of considerable importance in improving physical performance and preventing future disability, the group that may benefit the most from appropriately targeted interventions are those who are frail and living in some form of dependent care setting. Fiatarone and colleagues (1990, 1994) addressed this issue in their seminal work in very elderly nursing home residents. In the first study of 8 weeks duration (Fiatarone et al 1990), 10 frail volunteers aged 86–96 years undertook knee extensor training thrice weekly for three sets of eight repetitions at 80% of their 1 RM. Muscle strength improved by 174% and mid-thigh muscle area increased by 9%. These changes in muscle strength and size were accompanied by improved functional mobility. At the end of the study, tandem gait speed over 6 metres improved by 48%, while two subjects no longer used canes to walk and one subject who initially could not rise out of a chair without using her arms could now do so. In a subsequent study (Fiatarone et al 1994) in a larger cohort of frail nursing home residents, knee and hip extensors were trained three times per week for 12 weeks, resulting in an increase in muscle strength of 113% and thigh muscle CSA by 2.7%. Again, these changes were accompanied by clinically relevant improvements in functional performance as well as an increased level of spontaneous physical activity. Habitual gait velocity increased by 11.8% and stair-climbing ability, as determined by stair-climbing power, by 28.4%. In addition, several participants who required a walker at the commencement of the study only required a cane after the study.

Nutritional supplementation may also augment the skeletal muscle response to exercise. Fiatarone Singh et al (1999), in a report on a subgroup of frail elderly from an earlier study (Fiatarone et al 1994), found that muscle hypertrophy and strength were augmented when a nutritional supplement (360 kcal) and resistance training were combined compared with resistance training or supplement alone. Following the 10 weeks of thrice weekly high-intensity resistance training, the exercise and supplement group improved their maximal strength by ~250% compared with 100% in the exercise alone group, and no change in the supplement only or a control group. The increase in strength in the combined group was associated with a significant increase in type II fibre CSA of 10% with a similar trend for type I fibre area determined from vastus lateralis muscle biopsies. Moreover, there was evidence of significant regeneration within the muscle with increases in developmental myosin and IGF-1 immunoreactivity.

It is evident from these studies that muscle hypertrophy does not account for all of the changes in muscle strength with training. As with younger adults, significant neural adaptations, especially in the initial stages, appears to be the main response to resistive training, and is mediated to a variable extent by fibre hypertrophy (Lexell et al 1995). These adaptations include enhanced neural drive, motor unit recruitment and synchronization, and improved skill and coordination (Rogers and Evans 1993, Sale 1988). The magnitude of neural contributions is evident when muscle strength is assessed on the equipment used for training compared with testing on novel or unfamiliar equipment. In the 12-week study by Frontera and colleagues (1988), dynamic concentric strength (1 RM) increases for the knee extensors and flexors when assessed on the same devices as used for training and using the same motor patterns was approximately 10-fold greater than when assessed using isokinetic testing. Moreover, training appeared to have the greatest effect at movement speeds that were similar to those used in training, illustrating the specificity of training. Similarly, smaller increases have been reported by other investigators for isometric (Hunter et al 1995, Sipilä et al 1996) and isokinetic (Lexell et al 1995) muscle strength after dynamic resistance training compared with 1 RM testing on training equipment utilized in these studies.

The results gained from training are transient and removal of the training stimulus will result in a gradual loss of muscle strength and size. Strength change is typically minor for the first several weeks following the discontinuation of training and training as infrequently as once every 2 or 4 weeks may be sufficient to largely maintain muscle strength (Lexell et al 1995, Taaffe and Marcus 1997). Moreover, strength that is lost with detraining is rapidly recouped with resumption of training. These adaptations to detraining and retraining can be seen in Figure 8.6. In this 44-week study (Taaffe and Marcus 1997), participants underwent resistive exercise training for several upper and lower body muscle groups thrice weekly for 24 weeks; this resulted in a rapid improvement in maximal strength in the first 10 weeks, which was maintained through week 24. The strength gains varied from 26% for the

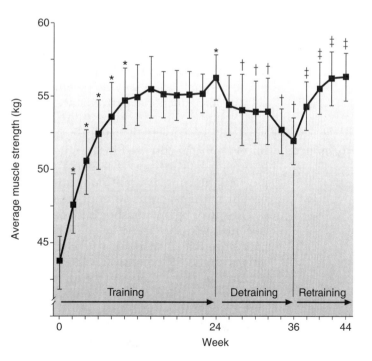

Figure 8.6 Alterations in muscle strength with training, detraining and retraining in older men. *Improvement in muscle strength from the preceding test during the training phase. †Different from peak muscle strength. ‡Improvement in strength with retraining. (Reprinted with permission of Blackwell Publishing, from Taaffe D R, Marcus R (1997) Dynamic muscle strength alterations to detraining and retraining in elderly men. Clinical Physiology, 17, 311–324.)

bench press (upper body exercise) to 84% for the knee extensors, and were accompanied by hypertrophy of type I and II muscle fibres of 17% and 26%, respectively. Following 12 weeks of detraining, a substantial portion (70%) of the strength gained in the first 24 weeks remained, but muscle fibre CSA reverted to pre-training levels. However, the strength that was lost with detraining was recouped within 4–6 weeks of retraining. These findings are important for individuals who anticipate a period of reduced activity following illness or limited periods of disability. Consequently, resistance training prior to the anticipated period of inactivity or hospitalization will provide a greater safety margin for performing activities of daily living following inactivity.

Apart from muscle strength, muscle power is also increased with resistance training. This may not seem surprising given that power is a function of force and the velocity of movement. Jozsi and colleagues (1999) found comparable increases in young and older men and women for arm pull and leg extensor power of ~20–30%, as they did for muscle strength, following 12 weeks of thrice weekly exercise. Similar findings were also observed by Izquierdo et al (2001) for arm and leg muscle power following 16 weeks of strength training in middle-aged and older men, and Skelton and colleagues (1995) for power of the leg extensors in women. Recently, two studies examined the beneficial effects of high-velocity training, in comparison to conventional resistance training that uses slow movement speeds, in the elderly. Earles et al (2001) subjected volunteers aged greater than 70 years to high-velocity resistance training for the legs thrice weekly for 12 weeks and found a 22% increase in peak muscle power. In contrast, there was no change in muscle power in individuals randomized to a walking group for 12 weeks. In older women with self-reported disability, Fielding and colleagues (2002) found that although leg press and knee extensor strength was similar between those undertaking high-velocity compared with low-velocity training for 16 weeks, leg press power increased substantially more in the high-velocity group. It is clear that this is an important area for future research, especially its potential effect on improving movement velocity and functional performance.

Physical performance benefits

Importantly, as observed in the studies by Fiatarone et al (1990, 1994), improvements in muscle strength may have a substantial effect on physical function in frail older adults. Indeed, this population may benefit the most from appropriate interventions as these individuals lie close to or below thresholds for the performance of many daily tasks. In contrast, less impact may be seen in well-functioning individuals as they have adequate muscle function for undertaking daily activities. This is due to the non-linear relationship between muscle strength and performance (Buchner et al 1996), where a certain amount of strength is required for successful performance and strength above that level may have minimal additional effect. However, even in well-functioning older adults, training will result in a greater reserve capacity that would place them further above the threshold for performance of activities, thereby prolonging independence, and may also be of value in the short-term in regard to recovery following a prolonged illness or hospitalization.

Nevertheless, even in healthy volunteers recruited to participate in exercise trials, functional performance benefits are accrued. Several of the studies listed in Table 8.1 included performance tasks as an outcome, and improvements in physical function were observed for some of these tasks. An essential component of independent functioning is walking ability, both the velocity of movement as well as the ability to move without stumbling or falling. Maximal walking velocity has been shown to increase by 18% after 16 weeks (Hunter et al 1995) and 11.6% following 18 weeks (Sipilä et al 1996) of strength training in older women. In addition to maximal walking velocity, usual gait velocity was also improved by 8% following 12 weeks of resistance training, although the mean age for this group was 82 years (Judge et al 1993). Apart from gait speed, walking endurance has also been shown to improve in community-dwelling elderly people following weight training. Following 12 weeks of training in men and women aged 65 years and older, leg strength improved as did walking endurance, determined as walking time at 80% of baseline peak aerobic capacity, from 25 ± 4 to 34 ± 9 minutes (Ades et al 1996). The relation between change in leg strength and walking endurance was significant ($r = 0.48$). This association between change in leg strength and walking endurance is important for elderly persons who are at an increased risk for mobility disability.

In addition, the ability to rise from a chair (Taaffe et al 1999) and dynamic balance (Nelson et al 1994) have been reported to improve following prolonged training in men and women. Hunter et al (1995) also found that the ability to rise from a seated position and carry groceries was easier subsequent to strength training. In a longitudinal exercise trial conducted by McCartney and colleagues (1996), significant improvements were found for symptom-limited endurance in cycling, walking and stair climbing of 6%, 29% and 57% respectively.

As mentioned previously, steadiness declines with ageing of the neuromuscular system, reducing the ability to perform fine motor skills. A 12-week strength training programme in elderly subjects has also been shown to decrease the magnitude of submaximal force fluctuations (Keen et al 1994). Subjects trained thrice weekly with six sets of 10 repetitions at 80% of their 1 RM. Dynamic muscle strength increased by 137% and isometric force of the first dorsal interosseous muscle by 39%, accompanied by a decline in normalized force fluctuations from 9.5% to 5.8%, resulting in improved steadiness. However, the ability of resistance training to improve steadiness may be dependent on the muscle group examined. Recently, Bellow (2002) examined the ability to control submaximal force of the quadriceps following 12 weeks of high intensity strength training in men and women aged 59–83 years. Although training resulted in significant improvements in quadriceps strength, there was no change in the ability to control submaximal forces. Therefore, it is unclear whether resistance training can improve the modulation of muscle forces involved in the control of balance and postural sway.

Prevention of falls and fracture

A significant problem in elderly people that can lead to morbidity, mortality and loss of independence is falls. About a third of the community-dwelling elderly suffer a fall each year, and about 40–50% of fallers have multiple events (Fuller 2000, Nevitt et al 1989). Importantly, fracture risk in older adults, especially that for the hip, is dependent not only on bone strength, but also on the propensity to fall, with about 80–90% of hip fractures due to a fall (Cummings and Nevitt 1989). Although risk factors for falls are multifactorial, and include balance disorders, visual acuity, cognitive impairment, medication usage, postural hypotension and environmental hazards, a major factor for falls is muscle weakness (Fuller 2000, Nevitt et al 1989, Wolfson et al 1995). Several studies have demonstrated that muscle strength of the lower extremity is compromised in fallers compared with non-fallers (Gehlsen and Whaley 1990, Lord et al 1994, Whipple et al 1987). For instance, Whipple and colleagues (1987) compared muscle strength and power of the knees and ankles in nursing home residents with a history of falls to non-fallers. Overall, strength and power of the flexors and extensors at both joints in non-fallers was approximately twice that of the fallers, with dorsiflexion power in fallers being over 7-fold lower than in non-fallers.

Several intervention trials have indicated that exercise may have a protective effect on risk of falling (Buchner et al 1997, Campbell et al 1997, Lord et al 1995). Campbell et al (1997) used a home exercise programme of strength and balance training in 116 women aged 80 years and older. Muscle strengthening exercises for the lower extremity were of a moderate intensity using body weight and ankle cuff weights as resistance. Balance activities included tandem walking, walking on the toes and walking on the heels, walking backwards, sideways and turning around. After one year, there was an improvement in physical function and a substantial reduction in the number of falls, with 88 falls in the exercise group compared with 152 falls in a control group ($n = 117$). A subgroup of exercisers and control women continued after the one year, with benefits continuing over a 2-year period (Campbell et al 1999). A meta-analysis of the effect of four randomized intervention trials conducted by Campbell's research group indicated that individually prescribed muscle strengthening and balance retraining reduces the number of falls and fall-related injuries in elderly people by 35% (Robertson et al 2002).

Once a fall does occur, several factors probably determine whether a hip fracture will result. These factors include the orientation of the fall, lack of protective responses, insufficient local soft tissue to absorb substantial energy of the impact, and insufficient or low bone strength (Cummings and Nevitt 1989). Bone strength is dependent on bone density, which accounts for 50–80% of the variance in bone strength (Genant et al 1994), as well as bone geometry and its microarchitecture. Exercise that involves increased weight-bearing activity or resistance training may also increase bone mineral density, although the gains are modest, generally in the order of 1–3% and are site-specific (Kelley 1998a, 1998b, Wolff et al 1999). Consequently, of the primary risk factors for falls and fracture, muscle strength is most subject to improvement in older persons; therefore improving muscle strength may prove an effective strategy to reduce fracture risk and should form an integral part of a multi-faceted falls and fracture prevention programme.

Exercise prescription

If the goal is to repair deficits in muscle mass, muscle function and physical performance that occur with advancing age, then resistance training is an appropriate exercise mode. However, apart from the training mode, the exercise prescription encompasses the frequency, intensity and duration of activity. In addition, for benefits to accrue, the programme must be progressive in nature.

Apart from the exercise principle of progressive overload to induce adaptation, the programme has to abide to the principle of specificity, that is, 'you only get what you train for'. As a result, the programme should target the major muscle groups of the body as this will augment/maintain muscle mass of the exercised muscles and all-round body strength which is important for general functioning. This principle also relates to whether the individual is training for muscle strength/power or muscle endurance. If strength and power is the goal then heavier weights with few repetitions, such as 6–8, are recommended, whereas a lighter resistance with higher repetitions are performed for muscle endurance. During the performance of these exercises, movements should be taken through the full range of motion, as training is also specific to the range of motion utilized (ACSM 1998a).

The American College of Sports Medicine (ACSM) has published position stands on the recommended quantity and quality of exercise for healthy adults (ACSM 1998a) and exercise and physical activity for older adults (ACSM 1998b) that include guidelines for strength training. Training guidelines for elderly people have also been published by others (Christmas and Andersen 2000, Evans 1999). In general, the guidelines in these various reports are very similar to those recommended for well-functioning adults. However, in prescribing exercise for older adults, chronic conditions need to be taken into account to ensure that adverse outcomes do not eventuate. Nevertheless, resistance training has been repeatedly shown to be safe for the older adult, including the very old (Fiatarone et al 1990, 1994, Lexell et al 1995, Pyka et al 1994, Taaffe et al 1999).

Prior to the commencement of a vigorous exercise regimen, ACSM recommends that a medical evaluation and appropriate stress testing be undertaken (ACSM 2000). In general, stress testing involves a symptom limited treadmill or cycle ergometer test with monitoring of the electrocardiograph (ECG), heart rate and blood pressure. However, for strength training programmes, a weight-lifting stress test has also been used where participants perform three sets of eight repetitions at 80% of their 1 RM, with the monitoring of ECG and blood pressure responses during the exercise test (Evans 1999). As an alternative to a physician-supervised stress test, Evans (1999) maintains that for those contemplating the commencement of a walking or resistance training programme, a brief questionnaire developed by Fiatarone for a community-based exercise programme may be sufficient to determine who requires physician evaluation prior to exercise (see Evans 1999).

In addition to some form of screening and evaluation, consultation with the participant is critical to ensure that the exercise programme will be successful. Barriers to exercise, real and perceived, need to be addressed, and information regarding past and current activity, level of interest, motivation and social preferences regarding exercise need to be obtained and taken into account in developing the prescription (Christmas and Andersen 2000).

The following are general guidelines for a resistance training programme for healthy older people that uses resistance equipment such as weight machines. All sessions commence with a warm-up and conclude with a cool-down of 5–10 minutes each that combine low level activity and stretching.

Exercises

Exercise should target the major muscle groups of the upper and lower limbs and trunk, which may entail 8–10 separate exercises. Exercises for the lower limb are especially important for mobility, balance and the prevention of falls. A sample programme may include the leg press (quadriceps), knee extension (quadriceps), knee flexion (hamstrings) and calf raise for the lower limbs, triceps extensions and biceps curls for the upper limbs, and bench press (chest), shoulder press, and seated row (back musculature) for the trunk. In addition, exercises for the abdominal and lower back muscles would be undertaken. The sequence of exercises would commence with large muscle groups and end with smaller muscle groups, so that exercises such as the bench press would be performed before triceps extension or biceps curls.

Intensity

High-intensity training where the weight can be lifted (concentric contraction) and lowered (eccentric contraction) only 8–10 times (RM) is recommended. As a percentage of 1 RM, this will be approximately 70–80%. The repetitions are performed in a smooth controlled manner through a full range of motion, taking approximately 2–3 seconds for the concentric and 3 seconds for the eccentric portion of the movement. However, as discussed above, studies indicate that high-velocity movements are more beneficial for increasing muscle power. It should be noted that significant strength increases in older adults have also been reported with low-intensity training (14 repetitions at 40% 1 RM), and that this was accompanied by muscle fibre hypertrophy (Taaffe et al 1996). These gains may be possible due to the relatively untrained state of many elders. As a result, for those apprehensive about their ability to undertake a strength training programme, a low-intensity, high-repetition regimen may prove effective in addressing deficits in muscle function and also assist in developing confidence in their ability to undertake more intense training. The number of sets undertaken may vary from 1 to 3 sets (a set being a group of repetitions). Evidence is conflicting as to whether multiple-sets are superior to single-sets. If time is a constraint, then one set is sufficient to induce positive changes in muscle function.

Frequency

It is generally recommended that resistance exercise sessions be performed 2–3 days per week. However, as with the number of sets, there is conflicting evidence regarding the superiority of more frequent training compared with training only 1 or 2 days per week. In a 6-month study comparing high-intensity strength training 1, 2 and 3 days per week, strength gains for both the upper and lower body were similar, regardless of training frequency (Figure 8.7). In addition, strength gains were accompanied by modest increases in lean mass and functional performance, with no difference among the three exercise groups (Taaffe et al 1999). Consequently, if time is a limitation, then significant benefits can be derived from a high-intensity resistive programme of only one session per week.

Duration

To facilitate adherence to the programme, individual exercise sessions should not take longer than an hour. Regarding programme duration, the longer the better. As discussed above, 'if you don't use it you lose it', so some form of resistive training should always form part of the older adult's activity programme. After approximately 6 months of training, the frequency could be reduced to once every 1 or 2 weeks to largely maintain muscle function levels.

Many resistance exercises that are commonly performed in a gymnasium using exercise machines can also be undertaken with the use of commercially available elastic bands (Theraband), which can be adjusted to modify the resistance so that an appropriate stimulus can be applied. The use of elastic bands as a resistance seems well suited to home and community settings where exercise machine equipment is unavailable. Moreover, because of a lack of access to exercise facilities or pre-existing conditions that prevent older adults from travelling or using private/public transportation, exercise at home may be the only option. Home-based exercise programmes using these bands have been successfully undertaken in the elderly, with significant improvements in muscle strength (Capodaglio et al 2002, Jette et al 1996). Importantly, in a 6-month trial using these bands, adherence to the home-based programme was high at 89% (Jette et al 1999).

Another method to provide resistance in a home- or community-based programme is by the use of weighted vests. This form of resistance for the lower body in conjunction with exercise has proved to be safe and effective in improving indices of fall risk and prevention of hip bone loss in postmenopausal women (Shaw and Snow 1998, Snow et al 2000). Recently, it has been used in older adults with mobility limitations to improve muscle power and stair-climbing power (Bean et al 2002). The programme used by Bean and colleagues (2002) in mobility-limited older adults simply consisted of participants ascending and

Figure 8.7 Similar gains in upper (UB) and lower (LB) body strength with training 1 (EX1), 2 (EX2) or 3 (EX3) days per week. WB = whole body muscle strength. (Reprinted with permission of Blackwell Publishing, from Taaffe D R, Duret C, Wheeler S, Marcus R (1999) Once-weekly resistance exercise improves muscle strength and neuromuscular performance in older adults. Journal of the American Geriatrics Society, 47, 1208–1214.)

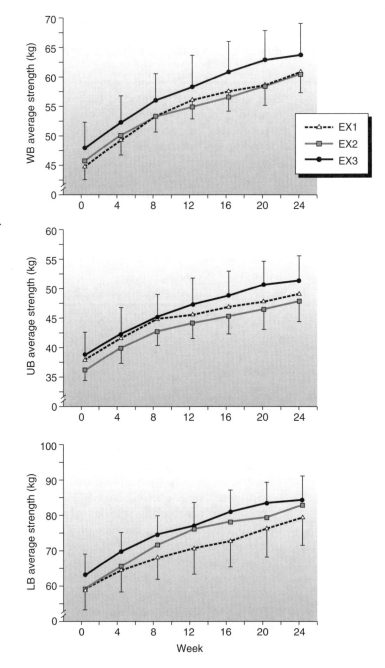

descending 12 flights (126 steps), divided into three sets of four flights, three times per week for 12 weeks. The sessions were brief, lasting no longer than 10 minutes (excluding warm-up and cool-down). The programme was progressive in nature by weights (as a percentage of body mass) being added when a target pace was achieved. Following training, leg press peak power significantly increased by 17% and stair-climbing power by 12%.

Apart from these devices and wrist and ankle weights, home-made equipment, such as drink bottles containing sand or pebbles, provide resistance which can be adjusted as muscle strength and endurance improves. Similarly, callisthenic exercises using body weight also provide an adequate resistance for maintaining and improving muscle function, as can the resistance applied by a partner.

Conclusion

Ageing is characterized by a decline in muscle mass and muscle function. Associated with the decline in muscle function is reduced physical performance that compromises the ability to undertake daily activities and maintain independence. Exercise, specifically resistance training, can reliably and substantially enhance muscle function in the older adult. The components of the training programme are similar to those prescribed for young and middle-aged adults with a frequency of once or twice per week sufficient to significantly improve muscle performance. This form of training is well tolerated in older adults, even the very old, and can result in improved functional performance. By repairing the age-related deficits in muscle function with appropriate exercise regimens, the maintenance of independent living and quality of life can be extended for older adults.

References

Ades P A, Ballor D L, Ashikaga T, Utton J L, Nair K S 1996 Weight training improves walking endurance in healthy elderly persons. Annals of Internal Medicine 124:568–572

Aloia J F, McGowan D M, Vaswani A N, Ross P, Cohn S 1991 Relationship of menopause to skeletal and muscle mass. American Journal of Clinical Nutrition 53:1378–1383

American College of Sports Medicine Position Stand 1998a The recommended quantity and quality of exercise for developing and maintaining cardiorespiratory and muscular fitness, and flexibility in healthy adults. Medicine and Science in Sports and Exercise 30:975–991

American College of Sports Medicine Position Stand 1998b Exercise and physical activity for older adults. Medicine and Science in Sports and Exercise 30:992–1008

American College of Sports Medicine 2000 ACSM's guidelines for exercise testing and prescription, 6th edn. Lippincott Williams & Wilkins, Philadelphia

Aniansson A, Gustafsson E 1981 Physical training in elderly men with special reference to quadriceps muscle strength and morphology. Clinical Physiology 1:87–98

Aniansson A, Hedberg M, Henning G-B, Grimby G 1986 Muscle morphology, enzymatic activity, and muscle strength in elderly men: a follow-up study. Muscle and Nerve 9:585–591

Avlund K, Schroll A K, Davidsen M, Løvborg B, Rantanen T 1994 Maximal isometric strength and functional mobility in daily activities among 75-year-old men and women. Scandinavian Journal of Medicine and Science in Sports 4:32–40

Bassey E J, Harries U J 1993 Normal values for handgrip strength in 920 men and women aged over 65 years, and longitudinal changes over 4 years in 620 survivors. Clinical Science 84:331–337

Bassey E J, Bendall M J, Pearson M 1988 Muscle strength in the triceps surae and objectively measured customary walking activity in men and women over 65 years of age. Clinical Science 74:85–89

Bassey E J, Fiatarone M A, O'Neill E F, et al 1992 Leg extensor power and functional performance in very old men and women. Clinical Science 82:321–327

Bassey E J, Mockett S P, Fentem P H 1996 Lack of variation in muscle strength with menstrual status in healthy women aged 45–54 years: data from a national survey. European Journal of Applied Physiology 73:382–386

Bean J, Herman S, Kiely D K, et al 2002 Weighted stair climbing in mobility-limited older people: a pilot study. Journal of the American Geriatrics Society 50:663–670

Bellew J W 2002 The effect of strength training on control of force in older men and women. Aging Clinical and Experimental Research 14:35–41

Bortz W M 1982 Disuse and aging. JAMA 248:1203–1208

Bosco C, Komi P V 1980 Influence of aging on the mechanical behavior of leg extensor muscles. European Journal of Applied Physiology 45:209–219

Brooks S V, Faulkner J A 1994 Skeletal muscle weakness in old age: underlying mechanisms. Medicine and Science in Sports and Exercise 26:432–439

Buchner D M, Larson E B, Wagner E H, Koepsell T D, de Lateur B J 1996 Evidence for a non-linear relationship between leg strength and gait speed. Age and Ageing 25:386–391

Buchner D M, Cress M E, de Lateur B J, et al 1997 The effect of strength and endurance training on gait, balance, fall risk, and health services use in community-living older adults. Journal of Gerontology Medical Sciences 52A:M218–224

Campbell A J, Robertson M C, Gardner M M, et al 1997 Randomised controlled trial of a general practice programme of home based exercise to prevent falls in elderly women. British Medical Journal 315:1065–1069

Campbell A J, Robertson M C, Gardner M M, Norton R N, Buchner D M 1999 Falls prevention over 2 years: a randomized controlled trial in women 80 years and older. Age and Ageing 28:513–518

Campbell W C, Trappe T A, Wolfe R R, Evans W J 2001 The recommended dietary allowance for protein may not be adequate for older people to maintain skeletal muscle. Journal of Gerontology Medical Sciences 56A:M373–380

Capodaglio P, Facioli M, Burroni E, et al 2002 Effectiveness of a home-based strengthening program for elderly males in Italy. A preliminary study. Aging Clinical and Experimental Research 14:28–34

Castaneda C, Charnley J M, Evans W J, Crim M C 1995 Elderly women accommodate to a low-protein diet with losses of body cell mass, muscle function, and immune response. American Journal of Clinical Nutrition 62:30–39

Charette S L, McEvoy L, Pyka G, et al 1991 Muscle hypertrophy response to resistance training in older women. Journal of Applied Physiology 70:1912–1916

Christmas C, Andersen R A 2000 Exercise and older patients: guidelines for the clinician. Journal of the American Geriatrics Society 48:318–324

Cohen H J, Pieper C F, Harris T, Rao K M K, Currie M S 1997 The association of plasma IL-6 levels with functional disability in community-dwelling elderly. Journal of Gerontology Medical Sciences 52A:M201–208

Cummings S R, Nevitt M C 1989 A hypothesis: the causes of hip fractures. Journal of Gerontology Medical Sciences 44:M107–111

Davis J W, Ross P D, Preston S D, Nevitt M C, Wasnich R D 1998 Strength, physical activity, and body mass index: relationship to performance-based measures and activities of daily living among older Japanese women in Hawaii. Journal of the American Geriatrics Society 46:274–279

De Vito G, Bernardi M, Forte R, et al 1998 Determinants of maximal instantaneous muscle power in women aged 50–75 years. European Journal of Applied Physiology 78:59–64

Delbono O, O'Rourke K S, Ettinger W H 1995 Excitation-calcium release uncoupling in aged human skeletal muscle fibers. Journal of Membrane Biology 148:211–222

Doherty T J, Vandervoort A A, Brown W F 1993a Effects of ageing on the motor unit: a brief review. Canadian Journal of Applied Physiology 18:331–358

Doherty T J, Vandervoort A A, Taylor A W, Brown W F 1993b Effects of motor unit losses on strength in older men and women. Journal of Applied Physiology 74:868–874

Doherty T J, Komori T, Stashuk D W, Kassam A, Brown W F 1994 Physiological properties of single thenar motor units in the F-response of younger and older adults. Muscle and Nerve 17:860–872

Earles D R, Judge J O, Gunnarsson O T 2001 Velocity training induces power-specific adaptations in highly functioning older adults. Archives of Physical Medicine and Rehabilitation 82:872–878

Ensrud K E, Nevitt M C, Yunis C, et al 1994 Correlates of impaired function in older women. Journal of the American Geriatrics Society 42:481–489

Evans W J 1995 What is sarcopenia? Journals of Gerontology 50A(special issue):5–8

Evans W J 1999 Exercise training guidelines for the elderly. Medicine and Science in Sports and Exercise 31:12–17

Fiatarone M A, Marks E, Ryan N D, et al 1990 High-intensity strength training in nonagenarians: effects on skeletal muscle. Journal of the American Medical Association 263:3029–3034

Fiatarone M A, O'Neill E F, Ryan N D, et al 1994 Exercise training and nutritional supplementation for physical frailty in very elderly people. New England Journal of Medicine 330:1769–1775

Fiatarone Singh M A, Ding W, Manfredi T J, et al 1999 Insulin-like growth factor I in skeletal muscle after weight-lifting exercise in frail elders. American Journal of Physiology 277:E135–143

Fielding R A, LeBrasseur N K, Cuoco A, et al 2002 High-velocity resistance training increases skeletal muscle peak power in older women. Journal of the American Geriatrics Society 50:655–662

Fischer J, Johnson M A 1990 Low body weight and weight loss in the aged. Journal of the American Dietetics Association 90:1697–1706

Foldavi M, Clark M, Laviolette L C, et al 2000 Association of muscle power with functional status in community-dwelling elderly women. Journal of Gerontology Medical Sciences 55A:M192–199

Frontera W R, Meredith C N, O'Reilly K P, Knuttgen H G, Evans W J 1988 Strength conditioning in older men: skeletal muscle hypertrophy and improved function. Journal of Applied Physiology 64:1038–1044

Fuller G F 2000 Falls in the elderly. American Family Physician 61:2159–2168

Gabay C, Kushner I 1999 Acute-phase proteins and other systemic responses to inflammation. New England Journal of Medicine 106:506–512

Gehlsen G M, Whaley M H 1990 Falls in the elderly: Part II, balance, strength, and flexibility. Archives of Physical Medicine and Rehabilitation 71:739–741

Genant H K, Glüer C C, Lotz J C 1994 Gender differences in bone density, skeletal geometry, and fracture biomechanics. Radiology 190:636–640

Giampoli S, Ferrucci L, Cecchi F, et al 1999 Hand-grip strength predicts incident disability in non-disabled older men. Age and Ageing 28

Greeves J P, Cable N T, Reilly T, Kingsland C 1999 Changes in muscle strength in women following the menopause: a longitudinal assessment of the efficacy of hormone replacement therapy. Clinical Science 97:79–84

Grimby G, Saltin B 1983 The ageing muscle. Clinical Physiology 3:209–218

Grimby G, Aniansson A, Zetterberg C, Saltin B 1984 Is there a change in relative muscle fibre composition with age? Clinical Physiology 4:189–194

Hagerman F C, Walsh S J, Staron R S, et al 2000 Effects of high-intensity resistance training on untrained older men. I. Strength, cardiovascular, and metabolic responses. Journal of Gerontology Biological Sciences 55A:B336–346

Hikida R S, Staron R S, Hagerman F C, et al S 2000 Effects of high-intensity resistance training on untrained older men. II. Muscle fiber characteristics and nucleo-cytoplasmic relationships. Journal of Gerontology Biological Sciences 55A:B347–354

Hunter G R, Treuth M S, Weinsier R L, et al 1995 The effects of strength conditioning on older women's ability to perform daily tasks. Journal of the American Geriatrics Society 43:756–760

Hyatt R H, Whitelaw M N, Bhat A, Scott S, Maxwell J D 1990 Association of muscle strength with functional status of elderly people. Age and Ageing 19:330–336

Institute of Medicine 1991 Disability in America: toward a national agenda for prevention. In: Pope A M, Tarlov A R (eds) Division of Health Promotion and Disease Prevention, National Academy Press, Washington, p 6–10

Izquierdo M, Aguado X, Gonzalez R, Lopez J L, Hakkinen K 1999 Maximal and explosive force production capacity and balance performance in men of different ages. European Journal of Applied Physiology 79:260–267

Izquierdo M, Hakkinen K, Ibanez J, et al 2001 Effects of strength training on muscle power and serum hormones in middle-aged and older men. Journal of Applied Physiology 90:1497–1507

Jette A M, Branch L G 1981 The Framingham disability study: II. Physical disability among the aging. American Journal of Public Health 71:1211–1216

Jette A M, Harris B A, Sleeper L, et al 1996 A home-based exercise program for nondisabled older adults. Journal of the American Geriatrics Society 44:644–649

Jette A M, Lachman M E, Giorgetti M M, et al 1999 Exercise – it's never too late: the strong-for-life program. American Journal of Public Health 89:66–72

Jozsi A C, Campbell W W, Joseph L, Davey S L, Evans W J 1999 Changes in power with resistance training in older and younger men and women. Journal of Gerontology Medical Sciences 54A:M591–596

Jubrias S A, Odderson I R, Esselman P C, Conley K E 1997 Decline in isokinetic force with age: muscle cross-sectional area and specific force. Pflügers Archives 434:246–253

Jubrias S A, Esselman P C, Price L B, Cress M E, Conley K E 2001 Large energetic adaptations of elderly muscle to resistance and endurance training. Journal of Applied Physiology 90:1663–1670

Judge J O, Underwood M, Gennosa T 1993 Exercise to improve gait velocity in older persons. Archives of Physical Medicine and Rehabilitation 74:400–406

Kallman D A, Plato C C, Tobin J D 1990 The role of muscle loss in the age-related decline in grip strength: cross-sectional and longitudinal perspectives. Journal of Gerontology Medical Sciences 45:M82–88

Keen D A, Yue G H, Enoka R M 1994 Training-related enhancement in the control of motor output in elderly humans. Journal of Applied Physiology 77:737–746

Kelley G 1998a Aerobic exercise and lumbar spine bone mineral density in postmenopausal women: a meta-analysis. Journal of the American Geriatrics Society 46:143–152

Kelley G A 1998b Exercise and regional bone mineral density in postmenopausal women: a meta-analytic review of randomized trials. American Journal of Physical Medicine and Rehabilitation 77:76–87

Klitgaard H, Mantoni M, Schiaffino S, et al 1990 Function, morphology and protein expression of ageing skeletal muscle: a cross-sectional study of elderly men with different training backgrounds. Acta Physiologica Scandinavica 140:41–54

Kuller L H 1999 Serum levels of IL-6 and development of disability in older persons. Journal of the American Geriatrics Society 47:755–756

Kurpad A V, Vaz M 2000 Protein and amino acid requirements in the elderly. European Journal of Clinical Nutrition 54 (Suppl 3):131–142

Larsson L, Karlsson J 1978 Isometric and dynamic endurance as a function of age and skeletal muscle characteristics. Acta Physiologica Scandinavica 104:129–136

Larsson L, Sjodin B, Karlsson J 1978 Histochemical and biochemical changes in human skeletal muscle with age in sedentary males, age 22–65 years. Acta Physiologica Scandinavica 103:31–39

Larsson L, Li X, Frontera W R 1997 Effects of aging on shortening velocity and myosin isoform composition in single human skeletal muscle cells. American Journal of Physiology 272:C638–649

Lexell J 1993 Ageing and human muscle: observations from Sweden. Canadian Journal of Applied Physiology 18:2–18

Lexell J, Taylor C C, Sjöström M 1988 What is the cause of the aging atrophy? Total number, size, and proportion of fiber types studied in whole vastus lateralis muscle from 15- to 83-year-old men. Journal of the Neurological Sciences 84:275–294

Lexell J, Downham D Y, Larsson Y, Bruhn E, Morsing B 1995 Heavy-resistance training in older Scandinavian men and women: short- and long-term effects on arm and leg muscles. Scandinavian Journal of Medicine and Science in Sports 5:329–341

Lord S R, Sambrook P N, Gilbert C, et al 1994 Postural stability, falls and fractures in the elderly: results from the Dubbo Osteoporosis Epidemiology Study. Medical Journal of Australia 160:684–691

Lord S R, Ward J A, Williams P, Strudwick M 1995 The effect of a 12-month exercise trial on balance, strength, and falls in older women: a randomized controlled trial. Journal of the American Geriatrics Society 43:1198–1206

Marcus R 1996 Should all older people be treated with growth hormone? Drugs Aging 8:1–4

McCartney N, Hicks A L, Martin J, Webber C E 1996 A longitudinal trial of weight training in the elderly: continued improvements in year 2. Journal of Gerontology Biological Sciences 51A:B425–433

Mitch W E, Goldberg A L 1997 Mechanisms of muscle wasting. The role of the ubiquitin–proteasome pathway. New England Journal of Medicine 335:1897–1905

Moritani T, deVries H A 1980 Potential for gross muscle hypertrophy in older men. Journal of Gerontology 35:672–682

Nagi S Z 1965 Some conceptual issues in disability and rehabilitation. In: Sussman M B (ed) Sociology and Rehabilitation. American Sociological Association, Washington, p 100–113

Nagi S Z 1979 The concept and measurement of disability. In: Berkowitz E D (ed) Disability Policies and Government Programs. Praeger, New York, p 1–15

Nelson M E, Fiatarone M A, Morganti C M, et al 1994 Effects of high-intensity strength training on multiple risk factors for osteoporotic fractures: a randomized controlled trial. Journal of the American Medical Association 272:1909–1914

Nevitt M C, Cummings S R, Kidd S, Black D 1989 Risk factors for recurrent nonsyncopal falls. Journal of the American Medical Association 261:2663–2668

Nichols J F, Omizo D K, Peterson K K, Nelson K P 1993 Efficacy of heavy-resistance training for active women over sixty: muscular strength, body composition, and program adherence. Journal of the American Geriatrics Society 41:205–210

Patten C 2000 Re-educating muscle force control in older persons through strength training. Topics in Geriatric Rehabilitation 15:47–59

Phillips S K, Rook K M, Siddle N C, Woledge R C 1993 Muscle weakness in women occurs at an earlier age than in men, but strength is preserved by hormone replacement therapy. Clinical Science 84:95–98

Posner J D, McCully K K, Landsberg L A, et al 1995 Physical determinants of independence in mature women. Archives of Physical Medicine and Rehabilitation 76:373–380

Pyka G, Lindenberger E, Charette S, Marcus R 1994 Muscle strength and fiber adaptations to a year-long resistance training program in elderly women. Journal of Gerontology Medical Sciences 49:M22–27

Rantanen T, Era P, Heikkinen E 1994 Maximal isometric strength and mobility among 75-year-old men and women. Age and Ageing 23:132–137

Rantanen T, Masaki K, Foley D, et al 1998 Grip strength changes over 27 yr in Japanese-American men. Journal of Applied Physiology 85:2047–2053

Ringsberg K 1993 Muscle strength differences in urban and rural populations in Sweden. Archives of Physical Medicine and Rehabilitation 74:1315–1318

Robertson M C, Campbell A J, Gardner M M, Devlin N 2002 Preventing injuries in older people by preventing falls: a meta-analysis of individual-level data. Journal of the American Geriatrics Society 50:905–911

Rogers M A, Evans W J 1993 Changes in skeletal muscle with aging: effects of exercise training. Exercise and Sport Sciences Reviews 21:65–102

Roos M R, Rice C L, Vandervoort A A 1997 Age-related changes in motor unit function. Muscle Nerve 20:679–690

Roubenoff R, Castaneda C 2001 Sarcopenia – understanding the dynamics of aging muscle. Journal of the American Medical Association 286:1230–1231

Rudman D, Kutner M H, Rogers C M, et al 1981 Impaired growth hormone secretion in the adult population: relation to age and adiposity. Journal of Clinical Investigation 67:1361–1369

Sale D G 1988 Neural adaptation to resistance training. Medicine and Science in Sports and Exercise 20:135–145

Salomon F, Cuneo RC, Hesp R, Sönksen P H 1989 The effects of treatment with recombinant human growth hormone on body composition and metabolism in adults with growth hormone deficiency. New England Journal of Medicine 321:1797–1803

Schroll M 1994 The main pathway to musculoskeletal disability. Scandinavian Journal of Medicine and Science in Sports 4:3–12

Seeley D G, Cauley J A, Grady D, et al 1995 Is postmenopausal estrogen therapy associated with neuromuscular function and falling in elderly women? Archives of Internal Medicine 155:293–299

Shaw J M, Snow C M 1998 Weighted vest exercise improves indices of fall risk in older women. Journal of Gerontology Medical Sciences 53A:M53–58

Sipilä S, Suominen H 1991 Ultrasound imaging of the quadriceps muscle in elderly athletes and untrained men. Muscle Nerve 14:527–533

Sipilä S, Suominen H 1993 Muscle ultrasonography and computed tomography in elderly trained and untrained women. Muscle Nerve 16:294–300

Sipilä S, Viitasalo J, Era P, Suominen H 1991 Muscle strength in male athletes aged 70–81 years and a population sample. European Journal of Applied Physiology 63:399–403

Sipilä S, Multanen J, Kallinen M, Era P, Suominen H 1996 Effects of strength and endurance training on isometric muscle strength and walking speed in elderly women. Acta Physiologica Scandinavica 156:457–464

Sipilä S, Elorinne E, Alen M, Suominen H, Kovanen V 1997 Effects of strength and endurance training on muscle fibre characteristics in elderly women. Clinical Physiology 17:459–474

Skelton D A, Greig C A, Davies J M, Young A 1994 Strength, power and related functional ability of healthy people aged 65–89 years. Age and Ageing 23:371–377

Skelton D A, Young A, Greig C A, Malbut K E 1995 Effects of resistance training on strength, power, and selected functional abilities of women aged 75 and older. Journal of the American Geriatrics Society 43:1081–1087

Snow C M, Shaw J M, Winters K M, Witzke K A 2000 Long-term exercise using weighted vests prevents hip bone loss in postmenopausal women. Journal of Gerontology Medical Sciences 55A:M489–491

Taaffe D R, Marcus R 1997 Dynamic muscle strength alterations to detraining and retraining in elderly men. Clinical Physiology 17:311–324

Taaffe D R, Pruitt L, Reim J, et al 1994 Effect of recombinant human growth hormone on the muscle strength response to resistance exercise in elderly men. Journal of Clinical Endocrinology and Metabolism 79:1361–1366

Taaffe D R, Pruitt L, Pyka G, Guido D, Marcus R 1996 Comparative effects of high- and low-intensity resistance training on thigh muscle strength, fiber area, and tissue composition in elderly women. Clinical Physiology 16:381–392

Taaffe D R, Duret C, Wheeler S, Marcus R 1999 Once-weekly resistance exercise improves muscle strength and neuromuscular performance in older adults. Journal of the American Geriatrics Society 47:1208–1214

Taaffe D R, Harris T B, Ferrucci L, Rowe J, Seeman T E 2000 Cross-sectional and prospective relationships of interleukin-6 and C-reactive protein with physical performance in elderly persons: MacArthur Studies of Successful Aging. Journal of Gerontology Medical Sciences 55A:M709–715

Tenover J L 1999 Testosterone replacement therapy in older adult men. International Journal of Andrology 22:300–306

Tomlinson B E, Irving D 1977 The numbers of limb motor neurons in the human lumbosacral cord throughout life. Journal of the Neurological Sciences 34:213–219

Tomonaga M 1977 Histochemical and ultrastructural changes in senile human skeletal muscle. Journal of the American Geriatrics Society 25:125–131

Van Heuvelen M J G, Kempen G I J M, Bouwer W H, De Greef M H G 2000 Physical fitness related to disability in older persons. Gerontology 46:333–341

Vellas B, Lauque S, Andrieu S, et al 2001 Nutrition assessment in the elderly. Current Opinion in Clinical Nutrition and Metabolic Care 4:5–8

Verbrugge L M, Jette A M 1994 The disablement process. Social Science and Medicine 38:1–14

Whipple R H, Wolfson L I, Amerman P M 1987 The relationship of knee and ankle weakness to falls in nursing home residents: an isokinetic study. Journal of the American Geriatrics Society 35:13–20

Wolff I, van Croonenborg J J, Kemper H C G, Kostense P J, Twisk J W R 1999 The effect of exercise training programs on bone mass: a meta-analysis of published controlled trials in pre- and postmenopausal women. Osteoporosis International 9:1–12

Wolfson L, Judge J, Whipple R, King M 1995 Strength is a major factor in balance, gait, and the occurrence of falls. Journal of Gerontology 50A(special issue):64–67

Yarasheski K E, Campbell J A, Smith K, et al 1992 Effect of growth hormone and resistance exercise on muscle growth in young men. American Journal of Physiology 262:E261–267

Young A 1986 Exercise physiology in geriatric practice. Acta Medica Scandinavica Supplementum 711:227–232

9

Therapeutic exercise guidelines for the rehabilitation of older people following fracture

Nicholas F Taylor and Tania Pizzari

CHAPTER CONTENTS

Introduction 187

Guidelines for prescription of exercises for older people after fracture 189

Increasing movement after fracture 192

Exercising muscles after fracture 199

Conclusion 205

References 206

Introduction

Health consequences of fractures in older people

Bone fractures are common in older people. More than half of all women and one-quarter of men will fracture a bone after the age of 60 years (Jones et al 1994). Fractures of the proximal femur are particularly common in older people, accounting for more than 40% of fractures in people aged over 80 years (Jones et al 1994). Fractures involving the proximal humerus, wrist and vertebrae also frequently occur in older people (Nguyen et al 2001). According to Masud et al (2001), one in seven women over the age of 50 years will fracture their distal radius.

Factors associated with ageing, such as falls and osteoporosis, make older people particularly susceptible to fractures. Around 30% of people aged 65 years and older fall each year and half of those in their eighties fall at least once every year (Campbell et al 1981). The increased rate of falls means that older people more often put 'at-risk' forces through their bones.

Ageing is also associated with a loss of bone strength, particularly in women. It is estimated that 13–21% of older women have osteoporosis and 37–50% have osteopenia, whilst 3–6% of older men have osteoporosis and 28–47% have osteopenia (Kanis et al 2000, Looker et al 1997). Osteoporosis refers to a pathological loss of bone mineral density that is more than 2.5 standard deviations (SD) below the mean for young adults. Osteopenia is bone loss where bone mineral density is more than one SD below the usual values for young adults (World Health Organization 1994). A force that might be considered trivial for a younger person, such as stumbling and catching oneself on an outstretched hand, might be sufficient to fracture an osteoporotic distal radius or neck of humerus in an older person.

Significant health consequences can occur as a result of fractures in older people. For example, following fracture of the proximal femur in older people, mortality was reported to be approximately 17% at 4 months (March et al 2000) and almost 35% at 12 months (Dzupa et al 2002). Other fractures in older people, such as vertebral fractures, are also associated with increased mortality (Center et al 1999).

Fractures in older people can lead to considerable disability. Approximately 50% of people who survive hip fracture are discharged to nursing homes and around 25% remain institutionalized 1 year later (Keene et al 1993). Only 40% of older people return to their pre-injury level of walking after fracture of the proximal femur (Koval and Zuckerman 1994). Fractures that are sometimes considered to be relatively trivial, such as fracture of the distal radius (Colles' fracture), can lead to long-term loss of range of motion, loss of grip strength, as well as a reduced capacity to carry out everyday tasks such as walking, dressing and shopping (de Bruijn 1987, MacDermid et al 2001).

Older people who have suffered a fracture are at increased risk of having further fractures (Cuddihy et al 1999, Ross et al 1991). For example, the risk for further vertebral or hip fractures increases after one or more vertebral fractures (Cuddihy et al 1999, Ross et al 1991). Also, after a fracture of the distal radius, an older person is twice as likely to fracture the neck of femur and five times as likely to sustain a compression fracture of a vertebra (Masud et al 2001).

Exercise and rehabilitation in the management of fractures in older people

The three principles of fracture management – to reduce the fracture if necessary, to hold or immobilize the fracture if necessary, and to move or rehabilitate the affected body part – are well established (Adams and Hamblen 1999). Clinical authorities have argued that rehabilitation is the most important of the three principles of fracture management (Adams and Hamblen 1999). Not all fractures need to be reduced and held (e.g. rib fractures, fractures of the phalanges). However, it is advocated that movement of the person and part is always necessary after a fracture.

Rehabilitation following fracture helps to regain range of motion and strength and prevents ongoing disability. Several studies have shown that exercise training after fracture of the proximal neck of the femur leads to improved strength and motor function (Hauer et al 2001, 2002,

Sherrington and Lord 1997). Furthermore, intensive inpatient rehabilitation following such fractures has been related to reduced length of hospital stay (Swanson et al 1998). After fracture of the distal radius, rehabilitation in the form of outpatient physiotherapy resulted in improved movement of the wrist (Wakefield and McQueen 2000, Watt et al 2000). These studies demonstrate the role of exercise in the rehabilitation of fractures that typically affect older people and highlight the need to establish guidelines for optimal exercise prescription.

Guidelines for prescription of exercises for older people after fracture

There are well-developed guidelines for exercise prescription in healthy adults. The American College of Sports Medicine (ACSM) has published authoritative and well-referenced position statements for the prescription of exercise (1998a). More recently, the ACSM published a further statement on exercise progression for strength training for healthy adults (American College of Sports Medicine 2002). The elements of these guidelines are summarized in Table 9.1.

These guidelines provide a good starting point for the prescription of exercises in healthy adults and can be utilized for the prescription of exercise in older people following fracture. When extrapolating the guidelines for use in the rehabilitation of older adults following fracture, four important factors should be considered:

- fracture healing
- pain
- client safety
- the aim of the exercise.

Table 9.1 Exercise guidelines for healthy adults (adapted from American College of Sports Medicine 1998a, 2002)

	Muscle strength	Cardiorespiratory fitness	Flexibility
Frequency	2–3 days/week	3–5 days/week	2–3 days/week
Intensity	8–12 RM 60–80% of 1 RM for 8–12 repetitions	55–90% of maximum heart rate	
Duration	1–3 sets with a 2–3 minute rest period between sets	20–60 minutes (minimum 10 minute bouts throughout the day)	Static holds for 10–30 seconds, at least 4 repetitions

Note: RM refers to repetition maximum, the maximal number of times a load can be lifted before fatigue using good form and technique.

Stage of fracture healing

The stage of fracture healing can influence the prescription of exercise with regard to exercise type, resistance and repetitions. For example, a conservatively managed (i.e. not surgically fixed) un-united fracture

Figure 9.1 Guidelines for exercise prescription, taking account of fracture healing.

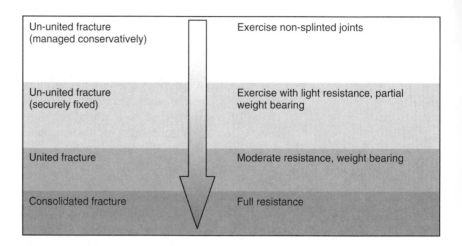

Un-united fracture (managed conservatively)	Exercise non-splinted joints
Un-united fracture (securely fixed)	Exercise with light resistance, partial weight bearing
United fracture	Moderate resistance, weight bearing
Consolidated fracture	Full resistance

should not be prescribed exercises that put external stress through the fracture (Hoppenfeld and Murthy 2000). At this stage the clinician may safely mobilize any non-splinted joints and prescribe static muscle contractions; but should not, as a guideline, prescribe any weight-bearing exercise or exercise using resistance (Figure 9.1).

Many fractures are now managed with open reduction and internal fixation. Open reduction refers to when the fracture fragments are placed into position under direct vision during surgery, and internal fixation is when devices such as screws, plates and nails are used to secure the fracture. With secure fixation, older people may be safely prescribed exercises with light resistance. Light resistance could take the form of exercising in an isometric manner or with elasticized tubing. Typically, patients with securely fixed fractures of the proximal femur, can weight-bear safely (Koval et al 1998).

At the stage of bony union, basic healing has occurred (Adams and Hamblen 1999, Apley and Solomon 1994, Solomon et al 2001) so that stress can be safely put through the fracture during exercise. Exercises in weight-bearing positions or with moderate resistance are appropriate at this stage. For example, after an ankle fracture, a weight-bearing lunge exercise could be prescribed to help the return of ankle dorsiflexion range or a bilateral heel raise exercise could be prescribed to help return of ankle plantar flexor strength. However, at the stage of early union the bone will not have sufficient strength to safely withstand high intensity loads. For this reason, strengthening exercises based on ACSM (1998a) guidelines of 8–12 repetition maximum (Table 9.1) might be unsafe for a person whose fracture is at the stage of early union.

It is only at the stage of fracture consolidation, when the bone is considered to have recovered full strength, that there are no exercise restrictions. Because there are no exercise restrictions at fracture consolidation, this is the stage when sports medicine exercise guidelines might be most appropriate (Table 9.1). However, many older clients with fractures will have been discharged from therapy before reaching the stage of fracture consolidation (Abraham et al 1995, Watt et al 2000). This might explain why sports medicine exercise guidelines are not observed commonly in clinical practice after fracture, since these guidelines do not take account of the restrictions associated with bone healing.

Pain

The presence of pain also governs exercise prescription after fracture. Pain can result directly from the fracture itself, from associated soft tissue injury, from operative procedures to reduce and immobilize the fracture, or as a result of a period of immobilization (Feldt and Finch 2002). Pain following fracture can limit the ability of a person to move the injured part, even in the presence of normal soft tissue structure and function.

Exercise for a person unable to move due to pain will most likely have a different focus than exercises to mobilize and strengthen where soft tissue changes are present. Exercise in the presence of pain might be aimed at modulating or reducing the effect of pain. There is some preliminary evidence from the literature on passive movement that oscillatory movements can be more effective than sustained stretches for increasing range early after wrist fracture where pain is the likely limiting feature (Coyle and Robertson 1998). Consistent with the gate control theory of pain (Melzack and Wall 1965), it is thought that movement may have an important role in pain relief by activating joint receptors (Wyke 1985) or possibly, by activating descending pain inhibitory systems (Wright 1995).

Client safety

Since older people are at high risk of falls and subsequent fractures, client safety also needs to be considered when prescribing exercise. Strategies that can be used by the clinician to ensure safety for the older person exercising after fracture include: starting the exercise with moderate loads (American College of Sports Medicine 1998a, 2002), using fixed equipment such as weight machines or elastic tubing that help stabilize the body rather than free equipment (American College of Sports Medicine 2002), and ensuring safety in exercise set-up, so that the person is not at risk of falling, by providing a nearby support, and by starting the exercise in a posture with a more stable base of support.

Exercise aim

Another important consideration in exercise prescription is the aim of the exercise. Often the aim is to improve muscle strength or muscle endurance, or to increase the range of movement of a joint or muscle. Based on the International Classification of Functioning (ICF) (World Health Organization 2001), these types of exercise target therapy at the level of impairment of body structure and function. This might be appropriate if the person's main problem is muscle weakness or joint stiffness. On the other hand, the person's main problem could be an inability to perform everyday tasks, or restricted societal participation. The assumption that a correlation exists between impairment and activity limitation has been questioned (Jette 1995). An exercise targeted at improving range of motion does not necessarily improve functional tasks. Exercise might be more meaningfully aimed at improving activity limitation if that is the person's main problem. The importance of determining the person's main problem emphasizes the importance of an accurate and thorough clinical assessment before exercise prescription.

To synthesize, a range of clinical reasoning skills are required for optimal exercise prescription after fracture. The exercises prescribed should be based on the clinician's assessment of the main problems affecting the older person, and on the finding of the most likely contributing factors to the main problem. With knowledge about fracture healing and the exercise guidelines from the sports medicine literature, the clinician is in a position to prescribe exercises that will be safe and of optimal benefit. The clinical reasoning approach, with its emphasis on thinking (working out the client's main problem based on assessment) as well as knowledge, is central to clinical practice (Higgs and Jones 1995, Jones 1997). In the following section we will present exercise guidelines suitable for fracture rehabilitation that incorporate a clinical reasoning approach and are based on a synthesis of the sports medicine and fracture literature.

Increasing movement after fracture

Loss of movement is common and substantial after fracture. In particular, a loss of range of movement frequently occurs after the immobilization phase of fracture management (Adams and Hamblen 1999). There may be loss of movement of a part (impairment) or loss of movement of a task (activity limitation) (World Health Organization 2001). Impaired movement can present as reduced range of joint movement or reduced muscle length. For example, immediately after cast removal, older people with a fracture of the distal radius demonstrated an average active range of wrist extension of just under 30–35° compared with 64° on the unaffected wrist (Tremayne et al 2002, Watt et al 2000). Activity limitations related to movement may present as limitations in using the hand for everyday tasks such as dressing, washing, meal preparation, or transfers.

Because movement is often restricted after a fracture, a common goal of exercise therapy is to restore movement. Figure 9.2 displays a decision algorithm for prescribing exercise for increasing movement after fracture whether the loss is of the movement of a part or movement of a task. The algorithm is based on a synthesis of sports medicine literature and evidence in the musculoskeletal and neurological literature and can be used to guide management.

The algorithm involves a decision on whether the main movement problem relates to a specific body part or whether it affects the person at the activity level. Traditionally in musculoskeletal rehabilitation there has been an emphasis on 'relieving pain and restoring full range' (Maitland et al 2001). This approach is based on the assumption that reducing movement impairment will reduce limitations in activity. As mentioned previously, the assumption that a relationship exists between impairment and activity limitation has been questioned (Jette 1995). For example,

Figure 9.2 Decision algorithm for increasing movement after fracture.

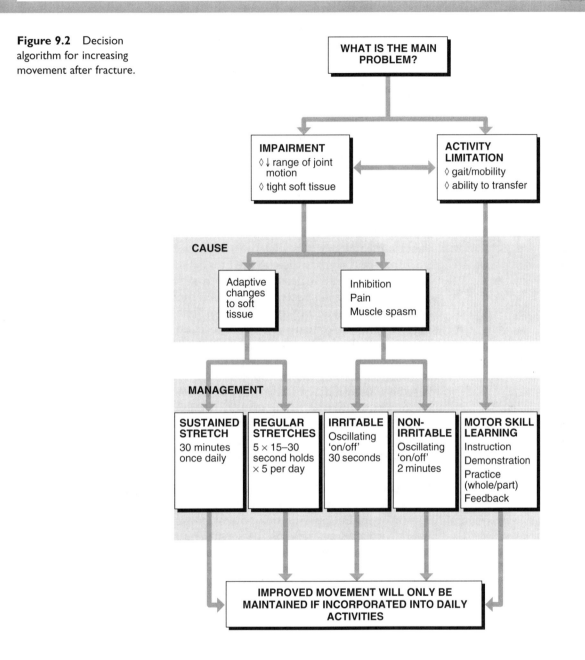

in older people after a fracture of the distal radius, it was shown that only a weak relationship existed between range of movement and functional activity ($0.17 < r_s < 0.55$), as measured by the Jebsen Test of Hand Function (Jebsen et al 1969, Tremayne et al 2002). If rehabilitation is limited to improving impairments, the opportunity to help clients improve the performance of functional activities might be missed (Stevens and Hall 1998).

If the clinician's assessment finds the main problem to be one of activity limitation, it is recommended that therapy be directed towards improving the relevant activities of daily living. Principles of motor skill learning (Schmidt 1999) can be applied to the management of musculoskeletal rehabilitation after fracture. Elements of a motor skill learning approach that may enhance outcome include the provision of information (instruction, demonstration and feedback) and practice (making practice task specific and with more emphasis on practice of the whole task rather than simply the components of the task). To date, a skill training approach has been proposed in the back-care literature (Jull and Richardson 2000, Stevens and Hall 1998), and advocated for musculoskeletal rehabilitation (Carr and Shepherd 1995, Schmidt 1988), but given little consideration in fracture rehabilitation. Despite a lack of empirical evidence, there are theoretical grounds for a motor skill learning approach to be trialled and evaluated in the management of fractures. While particularly relevant for the management of activity limitation, elements of the motor skill learning approach can also be used for exercises directed at impairment.

If assessment indicates that impaired movement is the main problem, or if the clinician suspects that impaired movement is directly related to activity limitations, therapy can be reasonably directed towards increasing range of movement. A crucial decision is whether reduced movement is mainly due to adaptive soft tissue changes or due to inhibition, pain and muscle spasm. As can be seen in Figure 9.2, management is variable depending on the cause of the impairment. This difference can best be illustrated with an example. Consider two older people with an impacted fracture of the neck of humerus, both presenting with an inability to elevate the shoulder beyond 70 degrees. The first person is only 7 days post-fracture and attending therapy for the first time, while the second person is 3 months post-fracture (Table 9.2). The main limitation to shoulder elevation for the first person is likely to be different to the second person. The first person, a few days after impacted fracture of the neck of humerus, is likely to be limited due to pain and muscle spasm or inhibition. For this patient, manipulation under anaesthesia would probably reveal close to normal range of movement, so that the inability to move the shoulder is not related to underlying adaptive soft tissue changes. For the second person, 3 months after impacted fracture of the neck of humerus, the main cause of the limitation is likely to be

Table 9.2 Profiles of two people following impacted fracture of neck of humerus

Person 1		Person 2
80 years old Impacted fracture neck of humerus 7 days ago	**Patient details**	80 years old Impacted fracture neck of humerus 3 months ago
Un-united	**Stage of healing**	Well-united/consolidated
Limited shoulder elevation to 70 degrees	**Main problem**	Limited shoulder elevation to 70 degrees

related to adaptive changes in the muscles and peri-articular structures of the shoulder. A hypothetical manipulation under anaesthesia for this person may well confirm underlying joint stiffness. The appropriate exercise prescription for these two people will be presented in the subsequent sections of this chapter to illustrate the benefit of the decision algorithm (Figure 9.2).

Movement limited by pain or inhibition

Where pain or inhibition limits movement, the algorithm directs the therapist to the performance of oscillatory exercise to increase range of motion. Sustained stretching exercises aimed at increasing soft tissue length are not appropriate, since pain rather than shortened soft tissues limits the movement at this stage. This guideline is based on principles of passive joint mobilizing (Maitland et al 2001).

Passive joint mobilization, as described by Maitland et al (2001), is where oscillatory movements are applied to a joint at various grades and durations depending on the joint's irritability. It has been suggested that passive joint mobilization acts via afferent mediated responses to moderate pain and mediate reflex relaxation, causing an immediate increase in range of movement (Vernon 2000, Wright 1995, Zusman 1992, 1994). The principles of passive joint mobilizing can arguably be applied to exercise prescription to assist in increasing range of motion where pain and inhibition are the limiting factors. There is some empirical evidence for this guideline in the fracture literature, where pain has been the main factor limiting movement. For example, the application of oscillatory movements after wrist fracture was shown to be more beneficial when there was significant pain in the early post-immobilization phase (Coyle and Robertson 1998). Further evidence for the pain moderating effects of oscillatory exercises exists in the back-care literature. Oscillatory exercises, as described by McKenzie (1981), can be of benefit in the management of acute back pain (Maher et al 1999) and passive spinal mobilization can lead to benefits in the acute to subacute phase of spinal pain (Accident Rehabilitation and Compensation Insurance Corporation (ACC) and the National Health Committee 1997, Bigos et al 1994).

Observation of clinicians prescribing exercises during early fracture rehabilitation, suggests that therapeutic exercises are often prescribed in an oscillatory or on/off fashion, rather than as a sustained stretch, as might be expected from the literature on stretching. It is possible that clinicians intuitively find that exercises to increase range may be more effective in the presence of pain, when performed in an oscillatory manner. There has been renewed interest in the role of oscillatory or cyclic stretching and it has been demonstrated that oscillatory stretching can be effective in decreasing short-term ankle stiffness (Bressel and McNair 2002, McNair et al 2001).

This algorithm includes the concept of irritability, central to the Maitland (2001) approach to manual therapy, to direct exercise prescription in the presence of pain. A joint with severe pain that is easily brought on by activity and lasts for a period after cessation of the activity is considered to be 'highly irritable'. If pain is only brought on by a

Figure 9.3 Performing pendular exercises to increase range of shoulder elevation 7 days after an impacted neck of humerus fracture.

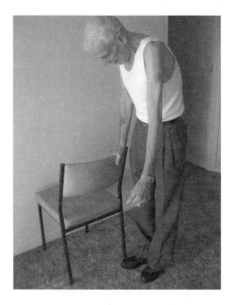

large amount of activity, and then stops immediately, the joint is considered to be non-irritable. A highly irritable joint should be treated for a shorter time (e.g. 30 seconds) by not pushing into resistance, whereas a non-irritable joint may be treated into resistance for longer periods (e.g. sets of 2 minutes) (Magarey 1985, Maitland et al 2001).

The concepts of exercise prescription in the presence of pain and inhibition can best be illustrated using the example of a person with an impacted neck of humerus fracture sustained only 7 days ago (Person 1, Table 9.2). Since the fracture was sustained only 7 days prior, the main limiting factor to shoulder movement would be pain and inhibition rather than soft tissue changes. If the shoulder was considered to be highly irritable, then an appropriate exercise could be pendular exercises, performed in an oscillatory on/off manner for a short time period (30 seconds), repeated a few times each day (Figure 9.3). A higher dosage or a dosage that pushes into range at this stage might prove counter-productive because it could increase pain and therefore increase the risk of ongoing avoidance of shoulder movement and activity limitation.

If the shoulder was determined to be non-irritable, for example if pain was only brought on towards the end of range and was eased immediately, an appropriate exercise might involve oscillatory elevation into resistance for sets of about 2 minutes, as seen in end-of-range pendular exercises.

Movement limited due to adaptive soft tissue changes

Where movement is limited by adaptive changes in the muscles and peri-articular structures of a joint, sustained stretching can be appropriately prescribed to increase movement. The main aim of stretching is to provide sufficient stimulus to cause adaptive changes in the soft tissues limiting the movement (De Deyne 2001, Herbert 1993b). It is important to note that people with such adaptive shortening of soft tissue will also experience discomfort with movement; however, pain will not be the limiting factor.

Short-term or one-off stretching leads only to viscous deformation of tissues (Herbert 1993b) and does not provide sufficient stimulus to make lasting changes to soft tissue. Whether the one-off stretch is maintained for 15, 45 or 120 seconds appears to have little effect on the immediate change in tissue length or viscous deformation (Madding et al 1987). After a one-off stretch soft tissues return to resting length over time, typically within a few hours (Best et al 1994, Magnusson et al 2001, McCarter et al 1971, Moller et al 1985, Zito et al 1997).

The decision algorithm for increasing movement in the presence of soft tissue adaptation (Figure 9.2) includes two possible approaches to providing sufficient stimulus to increase the length of soft tissue: sustained stretching, where a person maintains a stretch for approximately 30 minutes a day, and regular stretching, where a person performs a stretch for a shorter time but performs the exercise a number of times a day. The selection of the most appropriate method is often dependent on the type of exercise (i.e. can it feasibly be sustained for 30 minutes) and the person (i.e. willingness to perform the exercise for sustained periods).

Low load sustained stretching can provide sufficient stimulus to cause adaptive lengthening of soft tissues. Light et al (1984) found that a sustained low load in the form of 5–12 pounds of skin traction for one hour each day was more effective than 15 minutes of high load stretch and passive movement for increasing range of knee extension in people with knee flexion contractures. Sustained stretch for 30 minutes daily has also been demonstrated to increase range of ankle dorsiflexion in patients with neurological disorders (Bohannon and Larkin 1985, Bressel and McNair 2002) and to prevent shortening on otherwise immobilized muscle in an animal model (Williams 1988, 1990). Based on the same principle, sustained increases in range of movement can be accomplished with serial casts (Brouwer et al 2000, Johnson and Siverberg 1995, Moseley 1997) or dynamic splints (Bonutti et al 1994, Flowers and LaStayo 1994, Jansen et al 1996).

The other approach to providing a sufficient stimulus to make adaptive changes in soft tissues is to stretch regularly, so that the soft tissues do not return to resting length (Flowers and LaStayo 1994). Despite considerable research, there is still no consensus on optimal protocols for stretch-induced gains in range of motion (Kisner and Colby 2002). It is proposed that five times 15–60 second holds every 2 hours or five times per day might be expected to effectively keep soft tissues out to length to stimulate adaptive changes (Figure 9.2). Consistent with this, it has been demonstrated that a 15 second hold repeated 10 times through the day is effective in making sustained increase to hamstring muscle length (Gajdosik 1991).

Other protocols have demonstrated sustained gains in muscle length with less frequent stretching. Felund et al (2001) found that four repetitions of 60 seconds of passive stretch applied to the hamstrings of older people five times a week was effective for obtaining sustained changes in

Figure 9.4 Performing wall walk exercise to increase range of shoulder elevation 3 months after an impacted neck of humerus fracture.

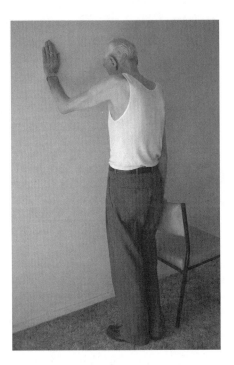

muscle length. A protocol of 30 to 60 seconds of passive stretching completed five times per week has also been effective in increasing muscle length in younger adults (Bandy and Irion 1994, Bandy et al 1997, 1998).

Prescribing an exercise for a person 3 months after an impacted fracture of the neck of humerus (Person 2, Table 9.2) will illustrate the use of the decision algorithm (Figure 9.2) for people with soft tissue adaptation. An appropriate exercise for this person could be five times 30 second holds at end of range of the wall walk exercise to be completed up to five times per day (Figure 9.4). At this stage the fracture would be well healed so there would be little concern about putting too much force through the fracture. This dosage might be expected to provide sufficient stimulus to prevent the soft tissues returning to resting length and so produce adaptive changes. However, based on the findings of Felund et al (2001), exercise frequency of as little as once daily could also be expected to sustain improvement. The exercise could be accompanied by advice to reinforce the improved range in everyday tasks involving the shoulder. In the execution of this exercise, appropriate support should be provided for client safety. Support could be provided by a stable chair or a bench positioned close to the client.

Adaptive changes to soft tissues, either contractile or non-contractile, are achieved in the same manner, with tissues being held out in a lengthened position for a sustained time. When muscles are held in a lengthened position for several weeks, sarcomeres are added in series; that is, structural changes are made (De Deyne 2001). Also, when non-contractile tissues such as peri-articular structures are maintained in stretch, the length of connective tissues increase with adaptive changes (Cummings and Tillman 1992, Kottke et al 1966, Tardieu et al 1982). For the clinician, the distinction between whether joint or muscle is limiting range may not be crucial or change the exercise prescribed.

Apart from static and oscillatory exercises for increasing movement, other techniques such as those based on the proprioceptive neuromuscular facilitation approach have been proposed (Voss et al 1985). These active inhibition techniques such as 'hold–relax' focus on obtaining muscle relaxation just before or during the stretch. Typically therapist controlled, these techniques may lead to short-term lengthening due to elastic changes in actin–myosin overlap (e.g. Cornelius et al 1992). However, on theoretical grounds, it is difficult to see how these short-term therapist intensive techniques, alone, could lead to long-term changes in a person with adaptive soft tissue changes. Moreover, there is a lack of evidence demonstrating the efficacy of these techniques in effecting long-term changes.

In summary, the decision algorithm in Figure 9.2 provides a guide to prescribing exercise to increase movement after fracture. There is still a need for high quality randomized studies to evaluate the lasting effects of stretching exercises on people with restricted movement after fracture (Harvey et al 2002). Issues concerning the stage of fracture healing and client safety must also be taken into account when using the algorithm to guide exercise prescription. Importantly, any gains in movement achieved through exercising need to be incorporated into daily activities to ensure they are maintained.

Exercising muscles after fracture

Older people, as part of normal ageing, demonstrate a significant loss of muscle strength and muscle mass. Muscle strength declines by approximately 15% per decade in the 6th and 7th decade and about 30% thereafter (American College of Sports Medicine 1998b). The effects of fracture and disuse in the form of cast immobilization can lead to further loss of strength for the already weakened older person. Cast immobilization for 6 weeks can lead to strength losses of 60%, and these strength losses are greater if the immobilization follows injury, such as fracture (Bloomfield 1997, Herbert 1993a). Furthermore, strength losses after musculoskeletal injury and surgery can be persistent and long-lasting (Holder-Powell and Rutherford 1999, Reardon et al 2001).

Strength losses after fracture along with the normal decline in strength may have important activity consequences for older people. A strong relationship between quadriceps strength and walking speed in frail older men and women has been demonstrated (Fiatarone et al 1990). In addition, muscle weakness has been related to an increased incidence of falls in older people (Campbell et al 1989, Nevitt et al 1991, Tinetti et al 1988). For these reasons, exercise prescription to retrain muscle is often an important therapeutic goal after fracture in older people. Figure 9.5 displays a decision algorithm for prescribing exercise for retraining muscle after fracture in older people. Similar to the algorithm for restoring movement (Figure 9.2), this algorithm can be used to guide management

Figure 9.5 Decision algorithm for increasing muscle activation after fracture (dosage for muscle strength and muscle endurance adapted from American College of Sports Medicine 1998a, 2002).

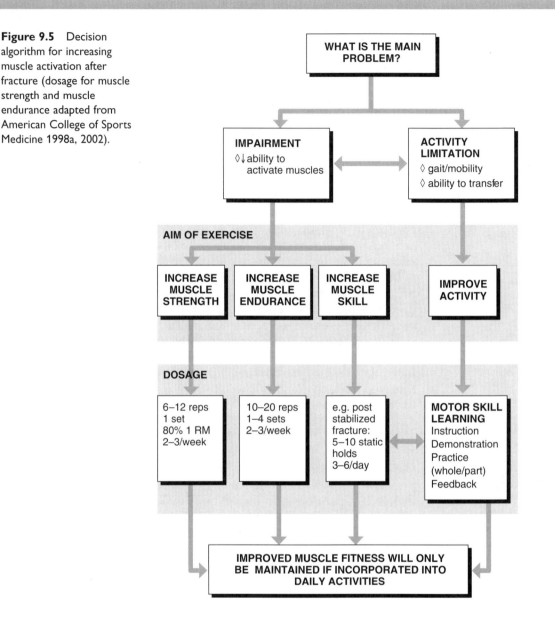

and is based on a synthesis of the sports medicine literature and evidence from the rehabilitation literature.

In retraining muscles after fracture, first, it must be decided whether the main problem is one of impairment or one of activity limitation (Figure 9.5). If the main problem is one of limited activity such as an inability to transfer or go up and down steps independently, the principles of motor skill learning can be applied, with instruction, demonstration, practice of the task and the provision of feedback.

The principle of specificity of training suggests that exercises for muscles will be most effective if closely allied to the task to be improved (American College of Sports Medicine 2002). The responses to strength

Table 9.3	Profiles of two people after fracture of the neck of femur	
Person 3		**Person 4**
77 years old	**Patient details**	77 years old
Fracture neck of femur 2 days ago		Fracture neck of femur 12 weeks ago
Open reduction and internal fixation with a Dynamic hip screw		Open reduction and internal fixation with a Dynamic hip screw
May partially weight-bear		Walking independently with single point stick
Hospital inpatient	**Setting**	Outpatient
Poor quadriceps control	**Main problem**	Poor quadriceps control

training are specific to the muscles trained, to the speed of movement (concentric, isometric, eccentric) (Dudley et al 1991), range of motion (Bandy and Hanten 1993), and even body posture in which the training is performed (Rasch and Morehouse 1957).

Isolated exercises in bed to strengthen the quadriceps and hip extensors may have little carryover to improving the task of rising from sitting (American College of Sports Medicine 2002, Negrete and Brophy 2000). For this reason, the role of generalized non-specific bed exercises in rehabilitation must be questioned (Jesudason and Stiller 2002). The principle of specificity, both from motor skills training principles and from strength training principles, suggests that the greatest benefit will follow from having the person practise the whole task of rising from sitting.

If the main problem is assessed to be one of impairment of the ability to activate muscles, the next decision to be made by the clinician is whether the aim of the exercise is to increase muscle strength, increase muscle endurance, or increase the skill of activating the affected muscles. The main differences at this stage can be illustrated with a clinical example of impaired quadriceps function after fracture of the neck of femur (Table 9.3).

Increasing the skill of muscle activation

For a person 2 days after surgery for a fractured neck of femur (Person 3, Table 9.3), a classic strength training protocol as outlined by the American College of Sports Medicine (2002) would be inappropriate. So soon after injury, the main reasons for poor quadriceps control are not likely to be related to changes in skeletal muscle morphology. Even though some changes in muscle morphology can occur within 3–5 days of injury or surgery (Crane 1977, Reardon et al 2001), the main difficulty at this stage is in activating the available muscle, due to pain and inhibition. Also, the forces and intensity required for a classic strengthening effect may be unsafe for a recently internally fixed, but un-united fracture. At this stage the aim is to improve the *skill* of contracting the quadriceps, rather than increasing the *strength* of the muscle.

Figure 9.6 Performing quadriceps control exercises with therapist assistance 2 days after surgery for fractured neck of femur.

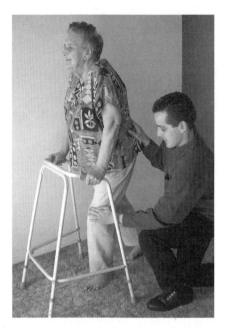

An appropriate exercise for a person 2 days after surgery for a fractured neck of femur would be to practise quadriceps control in stride standing. The quadriceps contraction could be stimulated by gentle weight transference onto the affected leg. To minimize inhibition due to pain the exercise should be timed to coincide with maximal pain cover from medication. For safety, the person would need to be supervised and would require support (e.g. from a walking frame) (Figure 9.6). Principles of skill training could be applied by the clinician with appropriate cueing by voice and touch, practice and feedback. There are no clear guidelines for the optimal dosage, although clinicians often prescribe 5–10 holds repeated a number of times throughout the day in this situation. The advantage of performing the exercises in a closed chain manner in standing means that there is likely to be greater carryover to functional activity (Negrete and Brophy 2000), assuming the clinician wants to improve quadriceps function so that the person can walk safely, without the affected leg collapsing.

Increasing muscle strength

For a person seen 3 months after a fracture of the neck of femur (Person 4, Table 9.3), also with impaired quadriceps function, the aim may be to increase the strength of the muscle. After three months there is likely to be disuse atrophy of the quadriceps. Also the fracture is likely to be well-healed (either well-united or consolidated), so that there are no contraindications to placing forces through the hip.

The key principles of strength training have essentially remained unchanged since the early work of DeLorme and Watkins (1948): apply sufficient resistance to get fatigue in 10 to 12 repetitions or less, and regularly progress or increase the resistance to provide enough stimulus for

Figure 9.7 Performing double quarter-squats to strengthen quadriceps 3 months after surgery for fractured neck of femur.

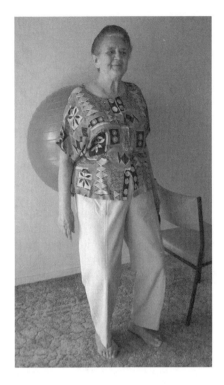

continued strengthening. Recent guidelines suggest that a person three months after surgery for a fractured neck of femur will achieve an optimal strengthening effect to the quadriceps from completing one set of 6–12 repetitions at 80% of 1 RM, with the exercise completed three days per week (American College of Sports Medicine 2002).

An appropriate exercise for a person 3 months after a fractured neck of femur would be a double quarter-squat, completing one set of 12 repetitions every second day (Figure 9.7). The load should be such that the person can only complete 12 repetitions of the exercise with good form. Load can be adjusted and progressed by using a weighted backpack or progressing to a single leg squat. Based on the principle of specificity, traditional open chain exercises such as knee extension on a weight machine or with ankle cuff weights are not as highly recommended; these may not be expected to carry over as much into weight-bearing tasks such as rising from sitting and walking (Negrete and Brophy 2000). Since the person may have a history of falls, safety remains an important consideration. The client should be supervised when first completing the exercise and should have hand support nearby.

It appears that the strength training protocols most often applied to young athletes can also be applied safely to older people with a well-healed fracture, with little modification required (Hauer et al 2001, 2002, Mitchell et al 2001). Hauer et al (2001, 2002) implemented a 12-week strength training programme for older people (mean 81.7 years) 6–8 weeks after hip fracture. Participants in the study completed two sets of leg press, hip abduction and plantar flexion exercises with resistance set at 70–90% of maximal workload. The patients in the intervention group increased muscle strength, and improved activity in walking, rising from sitting and stair climbing, compared with the control group. Importantly, the programme was completed with high adherence (93.1%) and it was noted that no major health problems occurred during testing or training, with minor problems such as aching muscles after initial training and scar aching resolved with adjustment of training and physiotherapy (Hauer et al 2001, 2002, Mitchell et al 2001). Although it has been recommended that to minimize the risk of injury older people might start their strengthening programmes with slightly lesser loads (10–15 RM) (American College of Sports Medicine 1998a), there have been surprisingly few injuries after strength training in older people (Pollock et al 1991). There has also been considerable debate over whether people should exercise with one or multiple sets. It appears, at least for the previously untrained person, that there may be little further strength gain from completing multiple sets of an exercise (American College of Sports Medicine 2002).

Isometric exercise may also have a role in exercise prescription after fracture in older people. Isometric exercise occurs when no change in muscle length accompanies tension development. An exercise dose of 5–10 isometric holds at 66% of maximal voluntary contraction (MVC) can be effective in increasing muscle strength (Moffatt and Cucuzzo 1993). The American College of Sports Medicine (1998a) recommends that dynamic strength training is preferable to isometric exercise, as the dynamic exercises best mimic everyday activities. The main limitation of isometric strength training is that the strengthening effect is limited to the joint angle at which the exercise is performed. However, in the situation where a muscle group acts as a stabilizer, rather than a prime mover, such as the hip abductors during walking, isometric exercises may be applicable. Also, isometric exercises may be appropriate if there are safety concerns with moving into a part of the range, such as the risk of early dislocation following a fractured neck of femur managed with a hemi-arthroplasty.

For a person 3 months after surgery for a fractured neck of femur (Person 4, Table 9.3), the clinician may also aim to increase muscle endurance. Muscle endurance is the ability to sustain repeated contractions of a given force over an extended time. The goal of muscular endurance may be relevant after fracture in older people in assisting with weakness associated with repetitive functional activities. For example, during the loading response phase of walking, the quadriceps act eccentrically for a short period. The limiting factor for a patient may be the ability to sustain repeated sub-maximal contractions (endurance) rather than the ability to generate a force against a given resistance (strength).

For optimal endurance, it has been recommended that increased repetitions with a slightly lesser load be used, e.g. 1–4 sets of 10–20 repetitions, completed 2–3 days each week (American College of Sports Medicine 2002). However, strength training dosages also improve muscle endurance. Strength training in older people produced significant increases in muscular endurance as assessed by activities such as walking endurance (Ades et al 1996, McCartney et al 1995, 1996) and specific muscle endurance (Adams et al 2001). Similar effects might also be found after fractures in older people. Therefore, the clinician aiming to improve muscle endurance can choose either a strengthening or endurance dosage (Figure 9.5).

Aerobic activities such as walking, swimming and cycling may have an important role to play during rehabilitation after fracture in older people. Aerobic exercise can have positive benefits on many of the chronic diseases that older people with a fracture often demonstrate as co-morbidities, such as coronary artery disease (American College of Sports Medicine 1994), hypertension (American College of Sports Medicine 1993), osteoporosis (American College of Sports Medicine 1995) and obesity (American College of Sports Medicine 1983). Aerobic activity is recommended for at least 20 minutes for 3–5 days per week at an intensity of at least 55% of maximum heart rate (American College of Sports Medicine 1998a). The absolute heart rate to achieve this training threshold may be as low as 105–115 beats per minute.

The focus in exercise prescription for older adults after fracture in clinical practice and in this chapter has been on recovery of function. The guidelines have been directed towards guiding the clinician to assist in *recovery of function*, by reducing impairment of movement or muscle weakness or in reducing activity limitation. This focus reflects clinical practice where patients are often discharged from therapy when safe for home discharge or after a small number of treatments aimed at impairments in an outpatient setting.

However, there are strong arguments that exercise may have an important role in *preventing future problems* for older people after fracture. Exercise may have an important role in addressing risk factors for subsequent fractures, through the prevention of falls and osteoporosis. Exercise, including strength and balance training, can be effective in lowering falls risk in older people (Campbell et al 1997, Gardner et al 2000). Also, there is evidence that exercise programmes involving both weight-bearing aerobic and strengthening components can help to preserve bone strength in older people (Kelley 1998, Kelley et al 2001). As the risk of fracture increases after the first fracture, and the initial fracture is often under-treated (Sambrook et al 2002), exercise may have an important role in managing the risk of future fracture and disability in older people.

Conclusion

These exercise guidelines are based on a synthesis of the sports medicine, fracture, and rehabilitation literature, emphasizing clinical reasoning. The guidelines are based on theory, available empirical evidence and reflect clinical practice, as we have observed it. It must be acknowledged that a relative dearth of quality experimental evidence exists to guide exercise prescription. The guidelines provide a model that can be applied in clinical practice as well as be formally tested and refined as new evidence becomes available.

References

Abraham B, d'Espaignet E, Stevenson C 1995 Australian health trends 1995. Australian Institute of Health and Welfare, Canberra

Accident Rehabilitation and Compensation Insurance Corporation (ACC) and the National Health Committee 1997 New Zealand acute low back pain guide. ACC, Wellington

Adams J C, Hamblen D L 1999 Outline of fractures including joint injuries, 11th edn. Churchill Livingstone, Edinburgh

Adams K J, Swank A M, Berning J M, et al 2001 Progressive strength training in sedentary, older African American women. Medicine and Science in Sports and Exercise 33(9):1567–1576

Ades P A, Ballor D L, Ashikaga T, Utton J L, Nair K S 1996 Weight training improves walking endurance in healthy elderly persons. Annals of Internal Medicine 124(6):568–572

American College of Sports Medicine 1983 Position stand: proper and improper weight loss programs. Medicine and Science in Sports and Exercise 15:9–13

American College of Sports Medicine 1993 Position stand: physical activity, physical fitness, and hypertension. Medicine and Science in Sports and Exercise 25:1–10

American College of Sports Medicine 1994 Position stand: exercise for patients with coronary artery disease. Medicine and Science in Sports and Exercise 26:1–5

American College of Sports Medicine 1995 ACSM position stand on osteoporosis and exercise. Medicine and Science in Sports and Exercise 27:1–7

American College of Sports Medicine 1998a Position stand: the recommended quantity and quality of exercise for developing and maintaining cardiorespiratory and muscular fitness, and flexibility in healthy adults. Medicine and Science in Sports and Exercise 30:975–991

American College of Sports Medicine 1998b Exercise and physical activity for older adults. Medicine and Science in Sports and Exercise 30:992–1008

American College of Sports Medicine 2002 Progression models in resistance training for healthy adults. Medicine and Science in Sports and Exercise 34:364–380

Apley A G, Solomon L 1994 Concise system of orthopaedics and fractures, 2nd edn. Butterworth-Heinemann, Oxford

Bandy W D, Hanten W P 1993 Changes in torque and electromyographic activity of the quadriceps femoris muscles following isometric training. Physical Therapy 73:455–467

Bandy W D, Irion J M 1994 The effect of time on static stretch on the flexibility of the hamstring muscles. Physical Therapy 74(9):845–850

Bandy W D, Irion J M, Briggler M 1997 The effect of time and frequency of static stretching on flexibility of hamstring muscles. Physical Therapy 77(10):1090–1096

Bandy W D, Irion J M, Briggler M 1998 The effect of static stretch and dynamic range of motion training on the flexibility of the hamstring muscles. Journal of Orthopaedic and Sports Physical Therapy 27(4):295–300

Best T M, McElhaney J, Garrett W E, Myers B S 1994 Characterisation of the passive responses of live skeletal muscle using the quasi-linear theory of viscoelasticity. Journal of Biomechanics 27:413–419

Bigos S, Bowyer O, Braen G 1994 Acute low back problems in adults. Clinical practice guideline no 14. Agency for Health Care Policy and Research, USA

Bloomfield S A 1997 Changes in musculoskeletal structure and function with prolonged bed rest. Medicine and Science in Sports and Exercise 29(2):197–206

Bohannon R W, Larkin P A 1985 Passive ankle dorsiflexion increases in patients after a regimen of tilt table-wedge board standing: a clinical report. Physical Therapy 65(11):1676–1678

Bonutti P M, Windau J E, Ables B A, Miller B G 1994 Static progressive stretch to re-establish elbow range of motion. Clinical Orthopaedics and Related Research 303:128–134

Bressel E, McNair P J 2002 The effect of prolonged static and cyclic stretching on ankle joint stiffness, torque relaxation, and gait in people with stroke. Physical Therapy 82(9):880–887

Brouwer B, Davidson L K, Olney S J 2000 Serial casting in idiopathic toe-walkers and children with spastic cerebral palsy. Journal of Pediatric Orthopedics 20(2):221–225

Campbell A J, Reinken J, Allan B C, Martinez G S 1981 Falls in old age: a study of frequency and related clinical factors. Age and Ageing 10(4):264–270

Campbell A J, Borrie M J, Spears G F 1989 Risk factors for falls in a community based prospective study of people 70 years and older. Journals of Gerontology. Series A. Biological Sciences and Medical Sciences 44:112–117

Campbell A J, Robertson M C, Gardner M M, et al 1997 Randomised controlled trial of a general practice programme of home-based exercise to prevent falls in elderly women. British Medical Journal 315:1065–1069

Carr J, Shepherd R 1995 Skill learning after musculoskeletal lesions. In: Gass E M (ed) Musculoskeletal physiotherapy: clinical science and practice. Butterworth-Heinemann, Oxford, p 32–44

Center J R, Nguyen T V, Schneider D, Sambrook P N, Eisman J A 1999 Mortality after all major types of osteoporotic fracture in men and women: an observational study. Lancet 353:878–882

Cornelius W L, Ebrahim K, Watson J, Hill D W 1992 The effects of cold application and modified PNF stretching techniques on hip joint flexibility in college males. Research Quarterly for Exercise and Sport 63(3):311–314

Coyle J A, Robertson V J 1998 Comparison of two passive mobilizing techniques following Colles' fracture: a multi-centre design. Manual Therapy 3(1):34–41

Crane C 1977 Protein turnover in patients before and after elective orthopaedic operations. British Journal of Surgery 64:129–133

Cuddihy M T, Gabriel S E, Crowson C S, O'Fallon W M, Melton L J 1999 Forearm fractures as predictors of subsequent osteoporotic fractures. Osteoporosis International 9:469–475

Cummings G S, Tillman L J 1992 Remodeling of dense connective tissue in normal adult tissues. In: Nelson R M (ed) Dynamics of human biologic tissues. F A Davis Company, Philadelphia

de Bruijn H P 1987 Functional treatment of Colles fracture. Acta Orthopaedica Scandinavica 58 (Suppl):1–90

De Deyne P G 2001 Application of passive stretch and its implications for muscle fibers. Physical Therapy 81(2):819–827

DeLorme T L, Watkins A L 1948 Techniques of progressive resistance exercise. Archives of Physical Medicine 29:263–273

Dudley G A, Tesch P A, Harris R T, Golden C L, Buchanan P 1991 Influence of eccentric actions on the metabolic cost of resistance exercise. Aviation Space and Environmental Medicine 62:678–682

Dzupa V, Bartonicek J, Skala-Rosenbaum J, Prikazsky V 2002 Mortality in patients with proximal femoral fractures during the first year after the injury. Acta Chirurgiae Orthopaedicae et Traumatologiae Cechoslovaca 69(1):39–44

Feldt K S, Finch M 2002 Older adults with hip fractures. Treatment of pain following hospitalization. Journal of Gerontological Nursing 28(8):27–35

Felund J B, Myrer J W, Schulthies S S, Fellingham G W, Meason G W 2001 The effect of duration of stretching of the hamstring muscle group for increasing range of motion in people aged 65 years or older. Physical Therapy 81(5):1111–1117

Fiatarone M A, Marks E C, Ryan N D, et al 1990 High-intensity strength training in nonagenarians: effects on skeletal muscle. JAMA 263: 3029–3034

Flowers K R, LaStayo P 1994 Effect of total end of range time on improving passive range of motion. Journal of Hand Therapy 7:150–157

Gajdosik R 1991 Effects of static stretching on the maximal length and resistance to passive stretch of short hamstring muscles. Journal of Orthopaedic and Sports Physical Therapy 14:250–255

Gardner M M, Robertson M C, Campbell A J 2000 Exercise in preventing falls and fall related injuries in older people: a review of randomised controlled trials. British Journal of Sports Medicine 34:7–17

Harvey L, Herbert R, Crosbie J 2002 Does stretching induce lasting increases in joint ROM? A systematic review. Physiotherapy Research International 7(1):1–13

Hauer K, Rost B, Rutschle K, et al 2001 Exercise training for rehabilitation and secondary prevention of falls in geriatric patients with a history of falls. Journal of the American Geriatrics Society 49:10–21

Hauer K, Specht N, Schuler M, Bartsch P, Oster P 2002 Intensive physical training in geriatric patients after severe falls and hip surgery. Age and Ageing 31:49–57

Herbert R 1983a Human strength adaptations – implications for therapy. In: McConnell J (ed) Key issues in musculoskeletal physiotherapy. Butterworth Heinemann, Oxford, p. 142–171

Herbert R 1993b Preventing and treating stiff joints. In: McConnell J (ed) Key issues in musculoskeletal physiotherapy. Butterworth-Heinemann, Oxford, p. 114–141

Higgs J, Jones M 1995 Clinical reasoning in the health professions. Butterworth-Heinemann, Oxford

Holder-Powell H M, Rutherford O M 1999 Unilateral lower limb injury: its long-term effects on quadriceps, hamstring, and plantarflexor muscle strength. Archives of Physical Medicine and Rehabilitation 80(6):717–720

Hoppenfeld S, Murthy V L 2000 Treatment and rehabilitation of fractures. Lippincott Williams & Wilkins, Philadelphia

Jansen C M, Windau J E, Bonutti P M, Brillhart M V 1996 Treatment of a knee contracture using a knee orthosis incorporating stress-relaxation techniques. Physical Therapy 76(2):182–186

Jebsen R H, Taylor N, Trieschmann R B, Trotter M J, Howard L A 1969 An objective and standardized test of hand function. Archives of Physical Medicine and Rehabilitation 63:335–338

Jesudason C, Stiller K 2002 Are bed exercises necessary following hip arthroplasty? Australian Journal of Physiotherapy 48(3):73–81

Jette A M 1995 Outcomes research: Shifting the dominant research paradigm in physical therapy. Physical Therapy 75(1):965–970

Johnson J, Siverberg R 1995 Serial casting of the lower extremity to correct contractures during the acute phase of burn care. Physical Therapy 75(4):262–266

Jones G, Nguyen T, Sambrook P N, Kelly P J, Eisman J A 1994 Symptomatic fracture incidence in elderly men and women: the Dubbo Osteoporosis Epidemiology Study (DOES). Osteoporosis International 4(5):277–282

Jones M 1997 Clinical reasoning: the foundation of clinical practice: part 1. Australian Journal of Physiotherapy 43(3):167–170

Jull G A, Richardson C A 2000 Motor control problems in patients with spinal pain: a new direction for therapeutic exercise. Journal of Manipulative and Physiological Therapeutics 23(2):115–117

Kanis J A, Johnell O, Oden A, et al 2000 Risk of hip fracture according to the World Health Organization criteria for osteopenia and osteoporosis. Bone 27(5):585–590

Keene G, Parker M, Pryor G 1993 Mortality and morbidity after hip fractures. British Medical Journal 307:1248–1250

Kelley G A 1998 Aerobic exercise and lumbar spine bone mineral density in post-menopausal women: a meta-analysis. Journal of the American Geriatrics Society 46:143–152

Kelley G A, Kelley K S, Tran Z V 2001 Resistance training and bone mineral density in women: a meta-analysis of controlled trials. American Journal of Physical Medicine and Rehabilitation 80:65–77

Kisner C, Colby L E 2002 Stretching, therapeutic exercise: foundations and techniques, 4th edn. F A Davis Company, Philadelphia, p 171–215

Kottke F J, Pauley D L, Ptak R A 1966 The rationale for prolonged stretching for correction of shortening of connective tissue. Archives of Physical Medicine and Rehabilitation 47(6):345–352

Koval K J, Zuckerman J D 1994 Functional recovery after fracture of the hip. Journal of Bone and Joint Surgery 76A(5):751–758

Koval K J, Sala D A, Kummer F J, Zuckerman J D 1998 Postoperative weight-bearing after a fracture of the femoral neck or an intertrochanteric fracture. Journal of Bone and Joint Surgery 80A(3):352–356

Light K E, Nuzik S, Personius W, Barstrom A 1984 Low-load prolonged stretch vs high-load brief stretch in treating knee contractures. Physical Therapy 64(3):330–333

Looker A C, Orwoll E S, Johnston C C, et al 1997 Prevalence of low femoral bone density in older U.S. adults from NHANES III. Journal of Bone Mineral Research 12(11):1769–1771

MacDermid J C, Richards R S, Roth J H 2001 Distal radius fracture: a prospective outcome study of 275 patients. Journal of Hand Therapy 14(2):154–169

Madding S, Wong J, Hallium A, Medeiros J 1987 Effect of duration of passive stretch on hip abduction range of motion. Journal of Orthopaedic and Sports Physical Therapy 8:409–416

Magarey M 1985 Selection of passive treatment techniques. Paper presented at the 4th Biennial Conference of the Manipulative Therapists Association of Australia, Brisbane

Magnusson S P, Aagaard P, Rosager S, Dyhre-Poulsen P, Kjaer M 2001 Load–displacement properties of human triceps surae aponeurosis in vivo. Journal of Physiology 531:277–288

Maher C, Latimer J, Refshauge K M 1999 Prescription of activity for low back pain: what works? Australian Journal of Physiotherapy 45:121–132

Maitland G D, Banks K, English K, Hengeveld E 2001 Maitland's vertebral manipulation, 6th edn. Butterworth-Heinemann, Oxford

March L M, Cameron I D, Cumming R G, et al 2000 Mortality and morbidity after hip fracture: can evidence-based clinical pathways make a difference? Journal of Rheumatology 27(9):2227–2231

Masud T, Jordan D, Hosking D J 2001 Distal forearm fracture history in an older community-dwelling population: the Nottingham Community Osteoporosis (NOCOS) study. Age and Ageing 30(3):255–258

McCarter R J, Nabarro F R, Wyndham C H 1971 Reversibility of the passive length-tension relation in mammalian skeletal muscle. Archives Internationales de Physiologie et de Biochimie 79(3):469–479

McCartney N, Hicks A, Martin J, Webber C E 1995 Long-term resistance training in the elderly: effects on dynamic strength, exercise capacity, muscle, and bone. Journal of Gerontology: Biological Sciences 50A(2):B97–104

McCartney N, Hicks A, Martin J, Webber C E 1996 A longitudinal trial of weight training in the elderly: continued improvements in year 2. Journal of Gerontology: Biological Sciences 51A(6):B425–433

McKenzie R A 1981 The lumbar spine; mechanical diagnosis and therapy. Spinal Publications, Waikanae

McNair P J, Dombroski E W, Hewson D J, Stanley S N 2001 Stretching at the ankle joint: viscoelastic responses to holds and continuous passive motion. Medicine and Science in Sports and Exercise 33(3):354–358

Melzack R, Wall P D 1965 Pain mechanisms: a new theory. Science 150:971–979

Mitchell S L, Stott D J, Martin B J, Grant S J 2001 Randomized controlled trial of quadriceps training after proximal femoral fracture. Clinical Rehabilitation 15(3):282–290

Moffatt R J, Cucuzzo N 1993 Strength considerations for exercise prescription, ACSM's resource manual for guidelines for exercise testing and prescription, 2nd edn. Lea & Febiger, Philadelphia

Moller M, Ekstrand J, Oberg B, Gillquist J 1985 Duration of stretching effect on range of motion in lower extremities. Archives of Physical Medicine and Rehabilitation 66(3):171–173

Moseley A M 1997 The effect of casting combined with stretching on passive ankle dorsiflexion in adults with traumatic head injuries. Physical Therapy 77(3):240–247

Negrete R, Brophy J 2000 The relationship between isokinetic open and closed chain lower extremity strength and functional performance. Journal of Sport Rehabilitation 9:46–61

Nevitt M C, Cummings S R, Hudes E S 1991 Risk factors for injurious falls: a prospective study. Journals of Gerontology. Series A Biological Sciences and Medical Sciences 46:154–170

Nguyen T V, Center J R, Sambrook P N, Eisman J A 2001 Risk factors for proximal humerus, forearm, and wrist fractures in elderly men and women: the Dubbo Osteoporosis Epidemiology Study. American Journal of Epidemiology 153(6):587–595

Pollock M L, Carroll J F, Graves J E, et al 1991 Injuries and adherence to walk/jog and resistance training programs in the elderly. Medicine and Science in Sports and Exercise 23(10):1194–1200

Rasch P J, Morehouse L E 1957 Effect of static and dynamic exercises on muscular strength and hypertrophy. Journal of Applied Physiology 11:29–34

Reardon K, Galea M, Dennett X, Choong P, Byrne E 2001 Quadriceps muscle wasting persists 5 months after total hip arthroplasty for osteoarthritis of the hip: a pilot study. Internal Medicine Journal 31:7–14

Ross P D, Davis J W, Epstein R S, Wasnich R D 1991 Pre-existing fractures and bone mass predict vertebral fracture in women. Annals of Internal Medicine 114:919–923

Sambrook P N, Seeman E, Phillips S R, Ebeling P R 2002 Preventing osteoporosis: outcomes of the Australian Fracture Prevention Summit. Medical Journal of Australia 176 (Suppl):1–16

Schmidt R A 1988 Motor control and learning: a behavioural emphasis, 2nd edn. Human Kinetics, Champaign, IL

Schmidt R A 1999 Motor control and learning: a behavioural emphasis, 3rd edn. Human Kinetics, Champaign, IL

Sherrington C, Lord S R 1997 Home exercise to improve strength and walking velocity after hip fracture. Archives of Physical Medicine and Rehabilitation 78:208–212

Solomon L, Warwick D, Nayagam S 2001 Apley's system of orthopaedics and fractures, 8th edn. Arnold, London

Stevens J, Hall K G 1998 Motor skill acquisition strategies for rehabilitation of low back pain. Journal of Orthopaedic and Sports Physical Therapy 28(3):165–167

Swanson C E, Day G A, Yelland C E, et al 1998 The management of elderly patients with femoral fractures. A randomised controlled trial of early intervention versus standard care. Medical Journal of Australia 169(10):515–518

Tardieu C, Tabary J C, Tabary C, Tardieu G 1982 Adaptation of connective tissue length to immobilization in the lengthened and shortened positions in the cat soleus muscle. Journal de Physiologie 78(2):214–220

Tinetti M E, Speechley M, Ginter S F 1988 Risk factors for falls among elderly persons living in the community. New England Journal of Medicine 319:1701–1707

Tremayne A, Taylor N F, McBurney H, Baskus K 2002 Correlation of impairment and activity limitation after wrist fracture. Physiotherapy Research International 7(2):90–99

Vernon H 2000 Qualitative review of studies of manipulative-induced hypoalgesia. Journal of Manipulative and Physiological Therapeutics 23(2):134–138

Voss D E, Ionla M K, Myers B J 1985 Proprioceptive neuromuscular facilitation, 3rd edn. Harper & Row, Philadelphia

Wakefield A E, McQueen M M 2000 The role of physiotherapy and clinical predictors of outcome after fracture of the distal radius. Journal of Bone and Joint Surgery 82B(7):972–976

Watt C F, Taylor N F, Baskus K 2000 Do Colles' fracture patients benefit from routine referral to physiotherapy following cast removal? Archives of Orthopaedic and Trauma Surgery 120(7/8):413–415

Williams P E 1988 Effect of intermittent stretch on immobilised muscle. Annals of the Rheumatic Diseases 47(12):1014–1016

Williams P E 1990 Use of intermittent stretch in the prevention of serial sarcomere loss in immobilised muscle. Annals of the Rheumatic Diseases 49:316–317

World Health Organization 1994 Assessment of fracture risk and its application to screening for osteoporosis: report of WHO study group. World Health Organization, Geneva

World Health Organization 2001 ICF: International Classification of Functioning, Disability and Health: short version. World Health Organization, Geneva

Wright A 1995 Hypoalgesia post-manipulative therapy: a review of a potential neurophysiological mechanism. Manual Therapy 1:11–16

Wyke B D 1985 Articular neurology and manipulative therapy. In: Glasgow E F (ed) Aspects of manipulative therapy. Churchill Livingstone, Edinburgh

Zito M, Driver D, Parker C, Bohannon R 1997 Lasting effects of one bout of two 15-second passive stretches on ankle dorsiflexion range of motion. Journal of Orthopaedic and Sports Physical Therapy 26(4):214–221

Zusman M 1992 Central nervous system contribution to mechanically produced motor and sensory responses. Australian Journal of Physiotherapy 38:245–255

Zusman M 1994 The meaning of mechanically produced responses. Australian Journal of Physiotherapy 40:35–39

10

Physical activity and exercise in people with osteoarthritis

Adrian M M Schoo and Meg E Morris

CHAPTER CONTENTS

Epidemiology, aetiology and symptoms 214

Therapeutic exercise in the management of osteoarthritis 217

Clinical recommendations 222

Conclusion 223

References 223

In this chapter we explore the epidemiology, aetiology and symptoms of osteoarthritis (OA) and evaluate the outcomes of physical activity programmes and therapeutic exercises for older adults with knee or hip OA. The factors that affect adherence to home exercise programmes in people with OA are also examined and recommendations are made for reducing impairments and activity limitations in people with this disabling condition.

Osteoarthritis is a common musculoskeletal condition in Western societies (Hill et al 1999, Odding et al 1998). It is estimated that around 68% of people in the USA who are over 55 years of age have radiographic signs of OA in one or more joints (Elders 2000). The 'Rotterdam Study' in the Netherlands showed evidence of hip OA in 14.1% of men and 16% of women aged 55 and over, and knee OA in 16% of the men and 29% of the women in this age group (Odding et al 1998). These findings are comparable with North American studies (Felson et al 1995, Oliveria et al 1995). As well as the costs to governments and communities, OA can be costly for individuals, both financially and in terms of disability. People with OA incur greater medical charges than do healthy people of similar age (Gabriel et al 1997). Medical charges are mainly for diagnostic and therapeutic procedures and for prescribed pharmaceuticals. The direct medical costs for OA are on average $US2650 per person annually, compared with only around US$1400 for those without the disease (Gabriel et al 1997). Pain, swelling, restricted range of movement and muscle weakness can limit physical activity and restrict participation in community life.

Physical activity and therapeutic exercises for people with OA have the potential to reduce pain (Kovar et al 1992, Van Baar et al 1998), delay the onset or rate of progression of impairments and disabilities (Ettinger et al 1997) and reduce healthcare costs (Gabriel et al 1997). The American College of Rheumatology guidelines for the management of OA recommend regular exercise and physical activity for people with this progressive condition (Hochberg et al 1995a, 1995b). Physical activity can be defined as 'any skeletal muscle activity that results in energy expenditure' (Casperen et al 1985, p. 129). Therapeutic exercises are 'planned, structured, repetitive movement designed to improve or maintain some component of physical fitness' (Casperen et al 1985, p. 129).

Epidemiology, aetiology and symptoms

Epidemiology and impact of osteoarthritis

Osteoarthritis is a leading cause of disability in North America (Badley and Crotty 1995, Gabriel 1996). In Canada, 18% of people 16 years and older have symptoms of arthritis (mainly OA) and 2.5% of the total Canadian population have long-term disability due to arthritis (Badley 1995). Similarly, for the USA, 15% of people 16 years and older are reported to have arthritis and 2.8% have long-term disabilities arising from the disease (Badley 1995).

Advanced age is a major predictor of lower limb OA, particularly for those 50 years and older (Felson et al 1997, Lethbridge-Cejku et al 1994, Oliveria et al 1995). Female gender is another factor associated with increased incidence (March et al 1998, Victorian Department of Human Services 2000). In a North American study, Felson et al (1995) found the incidence of OA to be 1.7 times higher in women than men. Felson et al found that 2% of women developed radiographic detectable OA annually and 4% experienced progression of earlier diagnosed OA.

Osteoarthritis is associated with reduced life expectancy due to its co-morbidities (Gabriel et al 1999). For example, there is a relationship between OA of the knees/hips and cardiovascular disease (Philbin et al 1996, Ries et al 1995). This appears to occur because people with advanced OA move less frequently and have lower levels of physical activity than able-bodied people (Bank et al 1997). The disease is also associated with gastrointestinal problems, possibly due to the use of non-steroid anti-inflammatory drugs (Gabriel et al 1999). An increased incidence of depression has been reported (Egberts et al 1997, Hopman-Rock et al 1997a), although it is not clear whether this is due to concomitant pain, disability, restrictions in societal roles or other factors.

Aetiology of osteoarthritis

Osteoarthritis is a disorder associated with focal destruction of articular cartilage followed by changes in subchondral bone structure (Imhof et al

1997). Bony sclerosis and formation of osteophytes are common (Dieppe et al 1997). Other joint changes can include joint space narrowing, micro-fractures and joint swelling (Dieppe 1997). There is growing evidence that a genetic predisposition to OA exists. For example, a study on twins found the heritable component of OA to be up to 65% for articular joints (Spector et al 1996). Mutations in type II collagen and alterations in cartilage or bone metabolism have also been associated with some forms of OA (Cicuttini and Spector 1996). Generalized 'nodal' OA (Heberden's, Bouchard's) also has a hereditary component (Marks et al 1979).

Obesity is a well-accepted risk factor for premature OA of the knees (Anderson and Felson 1988, Cicuttini et al 1997, Hochberg et al 1995c) and hips (Tepper and Hochberg 1993). Data from the Framingham study showed the risk of developing knee OA to increase four-fold in obese individuals (Felson 1995). Participants in the Framingham study were examined for the presence of OA from 1983 to 1985, and also between 1992 and 1993 (Felson et al 1988, 1992, 1995, 1997). The medical examination included an antero-posterior weight-bearing radiograph, measurement of body mass and quantification of knee pain. People were asked if they experienced: (i) knee pain in or around the joint on most days of the month; and (ii) if there was current pain. Osteoarthritis was defined as symptomatic when the roentgenogram showed OA changes greater than or equal to grade 2 on the Kellgren/Lawrence scale (definite osteophytes with possible joint space narrowing) and knee pain was present.

One of the criticisms of the Framingham study is that it measured outcome using the Kellgren/Lawrence scale which assumes a set sequence in the progression of OA. The scale also lacks sensitivity because it gives greater weight to the presence of osteophytes whilst attaching less value to joint space narrowing (Kallman et al 1989). Another criticism of the Framingham study relates to the definition of a 'symptomatic' joint, which Felson et al (1995) defined as the person experiencing pain in or around the knee on most days of the month. There is growing evidence that pain varies to a greater extent than this (Dieppe et al 1997). The relationships between clinical symptoms such as pain and radiographic changes at the knee joint also remain unclear (Dieppe et al 1997). For example, the Bristol 'OA500' study which documented the progression of OA over a 3-year period found that radiographic changes were not reliable indices of clinical outcome in OA.

Prolonged strenuous physical activity has also been shown to be a predictor of OA in several studies (Felson et al 1997, Simpson and Kanter 1997, Spector et al 1996b). Forces on articular cartilage arising from heavy or sustained physical activities or exercises can be substantial and may lead to joint damage and pain (Simpson and Kanter 1997). A large Swedish study on twins found that strenuous physical activity in the workplace increased the likelihood of joint pain (Charles et al 1999). It was assumed that joint pain was related to OA, even though the presence of OA had not been confirmed by a medical practitioner. Studies that examine the relationship between strenuous physical activity and OA need to include outcome measures such as roentgenograms because there is no clear relationship between joint pain and OA (Bagge et al 1991, Dieppe et al 1997).

The Framingham study showed that people who were very active had an increased risk of radiographically detectable OA (Felson et al 1997). This was in agreement with research conducted by Spector et al (1996b), who showed that women who were once elite athletes engaging in weight-bearing sports had a 2–3-fold increase in radiographically detectable OA. Workplace investigations also show that strenuous physical activities are associated with joint damage, particularly in older people. Cooper et al (1994) found that people with occupations that require squatting or kneeling for more than 30 minutes per day, or climbing more than 10 flights of stairs per day were 2.7–6.9 times more likely to have radiographic signs of OA than people whose main tasks required less strenuous activity. Their study, however, relied on recall of a lifetime occupational history with details of physical activities in the workplace, which may not have been completely accurate for every individual.

Symptoms of osteoarthritis

Osteoarthritis is associated with a slow and insidious development of intermittent discomfort in one or more joints, stiffness, surrounding muscle pain, swelling, crepitus and decreased function (Bagge et al 1991, Dieppe et al 1997). The most commonly reported symptoms of OA are 'pain, joint stiffness after rest, loss of movement, feelings of joint instability and functional limitations' (Bagge et al 1991, Dieppe et al 1997). Clinical signs include 'tender areas over and around the joint line, joint swelling, crepitus, locking, inflammation, reduced and painful range of motion with a tight end-feeling, and joint instability' (Bagge et al 1991, Dieppe et al 1997) (Table 10.1).

The relationship between clinical symptoms and radiographic changes at the knee over a 3-year period was examined in the Bristol 'OA500'

Table 10.1 Symptoms and signs of OA

Subjective symptoms	Objective signs
■ Slow and insidious onset	■ Destruction of articular cartilage
■ Intermittent activity-related joint discomfort	■ Changes in subchondral bone structure
	■ Increased intra-articular pressure
■ Joint stiffness after rest	■ Microfractures
■ Loss of function	■ Subchondral cyst formation
■ Muscle pain	■ Sclerosis
■ Joint pain	■ Osteophytes
■ Swelling	■ Joint space narrowing
■ Crepitus	■ Tender areas over and around the joint line
■ Joint locking	■ Inflammation
■ Feelings of instability	■ Swelling of the joint
	■ Joint instability
	■ Reduced and painful range of motion with a tight 'end-feeling'

study by Dieppe et al (1997). The majority of people in the Bristol sample reported joint deterioration and increased disability over time, although the severity of pain remained unchanged. Radiographic evaluation of their lower limbs showed degeneration in 30% of the tibiofemoral joints and 3.6% of patellofemoral joints. Strong positive relationships were found between joint space narrowing, the presence of osteophytes and subchondral bone sclerosis. No correlation was found between radiographic and clinical changes, which was consistent with earlier studies (Bagge et al 1991, Cobb et al 1957, Lawrence et al 1966). Outcome measures used in the Bristol 'OA500' study were not disease specific. Whereas instruments such as the Western Ontario and McMaster University Osteoarthritis Index (WOMAC) (Bellamy et al 1997, Sun et al 1997) and the Knee Pain Scale (KPS) (Rejeski et al 1995) measure disability in OA, Dieppe et al (1997) measured overall pain on a four-point Likert scale (none, mild, moderate or severe).

Therapeutic exercise in the management of osteoarthritis

Evidence is accumulating that therapeutic exercise is effective for people with OA, particularly of the knees and/or hips (Ettinger et al 1997, Van Baar et al 1998b). Exercise can be used to increase muscle strength (Røgind et al 1998), mobility (Van Baar et al 1998b) and endurance (Ettinger et al 1997). It has also been associated with positive changes in health and wellbeing (Bassett and Howley 1998, Coleman et al 1996, Ettinger et al 1997, Røgind et al 1998). Exercise programmes can be performed on an individual basis at home (Green et al 1993, Petrella and Bartha 2000), or in a clinic (Van Baar et al 1998b). They can also be performed within structured group sessions (Fisher and Pendergast 1994, Kovar et al 1992, O'Reilly et al 1999). Programmes may include a mixture of exercises that aim to improve variables such as mobility, muscle strength, endurance and aerobic capacity (Ettinger et al 1997) in order to reduce pain, inflammation, joint instability, deformity and disability (Ettinger et al 1997).

Physiological effects of exercise and physical activity

Exercise and physical activity have been associated with several positive physiological outcomes. Benefits can include weight control due to increased metabolism (Andersen et al 1999), normalization of glucose tolerance (Dunn et al 1999), increases in levels of high-density-lipid concentrations in the blood (Dunn et al 1999) and a reduction in blood pressure (Dunn et al 1999). Philbin et al (1996) found that people with OA of knees and/or hips had a greater mean body mass index (BMI), waist–hip ratio, systolic blood pressure, fasting blood glucose, and lower mean high-density lipoprotein cholesterol compared with a control group who did not have OA. The mean estimated risk for the development of coronary heart disease was also greater in people with OA compared with a control group (Philbin et al 1996). The study used the 'Hospital for Special Surgery Knee' and 'Harris Hip' surveys in addition to the Arthritis Impact Measurement Scale (AIMS) to measure the severity of deformity, pain and impact of OA on activities of daily living.

The latter two instruments have been found to be valid and reliable for people with OA (Sun et al 1997).

Ries et al (1996, 1997) found that, over a 2-year period, people with lower limb OA continued to show progressive reductions in exercise duration, maximum workload and workload at anaerobic threshold. In contrast, people with OA who underwent knee arthroplasty showed significant improvements in maximum oxygen consumption and oxygen uptake (Ries et al 1996). Likewise, after hip arthroplasty improvements were found in exercise duration, maximum workload, peak oxygen consumption and oxygen uptake (Ries et al 1997). Although the studies by Ries et al (1996, 1997) used small samples, they showed that physical activity and fitness improved following surgery. The increased cardiovascular fitness after arthroplasty may have resulted from the resumption of functional activities of daily living, such as walking, stair-climbing and home duties.

The roles of exercise and physical activity for osteoarthritis

Reductions in muscle strength, tendon strength and aerobic capacity can occur with both ageing and inactivity (Ansved and Larsson 1990, Åstrand 1992, Schoutens et al 1989). There is growing evidence that such changes can be delayed or slowed in the rate of progression by a more active lifestyle (Pocock et al 1986, Tipton and Vailas 1990). Several experiments have shown that exercise and physical activity can delay or retard the rate of sarcopenia and osteopenia with advancing age (Young et al 1984, 1985, Young 1997).

Engaging in weight-bearing activities such as aerobic walking can enable older people to maintain muscle strength and general fitness (Rejeski et al 1997). When performed at extreme levels, however, some physical activities can become dangerous for people with OA. Exercises involve joint loading, some exercises in single leg standing, very slow walking or prolonged isometric abduction exercises can produce high acetabular pressures (Tackson et al 1997). The increased pressure can predispose some people towards further cartilage damage and can sometimes affect bone (Bruns et al 1993). Despite the finding that excessive strenuous activities can increase the risk and rate of progression of OA (Spector et al 1996b), studies in animals have shown positive effects on chondrocyte activity from moderate intensity intermittent joint compression (Burton-Wurster et al 1993). The inclusion of non-weight-bearing exercises such as stretching exercises within an exercise programme reduces constant exposure to abnormal stresses exerted on the articulate surfaces of the joints. Joint loading usually has a positive effect although programmes for older people with OA are best designed to avoid marked joint loading, particularly when they have poor joint stability, weakness, severe articular degeneration or pain (Buckwalter 1995). Walking programmes (Ettinger et al 1997, Kovar et al 1992), low-intensity weight-bearing exercises (Bautch et al 1997), isokinetic muscle-strength training (Schilke et al 1996) and progressive resistance strength training (Ettinger et al 1997) involve joint loading yet have been shown to improve joint function and pain in people with OA (Van Baar et al 1999).

Research on the effects of exercises that aim to reduce joint loading in order to decrease pain associated with OA has yielded mixed results. One study by Mangione et al (1996) found that mechanical 'weight relief' using a body weight support device during treadmill training did not reduce knee pain in people with OA, even though aerobic capacity improved. Green et al (1993) reported no differences in hip pain between people with OA who participated in a home exercise programme that incorporated weight-bearing activities compared with those who attended hydrotherapy classes. Both of these studies utilized small samples and had insufficient control of concomitant interventions such as the use of medication.

Studies on the effects of 'weighted' (resistance) versus 'unweighted' (free) exercises for people with OA have yielded equivocal results. Petrella and Bartha (2000) compared the effects of 'sham exercises' and weighted exercises on movement function and pain in people with OA who used non-steroid anti-inflammatory drugs (NSAIDs). The control group received NSAIDs together with non-weight-bearing leg exercises and stretches. The experimental group received the same programme and two additional exercises that increased joint loading. Both groups improved with respect to function and pain relief, although the effect sizes were greater in the experimental group. The experimental group also exercised longer every week than the control group (78 ± 9 minutes versus 51 ± 3 minutes). It is therefore not clear whether greater pain relief in the experimental group was due to the weighted exercises or to the increased time spent exercising.

In contrast to the beneficial effects of exercise, deconditioning as a result of inactivity has been linked to an increase in the symptoms of OA (Slemenda et al 1997, Van Baar et al 1998a). Muscle weakness is also associated with increased disability (Hopman-Rock et al 1996, 1997b, Van Baar et al 1998a) and increased healthcare utilization in older people with OA (Hopman-Rock et al 1997a). In addition Van Baar et al found that muscle weakness was associated with increased pain and a reduction of mobility. A hospital-based study showed that reduced isokinetic strength of the quadriceps was associated with increased knee pain and functional impairment in people with knee OA (Madsen et al 1995). People with lower limb OA could benefit from maintaining a physically active lifestyle which may include therapeutic exercises, thereby reducing the risk of developing muscle weakness, functional impairment and the need for regular healthcare services.

Muscle strength can increase through exercise training, even in old age (Dodd et al, Chapter 7 this volume; Ettinger et al 1997, Fiatarone et al 1990, McMurdo and Burnett 1992). In a population-based study of people aged 68–85 years, Coleman et al (1996) found that exercise improved muscle strength without necessarily increasing pain. In some people with lower limb OA, pain and disability can be reduced in severity by increasing muscle strength (Ettinger et al 1997, Van Baar et al 1998b, 1999). For example, Van Baar et al found that exercise therapy incorporating strength training was associated with a reduction of knee and hip pain as well as disability. Although isokinetic muscle strength and pain can improve in people with lower limb OA, training is not always as effective when the disease is very severe (Fisher et al 1991, 1993, Maurer et al 1995, Røgind et al 1998).

Muscle strength, function and pain can improve with exercise programmes that include aerobic walking. In a randomized controlled trial Ettinger et al (1997) compared the effects of an aerobic walking programme with a progressive resistance strength training programme (dumbbells and cuff weights) and health education in 439 older adults with knee OA. The aerobic programme duration was 1 hour and started with a warm-up phase of 10 minutes which included slow walking and callisthenics. The core phase required walking for 40 minutes at 50–70% of the heart rate reserve, as measured from an initial treadmill test. Finally, the cool-down phase consisted of 10 minutes of slow walking and stretches of the shoulders, hamstrings and lower back. The resistance strength training also lasted for 1 hour per session and included 10-minutes of warm-up and cool-down. Resistance training incorporated 9 exercises performed in two sets of 12 repetitions. The resistance exercises included leg extension, leg curls, step ups, heel raises, chest flies, upright row, military press, biceps curls and pelvic tilt exercises. Both the aerobic walking and resisted exercises reduced pain and disability in people with OA and led to an increase in walking distance. In comparison to subjects who received only health education, participants in the aerobic walking group had 10% lower physical disability, 12% lower knee pain and superior performance on timed tests of functional tasks. Compared with the health education group, the muscle resistance training group had 8% lower physical disability, 8% lower pain, greater distance on the 6-minute walk, faster times on lifting and carrying tasks, and faster times getting in and out of a car. No adverse effects were detected in X-rays for the aerobic training or exercise group. The health education group showed an increase in disability over the 18-month period. Ettinger et al (1997) concluded that older people with knee OA can achieve modest reductions in disability, pain and physical performance from participating in an aerobic exercises or progressive resistance strength training programme.

Van Baar et al (1998b) compared the effects of an exercise programme that aimed to increase mobility and strength in people with lower limb OA with aerobic exercises and strength training in isolation. The training programme was developed by Oostendorp et al (1998) and included exercises to increase muscle strength, muscle length, joint mobility, coordination, and the performance of functional tasks of everyday living. The content (types of exercises), frequency (one to three sessions per week) and intensity of the combined programme were determined by a physiotherapist, based on the needs and tolerance of each individual. Sessions were delivered in a clinical setting lasting for approximately 30 minutes. Community-based medical practitioners also provided education on the benefits and limitations of rest and physical activities, although it is not clear if physical activity was encouraged. This programme resulted in greater pain reduction than aerobic walking or strength training alone, although aerobic walking produced the greatest reduction in disability.

The influence of exercise adherence on outcome

Adherence to exercise programmes is a major determinant of therapy outcomes in people with OA. It is well established that long-term adherence to exercise is essential for maintaining functional benefits (Sullivan et al 1998), particularly for progressive resistance strength training (Dodd et al, Chapter 7 this volume). Rejeski et al (1997) studied the predictors of adherence to exercise programmes in people with OA. Attendance at exercise sessions and the time spent exercising in the clinic or at home were examined as two different dimensions of adherence. Regression models showed that 26–46% of the variance in adherence could be explained by the time spent exercising. Fitness, health-related quality of life, performance-related disability and previous exercise behaviour were also investigated to establish whether they were predictors of adherence. Rejeski found that previous high levels of compliance with exercise programmes was a strong predictor of exercise adherence. This finding was replicated in a recent study by Schoo (2002). For an 8-week home exercise programme, exercise adherence during weeks 1–4 was the strongest predictor of home exercise adherence during weeks 5–8 (Schoo 2002). Other predictors of home exercise adherence were levels of physical activity performed outside the prescribed exercise programme and the perception of being physically active (Schoo 2002).

The effects of exercise adherence on pain and disability levels were also examined by Rejeski et al (1997). They found that the knee pain intensity in an aerobic group decreased with greater attendance at exercise sessions and increased with greater time spent exercising during these sessions. This effect was not found for a muscle resistance training group. Greater attendance at exercise sessions was associated with improved self-reported disability, particularly in the group that participated in aerobic exercises. The study by Rejeski et al (1997) has important ramifications for exercise delivery, showing that prescription of frequent bouts of activity (at least three times each week) of moderate duration (approximately 35 minutes) was beneficial for people with OA.

Influence of medication on the effect of exercise on pain

The use of analgesics and non-steroid anti-inflammatory drugs (NSAIDs) in addition to prescribed exercise can influence the outcome of exercise programmes, particularly in relation to pain (Petrella and Bartha 2000, Van Baar et al 1998b). Petrella and Bartha (2000) found that an exercise programme in addition to NSAIDs resulted in a greater decrease in pain than 'sham exercises' and NSAIDs. It was not clear whether the use of NSAIDs had a beneficial effect on pain or whether pain in the experimental group was positively influenced by longer accumulated exercise time per week. One of the disadvantages of analgesics is that they have been associated with increased varus loading in people with OA (Hurwitz et al 1999). Although not confirmed with controlled research, it remains possible that this could accelerate disease progression (see Chapter 5 this volume) even though pain levels might be concomitantly reduced.

Clinical recommendations

The clinical literature shows that therapeutic management of people with lower limb OA may include the following interventions:

1. *Patient education and self-management programmes.* Education and self-management have been associated with prolonged pain relief, reduced disability and reductions in the frequency of medical visits (Hirano et al 1994, Lindroth et al 1995, Lorig et al 1993).
2. *Weight loss.* Obesity is positively associated with premature OA of the hips and knees (Cicuttini et al 1997, Felson et al 1988, Tepper and Hochberg 1993). The Framingham study showed that weight loss of 5 kg over 10 years decreased symptoms of knee pain by more than 50% (Felson et al 1992). Theoretically, the combination of a reduction of calorie intake and expending energy through exercise should be more effective for improving weight loss than dieting alone (Bar-Or et al 1998, Epstein et al 1996) (see WHO classification in Appendix, p. 328).
3. *Physiotherapy and occupational therapy* can assist in improving or maintaining joint mobility, muscle strength, joint stability, inflammation, pain, functional independence and participation in societal roles (Fisher et al 1993, Fransen et al 1997, Puett and Griffin 1994, Rijken and Dekker 1998). Improved joint mechanics can also be achieved by therapeutic interventions such as taping or orthotics. For example, tracking of the patella can be facilitated by taping so that exercises or daily functional activities can be better tolerated (Cushnaghan et al 1994). Moreover, reduction of compression forces in the medial compartment of the knee can be achieved by providing a knee orthosis (Matsuno et al 1997) or a wedged heel insert.
4. *Exercise* has been associated with increased fitness, muscle strength, physical function, and decreased pain in individuals with lower limb OA (Ettinger et al 1997, Rejeski et al 1997, Van Baar et al 1999). Although exercise may occasionally increase joint effusion in some individuals (Coleman et al 1996, Røgind et al 1998), increased adherence to muscle strength training and aerobic walking has been associated with better health outcomes.
5. *Hydrotherapy* has recently gained popularity for the treatment of OA (Bálint and Szebenyi 1997), although it may not necessarily be more effective than other forms of exercise such as progressive resistance exercise training or home exercise regimens (Green et al 1993, Sjogren et al 1997). A reduction in joint loading experienced through buoyancy during water-based exercise programmes or the use of walking aids may benefit people with severe OA of the lower limbs, although several precautions need to be considered when hydrotherapy is prescribed for older people. These precautions are addressed by McBurney and Cook in Chapter 14.
6. *Pharmacological intervention* may assist in reducing pain and inflammation. Some types of medication, however, have been associated with medical problems such as stomach ulcers in some individuals (e.g. NSAIDs) (Gabriel et al 1999) or abnormal varus loading of the knees (Hurwitz et al 1999). The preferred medication may include

simple analgesics or NSAIDs with gastroprophylaxis (Cicuttini and Spector 1995, Gabriel 1996, Hochberg et al 1995a, 1995b).

7. *Nutriceuticals* such as glucosamine and chondroitin may also be effective in the treatment of symptoms in some people with OA and could assist with the performance of exercise therapy. Preliminary data suggest that glucosamine and chondroitin (sulphate or hydrochloride) may have disease-modifying effects (McAlindon et al 2000, Towheed et al 2001), although this needs to be verified with large-scale controlled clinical trials.

Conclusion

Osteoarthritis is common in older people. Although on the whole exercise is related to better functional outcomes and less pain in people with mild to moderate OA, its effects in people with severe lower limb OA still need to be investigated. Analgesic medication has been used in conjunction with exercise to enable people to perform their exercises without debilitating pain, although the long-term effects of this strategy on joint mechanics remains unclear. Low adherence to therapeutic exercises and physical activity programmes has been associated with poor exercise outcomes in people with OA. The main factors that predict adherence to therapeutic exercises in people with lower limb OA are attendance at exercise sessions, the time spent exercising in the clinic or at home, and previous patterns of exercise adherence. Further research needs to be conducted to clarify how adherence to physical activity and exercise programmes in people with OA can be increased, as well as the relative benefits of different types of physical intervention.

References

Andersen R E, Wadden T A, et al 1999 Effects of lifestyle activity vs structured aerobic exercise in obese women: a randomized trial. JAMA 281(4):335–340

Anderson J J, Felson D T 1988 Factors associated with osteoarthritis of the knee in the first National Health and Nutrition Examination Survey (HANES I): evidence for an association with overweight, race and physical demands of work. American Journal of Epidemiology 128:179–189

Ansved T, Larsson L 1990 Quantitative and qualitative morphological properties of the soleus motor nerve and the L5 ventral root in young and old rats. Journal of the Neurological Sciences 96:269–282

Åstrand P O 1992. Physical activity and fitness. American Journal of Clinical Nutrition 55(Suppl):1231–1236

Australian Bureau of Statistics 1997 National Health Survey: summary of results. Canberra, ACT. Australian Bureau of Statistics: 21

Badley E M 1995 The effect of osteoarthritis on disability and health care use in Canada. Journal of Rheumatology Supplement 43:19–22

Badley E M, Crotty M 1995 An international comparison of the estimated effect of the aging of the population on the major cause of disablement, musculoskeletal disorders. Journal of Rheumatology 22:1934–1940

Bagge E, Bjelle A, et al 1991 Osteoarthritis in the elderly: clinical and radiological findings in 79- and 85-year-olds. Annals of the Rheumatic Diseases 50:535–539

Bálint G, Szebenyi B 1997 Non-pharmacological therapies in osteoarthritis. Baillière's Clinical Rheumatology 11(4):795–815

Bank R A, Bayliss M T, et al 1997 Prevalence of leisure-time physical activity among persons with arthritis and other rheumatic conditions – United States, 1990–1991. MMWR Morbidity Mortality Weekly Report 46(18):389–393

Bar-Or O, Foreyt J, et al 1998 Physical activity, genetic, and nutritional considerations in childhood weight management. Medicine and Science in Sports and Exercise 30(1):2–10

Bassett D R, Jr, Howley E T 1998 American College of Sports Medicine Position Stand. Exercise and physical activity for older adults. Medicine and Science in Sports and Exercise 30(6):992–1008

Bautch J C, Malone D G, et al 1997 Effects of exercise on knee joints with osteoarthritis: a pilot study of biologic markers. Arthritis Care Research 10(1):48–55

Bellamy N, Campbell J, et al 1997 Validation study of a computerized version of the Western Ontario and McMaster Universities VA3.0 Osteoarthritis Index. Journal of Rheumatology 24(12):2413–2415

Bruns J, Volkmer M, Luessenhop S 1993 Pressure distribution at the knee joint. Influence of varus and valgus deviation without and with ligament dissection. Archives of Orthopaedic and Trauma Surgery 113(1):12–19

Buckwalter J A 1995 Osteoarthritis and articular cartilage use, disuse, and abuse: experimental studies. Journal of Rheumatology Supplement 43:13–15

Burton-Wurster N, Venier-Singer M, et al 1993 Effect of compressive loading and unloading on the synthesis of total protein, proteoglycan, and fibronectin by canine cartilage explants. Journal of Orthopaedic Research 11:717–729

Casperen C J, Powell K E, et al 1985 Physical activity, exercise, and physical fitness: definitions and distinctions for health related research. Public Health Reports 100:126–131

Charles S T, Gatz M, et al 1999 Genetic and behavioral risk factors for self-reported joint pain among a population-based sample of Swedish twins. Health Psychology 18(6):644–654

Cicuttini F M, Spector T, et al 1997 Risk factors for osteoarthritis in the tibiofemoral and patellofemoral joints of the knee. Journal of Rheumatology 24(6):1164–1167

Cicuttini F M, Spector T D 1995 Osteoarthritis in the aged. Epidemiological issues and optimal management. Drugs and Aging 6(5):409–420

Cicuttini F M, Spector T D 1996 Genetics of osteoarthritis. Annals of the Rheumatic Diseases 55:665–667

Cobb S, Merchant W R, et al 1957 The relation of symptoms to osteoarthritis. Journal of Chronic Diseases 5:197–204

Coleman E A, Buchner D M, et al 1996 The relationship of joint symptoms with exercise performance in older adults. Journal of the American Geriatrics Society 44(1):14–21

Cooper C, McAlindon T, et al 1994 Occupational activity and osteoarthritis of the knee. Annals of the Rheumatic Diseases 53(2):90–93

Cushnaghan J, McCarthy C, et al 1994 Taping the patella medially: a new treatment for osteoarthritis of the knee joint. British Medical Journal 308:753–755

Dieppe P A, Cushnagan J, et al 1997 The Bristol 'OA500' study: progression of osteoarthritis (OA) over 3 years and the relationship between clinical and radiographic changes at the knee joint. Osteoarthritis Cartilage 5(2):87–97

Dunn A L, Marcus B H, et al 1999 Comparison of lifestyle and structured interventions to increase physical activity and cardiorespiratory fitness: a randomized trial. JAMA 281(4):327–334

Egberts A C, Leufkens H G, et al 1997 Incidence of antidepressant drug use in older adults and association with chronic diseases: the Rotterdam Study. International Clinical Psychopharmacology 12(4):217–223

Elders M J 2000 The increasing impact of arthritis on public health. Journal of Rheumatology 60:6–8

Epstein L H, Coleman K J, et al 1996 Exercise in treating obesity in children and adolescents. Medicine and Science in Sports and Exercise 28(4):428–435

Ettinger W H, Jr, Burns R, et al 1997 A randomized trial comparing aerobic exercise and resistance exercise with a health education program in older adults with knee osteoarthritis. The Fitness Arthritis and Seniors Trial (FAST). JAMA 277(1):25–31

Felson D T 1995 Weight and osteoarthritis. Journal of Rheumatology Supplement 43:7–9

Felson D T, Anderson J J, et al 1988 Obesity and knee osteoarthritis. The Framingham Study. Annals of Internal Medicine 109:18–24

Felson D T, Zhang Y, et al 1992 Weight loss reduces the risk for symptomatic knee osteoarthritis in women. The Framingham Study. Annals of Internal Medicine 116:535–539

Felson D T, Zhang Y, et al 1995 The incidence and natural history of knee osteoarthritis in the elderly. The Framingham Osteoarthritis Study. Arthritis and Rheumatism 38(10):1500–1505

Felson D T, Zhang Y, et al 1997 Risk factors for incident radiographic knee osteoarthritis in the elderly: the Framingham Study. Arthritis and Rheumatism 40(4):728–733

Fiatarone M A, Marks E C, et al 1990 High-intensity strength training in nonagenarians. JAMA 263:3029–3032

Fisher N M, Gresham G E, et al 1993 Quantitative effects of physical therapy on muscular and functional performance in subjects with osteoarthritis of the knees. Archives of Physical Medicine and Rehabilitation 74:840–847

Fisher N M, Pendergast D R 1994 Effects of a muscle exercise program on exercise capacity in subjects with osteoarthritis. Archives of Physical Medicine and Rehabilitation 75(7):792–797

Fisher N M, Pendergast D R, et al 1991 Muscle rehabilitation: its effect on muscular and functional performance of patients with knee osteoarthritis. Archives of Physical Medicine and Rehabilitation 72(6):367–374

Fransen M, Margiotta E, et al 1997 A revised group exercise program for osteoarthritis of the knee. Physiotherapy Research International 2(1):30–41

Gabriel S E 1996 Update on the epidemiology of the rheumatic diseases. Current Opinion in Rheumatology 8(2):96–100

Gabriel S E, Crowson C S, et al 1997 Direct medical costs unique to people with arthritis. Journal of Rheumatology 24(7):719–725

Gabriel S E, Crowson C S, et al 1999 Comorbidity in arthritis. Journal of Rheumatology 26(11):2475–2479

Green J, McKenna F, et al 1993 Home exercises are as effective as outpatient hydrotherapy for osteoarthritis of the hip. British Journal of Rheumatology 32(9):812–815

Hill C L, Parsons J, et al 1999 Health related quality of life in a population sample with arthritis. Journal of Rheumatology 26(9):2029–2035

Hirano P C, Laurent D D, et al 1994 Arthritis patient education studies 1987–1991: a review of the literature. Patient Education and Counselling 24:9–54

Hochberg M C, Altman R D, et al 1995a Guidelines for the medical management of osteoarthritis. Part II. Osteoarthritis of the knee. American College of Rheumatology. Arthritis and Rheumatism 38:1541–1546

Hochberg M C, Altman R D, et al 1995b Guidelines for the medical treatment of osteoarthritis. Part I. Osteoarthritis of the hip. Arthritis and Rheumatism 38:1535–1540

Hochberg M C, Lethbridge Cejku M, et al 1995c The association of body weight, body fatness and body fat distribution with osteoarthritis of the knee: data from the Baltimore Longitudinal Study of Aging. Journal of Rheumatology 22(3):488–493

Hopman-Rock M, Odding E, et al 1996 Physical and psychosocial disability in elderly subjects in relation to pain in the hip and/or knee. Journal of Rheumatology 23(6):1037–1044

Hopman-Rock M, de Bock G H, et al 1997a The pattern of health care utilization of elderly people with arthritic pain in the hip or knee. International Journal for Quality Health Care 9(2):129–137

Hopman-Rock M, Odding E, et al 1997b Differences in health status of older adults with pain in the hip or knee only and with additional mobility restricting conditions. Journal of Rheumatology 2(12)4:2416–2423

Hurwitz D E, Sharma L, et al 1999 Effect of knee pain on joint loading in patients with osteoarthritis. Current Opinion in Rheumatology 11(5):422–426

Imhof H, Breitenseher M, et al 1997 Degenerative joint disease: cartilage or vascular disease? Skeletal Radiology 26(7):398–403

Kallman D A, Wigley F M, et al 1989 New radiographic grading scales for osteoarthritis of the hand. Arthritis and Rheumatism 32(12):1584–1591

Kovar P A, Allegrante J P, et al 1992 Supervised fitness walking in patients with osteoarthritis of the knee. A randomized, controlled trial. Annals of Internal Medicine 116(7):529–534

Lawrence J S, Bremner J M, et al 1966 Osteoarthritis: prevalence in the population and relationship between symptoms and X-ray changes. Annals of the Rheumatic Diseases 25:1–24

Lethbridge-Cejku M, Tobin J D, et al 1994 The relationship of age and gender to prevalence and pattern of radiographic changes of osteoarthritis of the knee: data from Caucasian participants in the Baltimore Longitudinal Study of Aging. Aging (Milano) 6(5):353–357

Lindroth S, Bauman A, et al 1995 A five year follow up of a controlled trial of an arthritis education programme. British Journal of Rheumatology 34:648–653

Lorig K R, Mazonson P D, et al 1993 Evidence suggesting that health education for self-management in patients with chronic arthritis has sustained health benefits while reducing health care costs. Arthritis and Rheumatism 36:439–446

Madsen O R, Bliddal H, et al 1995 Isometric and isokinetic quadriceps strength in gonarthrosis; inter-relations between quadriceps strength, walking ability, radiology, subchondral bone density and pain. Clinical Rheumatology 14(3):308–314

Mangione K K, Axen K, et al 1996 Mechanical unweighting effects on treadmill exercise and pain in elderly people with osteoarthritis of the knee. Physical Therapy 76(4):387–394

March L M, Schwarz J M, et al 1998 Clinical validation of self-reported osteoarthritis. Osteoarthritis Cartilage 6(2):87–93

Marks J S, Stewart I M, et al 1979 Primary osteoarthritis of the hip and Heberden's nodes. Annals of the Rheumatic Diseases 38:107–111

Matsuno H, Kadowaki K M, et al 1997 Generation II knee bracing for severe medial compartment osteoarthritis of the knee. Archives of Physical Medicine and Rehabilitation 78(7):745–749

Maurer B T, Moreno S I, et al 1995 A comparison of recruitment methods for an osteoarthritis exercise study. Arthritis Care Research 8(3):161–166

Maurer B T, Stern A G, et al 1999 Osteoarthritis of the knee: isokinetic quadriceps exercise versus an educational intervention. Archives of Physical Medicine and Rehabilitation 80(10):1293–1299

McAlindon T E, LaValley M P, et al 2000 Glucosamine and chondroitin for treatment of osteoarthritis: a systematic quality assessment and meta-analysis. JAMA 283(11):1469–1475

McMurdo M E, Burnett L 1992 Randomised controlled trial of exercise in the elderly. Gerontology 38:292–298

Odding E, Valkenburg H A, et al 1998 Associations of radiological osteoarthritis of the hip and knee with locomotor disability in the Rotterdam Study. Annals of the Rheumatic Diseases 57(4):203–208

Oliveria S A, Felson D T, et al 1995 Incidence of symptomatic hand, hip, and knee osteoarthritis among patients in a health maintenance organization. Arthritis and Rheumatism 38(8):1134–1141

Oostendorp R A B, van den Heuvel J H, et al 1998 Exercise therapy in patients with osteoarthritis: a protocol. Amersfoort/Utrecht, The Netherlands, NPI/NIVEL

O'Reilly S C, Muir K R, et al 1999 Effectiveness of home exercise on pain and disability from osteoarthritis of the knee: a randomised controlled trial. Annals of the Rheumatic Diseases 58(1):15–19

Petrella R J, Bartha C 2000 Home based exercise therapy for older patients with knee osteoarthritis: a randomized clinical trial. Journal of Rheumatology 27:2215–2221

Philbin E F, Ries M D, et al 1996 Osteoarthritis as a determinant of an adverse coronary heart disease risk profile. Journal of Cardiovascular Risk 3(6):529–533

Pocock N A, Eisman J A, et al 1986 Physical fitness as a major determinant of femoral neck and lumbar spine bone mineral density. Journal of Clinical Investigation 78:618–621

Puett D W, Griffin M R 1994 Published trials of nonmedicinal and noninvasive therapies for hip and knee osteoarthritis [see comments]. Annals of Internal Medicine 121(2):133–140

Rejeski W J, Brawley L R, et al 1997 Compliance to exercise therapy in older participants with knee osteoarthritis: implications for treating disability. Medicine and Science in Sports and Exercise 29(8):977–985

Ries M D, Philbin E F, et al 1995 Relationship between severity of gonarthrosis and cardiovascular fitness. Clinical Orthopaedics 313:169–176

Ries M D, Philbin E F, et al 1996 Improvement in cardiovascular fitness after total knee arthroplasty. Journal of Bone and Joint Surgery Am 78(11):1696–1701

Ries M D, Philbin E F, et al 1997 Effect of total hip arthroplasty on cardiovascular fitness. Journal of Arthroplasty 12(1):84–90

Rijken P M, Dekker J 1998 Clinical experience of rehabilitation therapists with chronic diseases: a quantitative approach. Clinical Rehabilitation 12(2):143–150

Røgind H, Bibow Nielsen B, et al 1998 The effects of a physical training program on patients with osteoarthritis of the knees. Archives of Physical Medicine and Rehabilitation 79(11):1421–1427

Schilke J M, Johnson G O, et al 1996 Effects of muscle-strength training on the functional status of patients with osteoarthritis of the knee joint. Nursing Research 45(2):68–72

Schoo A M M 2002 Exercise performance in people with osteoarthritis: Adherence, correctness and associated pain. Doctoral thesis, School of Physiotherapy, Bundoora, La Trobe University, Australia

Schoutens A, Laurent E, Poortmans J R 1989 Effects of inactivity and exercise on bone. Sports Medicine 7:71–81

Simpson K J, Kanter L 1997 Jump distance of dance landings influencing internal joint forces: I. Axial forces. Medicine and Science in Sports and Exercise 29(7):916–927

Sjogren T, Long N, et al 1997 Group hydrotherapy versus group land-based treatment for chronic low back pain. Physiotherapy Research International 2(4):212–222

Slemenda C, Brandt K D, et al 1997 Quadriceps weakness and osteoarthritis of the knee. Annals of Internal Medicine 127(2):97–104

Spector T D, Cicuttini F, et al 1996a Genetic influences on osteoarthritis in women: a twin study. British Medical Journal 312:940–943

Spector T D, Harris P A, et al 1996b Risk of osteoarthritis associated with long-term weight-bearing sports: a radiologic survey of the hips and knees in female ex-athletes and population controls. Arthritis and Rheumatism 39(6):988–995

Sullivan T, Allegrante J P, et al 1998 One-year follow-up of patients with osteoarthritis of the knee who participated in a program of supervised fitness walking and supportive patient education. Arthritis Care Research 11(4):228–233

Sun Y, Stürmer T, et al 1997 Reliability and validity of clinical outcome measurements of osteoarthritis of the hip and knee – a review of the literature. Clinical Rheumatology 16(2):185–198

Tackson S J, Krebs D E, et al 1997 Acetabular pressures during hip arthritis exercises. Arthritis Care Research 10(5):308–319

Tepper S, Hochberg M C 1993 Factors associated with hip osteoarthritis: data from the first National Health and Nutrition Examination Survey (NHANES-1). American Journal of Epidemiology 137:1081–1088

Tipton C M, Vailas A C 1990 Bone and connective tissue adaptations to physical activity. In: Bouchard C, Shephard R J, Stephens T S, Sutton J R, McPherson B D (eds) Exercise, fitness, and health. Human Kinetics Books, Champaign, IL, p 331–361

Towheed T E, Anastassiades T P, et al 2001 Glucosamine therapy for treating osteoarthritis. Cochrane Database of Systematic Reviews 1:CD002946

Van Baar M E, Dekker J, et al 1998a Pain and disability in patients with osteoarthritis of hip or knee: the relationship with articular, kinesiological, and psychological characteristics. Journal of Rheumatology 25(1):125–133

Van Baar M E, Dekker J, et al 1998b The effectiveness of exercise therapy in patients with osteoarthritis of the hip or knee: a randomized clinical trial. Journal of Rheumatology 25(1):2432–2439

Van Baar M E, Assendelft W J, et al 1999 Effectiveness of exercise therapy in patients with osteoarthritis of the hip or knee: a systematic review of randomized clinical trials. Arthritis and Rheumatism 42(7):1361–1369

Victorian Department of Human Services 2000 The burden of disease in Victoria, 1996. Volume 1. The mortality burdens of disease, injury and risk factors and projections to 2016. Department of Human Services, Melbourne

World Health Organization 2000 WHO Obesity Classification. Obesity: preventing and managing the global epidemic. Report of a WHO consultation. WHO Technical Report Series 894, Geneva

Young A 1997 Ageing and physiological functions. Philosophical Transactions of the Royal Society of London B: Biological Sciences 352:1837–1843

Young A, Stokes M, et al 1984 Size and strength of the quadriceps muscle of old and young women. European Journal of Clinical Investigation 14:282–287

Young A, Stokes M, et al 1985 The size and strength of the quadriceps muscle of old and young men. Clinical Physiology 5:145–154

11

Common foot problems that can impair performance of regular physical activity and exercise in older people: prevention and treatment

Hylton B Menz

CHAPTER CONTENTS

Introduction 229

Prevalence of foot problems in older people 230

The effect of foot problems on mobility 231

Effects of ageing on the foot 231

Common foot problems and their management 233

Can foot problems be prevented? 239

Can treatment of foot problems improve mobility and quality of life? 240

Conclusion 240

References 241

Introduction

The human foot plays an important role in all weight-bearing tasks. As the foot provides the only direct source of contact between the body and the supporting surface, impaired foot function may significantly influence an individual's ability to perform normal activities of daily living. With advancing age, the likelihood of developing a foot problem increases (Menz and Lord 1999). Unfortunately, many older people consider foot pain to be an unavoidable consequence of ageing (Williamson et al 1964), and subsequently may not consider volunteering foot problems when reporting their medical history to healthcare professionals (Munro and Steele 1998). As a consequence, older people may needlessly endure pain and disability despite evidence that most foot ailments can be prevented or effectively managed with conservative interventions (Freeman 2002, Prud'homme and Curran 1999, Redmond et al 1999). This chapter provides an overview of the prevalence and consequences of foot problems in older people, discusses the causes and treatment options for some of the more common foot complaints, and outlines simple strategies to prevent foot problems in this age group.

Prevalence of foot problems in older people

Foot problems have long been considered to be highly prevalent in older people, based largely on the observation that older people comprise the largest sector of the community who seek podiatric care (Australian Institute of Health and Welfare 2002, Greenberg 1994). However, reliable epidemiological data on the prevalence of foot problems in large samples of older people are lacking. One of the main barriers to the establishment of accurate figures is defining what actually constitutes a foot 'problem'. While some studies have used clinicians to assess and document a range of foot conditions, others have relied on subjective reports by older people. Clinicians will generally document more subtle foot conditions (such as dry skin) than older people will themselves report, and subsequently, there are considerable discrepancies in the reported rates of foot problems between different studies. The other main consideration in relation to foot problem prevalence data is sample bias. Studies conducted in hospitals or clinical settings often report very high rates of foot problems – up to 80% of older people (Crawford et al 1995, Ebrahim et al 1981, Hung et al 1985), whereas larger community studies (often involving telephone interviews) report much lower rates of foot problems – generally in the range of 30–40% (Greenberg 1994). Despite these discrepancies, most investigations have reported that women are more likely to suffer from foot problems than men, possibly due to the detrimental influence of wearing ladies' fashion footwear (Burns et al 2002, Frey et al 1993, Gorecki 1978). The prevalence of foot problems has been shown to increase with age. However, in the very old, foot problems become less prevalent as a consequence of reduced mobility and the increased number of older people who are confined to bed (Menz and Lord 1999).

The most commonly reported foot problems in older people are generally chronic in nature and reflect the long-term physiological changes that occur to the sensory, muscular, articular, neurological and vascular systems with advancing age. The most commonly observed and reported problems are hyperkeratotic lesions (corns and calluses), followed closely by nail disorders and structural deformities such as hallux valgus (bunions) and lesser toe deformities (hammertoes and clawtoes) (Menz and Lord 1999). However, a number of other conditions commonly diagnosed in the clinical setting (such as plantar heel pain) are rarely included in epidemiological surveys, and as a consequence, the prevalence of some of the more complex foot disorders in older people is unknown.

The effect of foot problems on mobility

Numerous investigations conducted in a range of different countries have shown that foot problems contribute to impaired physical functioning and ability to perform basic activities of daily living. In an epidemiological study of 459 elderly residents in a small Italian town, Benvenutti et al (1995) reported significant associations between the presence of clinically assessed foot problems and self-reported difficulty in performing housework, shopping and walking 400 metres. An evaluation of gait patterns also revealed that those with foot pain required a greater number of steps to walk 3 metres than those free of foot problems. A similar study of 1002 elderly women in the USA reported that women with chronic and severe foot pain (defined as pain lasting one month or longer in the past year and rated as severe) walked more slowly and took longer to rise from a chair. After controlling for age, body mass index, co-morbidities and pain in other sites, severe foot pain was independently associated with increased risk for walking difficulty and disability in activities of daily living (Leveille et al 1998). More recently, a population-based cross-sectional survey conducted in the Netherlands of 7200 people aged 65 years and older reported that the 20% of subjects with foot problems were more likely to suffer from limited mobility and poor perceived well-being (Gorter et al 2000).

Foot problems may also contribute to impaired balance and increase the risk of suffering a fall. A recent cross-sectional study of 135 older people reported that people with foot problems performed poorly in functional tasks and balance tests, the most detrimental foot conditions being the presence of pain and hallux valgus (Menz and Lord 2001a, 2001b). Three retrospective studies have shown that older people who suffer from foot problems are more likely to have a history of recurrent falls (Blake et al 1988, Dolinis and Harrison 1997, Wild et al 1980), and prospective studies have confirmed this association. Gabell et al (1985) reported that 'foot trouble' was associated with a threefold increased risk of falling in a sample of 100 older people, Tinetti et al (1988) found that the presence of a 'serious foot problem' (defined as a bunion, toe deformity, ulcer or deformed nail) doubled the risk of falling, and Koski et al (1996) found that older people with bunions were twice as likely to fall as those without. More recently, a study of musculoskeletal pain in 1002 elderly women found that foot pain was the only site of pain that was significantly associated with an increased risk of falling (Leveille et al 2002). These results indicate that foot problems are a falls risk factor, presumably mediated by impaired balance and ability to perform daily functional tasks.

Effects of ageing on the foot

There are a number of well-reported consequences of advancing age on foot structure and function. As with the rest of the body, the skin on the foot becomes drier due to the decreased number and output of sweat and sebaceous glands. The epidermis on an older person's foot is significantly thinner and less resilient than that on a younger person's foot, leading to an increased likelihood of fissuring (Muehlman and Rahimi 1990). Sensory receptors in the skin are degraded, leading to impaired tactile and vibration sensitivity (Rosenberg 1958, Stevens and Choo 1996). The gradual flattening of the dermo-epidermal junction with age decreases the mechanical resistance of the skin to shearing forces, and the subsequent reduction in penetration of capillary loops leads to reduced epidermal blood supply (Gilchrest 1996, Glogau 1997, Jenkins 2002, Muehlman and Rahimi 1990).

Reduced peripheral blood supply associated with advancing age is particularly evident in the foot, and leads to an increased prevalence of peripheral arterial disease and its associated complications, such as impaired healing, ulceration and intermittent claudication (Beard 2000). Similarly, impaired venous return often manifests in the foot and ankle, commonly producing ankle oedema, telangiectasia (permanent dilation of superficial capillaries), haemosiderosis (deposition of iron deposits in superficial tissues), varicose veins and ulceration in the medial ankle region (London and Nash 2000). Chilblains, itchy and often painful lesions on the toes caused by abnormal vascular reaction to warming the tissues, are also common in older people with impaired peripheral circulation who live in cold environments (Spittell and Spittell 1992).

The flexibility of the many joints in the foot also decreases with age. Nigg et al (1992) reported significantly smaller ranges of plantarflexion, inversion, abduction and adduction in subjects aged 70–79 years compared with subjects aged 20–39 years. Similarly, both James and Parker (1989) and Vandervoort et al (1992) reported smaller ranges of ankle dorsiflexion in older subjects. These changes may be functionally important, as restricted range of motion in the foot makes it more difficult for an older person to maintain balance when walking on irregular terrain (Fogel et al 1982, Johansson et al 1982) and may impair the ability of the lower limb to absorb shock (Saltzman and Nawoczenski 1995).

Ligamentous changes with advancing age are of particular importance to the structure and function of the foot. As a consequence of collagen cross-linking and reduction in elastin content, ligaments in the foot become stiffer but less resilient, and therefore less able to maintain the bony architecture of the foot. This commonly affects the plantar calcaneonavicular ligament, which is partly responsible for maintaining the medial arch of the foot (Kitaoka et al 1997).

The effect of ageing on the strength of foot muscles has not been evaluated in detail. Although numerous studies indicate that age-related changes in muscle strength are more pronounced in the lower limb than the upper limb (Jennekens et al 1971, McDonagh et al 1984), practical considerations have limited most investigators to muscle groups that are easily measured, such as ankle dorsiflexors and plantarflexors. The strength, speed of onset and resistance to fatigue of these muscle groups has been found to reduce with age (Davies and White 1983, McDonagh et al 1984, Vandervoort and McComas 1986), so it is likely that this also occurs in the smaller muscles of the foot. The only study that has directly evaluated age-related differences in the strength of toe muscles reported that older people had 29% less strong toe plantarflexor muscles than young controls, and older women were 39% less strong than older men (Endo et al 2002). This decreased toe strength may be functionally significant, as plantarflexion of the toes plays an important role in controlling sway when standing (Tanaka et al 1996), and stabilizing the foot during the propulsive phase of gait (Hughes et al 1990).

Common foot problems and their management

Nail disorders

Nail disorders are one of the most common foot complaints affecting older people. While often considered trivial conditions, nail disorders can be extremely painful, and in immunocompromised patients can predispose to quite serious secondary infection. The following section discusses the cause and treatment of the most common nail conditions affecting older people: onychauxis, onychocryptosis and onychomycosis.

Onychauxis

Onychauxis is the name given to hypertrophy (abnormal thickening) of the nail, which may result from a wide range of causes, including injury, trauma from ill-fitting shoes, infection, peripheral vascular disease, diabetes and nutritional deficiency (Cohen and Scher 1992). A more severe form of the condition, often called onychogryphosis or 'Ram's horn nail', results from long-term neglect (Mohrenschlager et al 2001) and is characterized by thickening in conjunction with pronounced curvature. Onychauxis and onychogryphosis are often accompanied by onychophosis, the formation of hyperkeratosis (callus) in the nail grooves. In some cases of onychauxis, pressure from bedclothes or tight hosiery can lead to quite severe pain, and if left untreated, subungual haematomas (blood blisters) may form under the nail, creating a potential site for infection. Regular maintenance of basic foot hygiene, including regular filing of nails, may be able to prevent excessive build-up. However, some cases may require treatment by a podiatrist, who will use a special drill to reduce the thickness of the nail. Surgical removal is occasionally indicated (Bartolomei 1995).

Onychocryptosis

The term onychocryptosis refers to 'ingrown' toenails, where a spicule of nail penetrates the skin, leading to inflammation, pain and increased risk of secondary infection. People with abnormally curved nails or over-riding toes are more likely to develop onychocryptosis. However, in many cases the condition is simply caused by inappropriate nail cutting and/or ill-fitting footwear. Toenails should be cut straight across, and shoes should have sufficient room in the toe-box to prevent constriction. Applying topical antiseptics and allowing the nail to grow out normally can successfully manage some cases. However, recurrent cases often require a minor surgical procedure performed by a podiatrist. This involves removing the offending portion of nail under local anaesthetic, and applying phenol to destroy some of the cells that produce the nail plate. This makes the nail narrower and prevents regrowth (Zuber 2002). A recent Cochrane review concluded that simple nail avulsion combined with phenolization is more effective in preventing recurrence compared to surgical excision, at the cost of increased risk of postoperative infection (Rounding and Hulm 2001).

Onychomycosis

The term onychomycosis refers to fungal nail infection, usually caused by dermatophyte, saprophyte and yeast organisms (Scherer and Kinmon 2000, Scherer et al 2001). Fungal infection of the nail is extremely common in older people, and results in yellow-brown discoloration, thickening, crumbling and offensive odour. While often considered a trivial complaint (Harris 1999), onychomycosis is by no means purely a cosmetic problem. Almost all people with onychomycosis report that the condition produces adverse psychosocial and physical effects that impact on their quality of life (Elewski 1997, Scher 1994). Furthermore, fungal nail infection increases the risk of onychocryptosis, which often leads to quite severe pain and secondary infection.

Conscientious management of foot hygiene, including washing the feet with soap and water and remembering to dry thoroughly, can prevent many fungal nail infections. Shoes, socks or hosiery should be changed daily to prevent excess moisture build-up. Once the condition has developed, it may take some time to achieve a complete cure. A wide range of treatments have been used to treat the condition; however, the 'gold standard' treatment is terbinafine (Lamisil), an oral medication that has been shown to cure the condition in 3–6 months (Crawford et al 2002a). In the presence of contraindications to oral medication, topical treatments (such as azoles, tolnaftate or undecenoic acid preparations) may be used. However, topical treatment takes much longer, requires considerable compliance, and complete cure rates are significantly lower (Hart et al 1999).

Skin disorders

Hyperkeratosis (calluses and corns)

Hyperkeratosis (epidermal thickening) is a normal physiological response to friction applied to the skin, and develops as a protective mechanism to prevent damage to deeper tissues. Skin affected by hyperkeratosis exhibits a range of histological differences from normal skin that are representative of increased epidermal cell production (Thomas et al 1985). The foot is a common site for the development of hyperkeratosis due to both its weight-bearing function and because the skin on the foot is subjected to friction from footwear. When the friction applied to the skin becomes excessive, the resultant focal thickening can become extremely painful, increasing the pressure on the underlying dermis and predisposing to ulceration. There are two types of hyperkeratosis: *calluses*, which generally develop on the plantar surface of the foot and appear as a diffuse thickening, and *corns*, which are more common on the toes and can be differentiated from a callus by the presence of a sharply demarcated central core. Corns can also develop in between the toes, and due to the associated moisture, are often soft and macerated (Coughlin 1984, Freeman 2002, Singh et al 1996).

Calluses and corns are caused by a range of factors: ill-fitting footwear, bony prominences, malunited fractures, short or long metatarsals and faulty foot biomechanics (Coughlin 1984, Singh et al 1996, Woodburn and Helliwell 1996). Probably the most common cause of calluses and corns in older people, particularly older women, is the wearing of shoes with an excessively tight toe-box (Burns et al 2002, Frey et al 1993, Frey 2000). A survey of 356 women conducted by the American Orthopedic Foot and Ankle Society reported that 88% wore shoes that were too small for their feet, and of these 58% reported pain in their toes (Frey et al 1993). Similarly, Burns et al (2002) reported that 72% of older people attending a rehabilitation ward who wore shoes that were too short and narrow were more likely to suffer from foot pain. Although intervention studies are yet to be performed, it is likely that changing shoe-wearing habits could have a considerable impact on reducing the prevalence of hyper-keratotic lesions. The inherent difficulty in changing footwear behaviour cannot be understated, as fashion requirements in many cases outweigh practical considerations (Joyce 2000, Rossi 1980, Seale 1995). Even if older people do seek appropriately fitting footwear, a recent study indicates that they may have some difficulty, as two-thirds of a sample of 100 older people were found to have feet too broad to comfortably fit into currently available casual footwear (Chantelau and Gede 2002).

In addition to the selection of more appropriate footwear, calluses and corns should be debrided and enucleated by a podiatrist. In most cases, this will lead to immediate relief of pain (Redmond et al 1999), increase the bearable pressure threshold of the foot (Prud'homme and Curran 1999), and decrease the pressures borne by the metatarsal heads when walking (Pitei et al 1999). These benefits are generally only short-term (Woodburn et al 2000), particularly if the underlying causes are not fully addressed. Simple foam and silicon pads can offer effective (if only tem-porary) relief (Bedinghaus and Niedfeldt 2001, George 1993). Medicated 'corn pads' should be avoided, as they contain acid preparations to break down the excessive build-up of skin (Freeman 2002). While this may not pose a problem for people with good skin integrity, in older people with frail skin and/or impaired peripheral vascular supply (such as older people with diabetes), these preparations can cause considerable dam-age – in some cases ulceration (Foster et al 1989). Longer-term manage-ment includes foot orthoses (Caselli et al 1997, Colagiuri et al 1995) and surgery; however, surgical intervention should be very carefully consid-ered. Metatarsal osteotomy is commonly associated with the development of new lesions at previously lesion-free sites due to the postoperative alteration in foot mechanics (Idusuyi et al 1998).

Dry skin (xerosis)

Dehydration of the skin is a common accompaniment of advancing age, and is particularly prevalent in older people with diabetes or peripheral vascular disease. Dry skin around the heels often leads to the develop-ment of fissures that may extend to the dermis, resulting in pain and risk of infection. A wide range of emollient preparations (including urea, alpha hydroxy acids, lactic acid and ammonium lactate) have been shown to be effective in rehydrating the skin (Ademola et al 2002, Jennings et al 1998, Jennings et al 2002, Uy et al 1999). However, it would appear that the frequency of application is as important as the active ingredient in the preparation. Soaking the feet in baths containing mois-turizing lotions may also be effective (Hopp and Sundberg 1974).

Structural foot problems

Hallux valgus

More commonly referred to as 'bunions' (from the Greek *bunios*, meaning 'turnip'), hallux valgus is the most common deformity of the first ray segment of the foot and refers to the abnormal medial prominence of the first metatarsal head. Although the most visible consequence of the deformity is the bulbous, often inflamed great toe joint, the condition is rather more complex and often involves the progressive structural deformation of the entire forefoot. Hallux valgus is a multifactorial condition, caused by muscle imbalance, structural deformity of the metatarsals (which is sometimes an inherited trait), faulty foot mechanics and the detrimental effects of ill-fitting footwear (Kilmartin and Wallace 1993).

The enlarged first metatarsal head creates problems with finding suitable footwear, and the friction created by the shoe often leads to the formation of a bursa (fluid-filled sac) over the site. Treatment of hallux valgus includes changing footwear to that with a broader forefoot, the application of foam or silicon pads over the joint, foot orthoses and surgery. Surgery has been shown to provide better long-term results than foot orthoses (Torkki et al 2001). However, there are a wide range of surgical techniques which may not all provide similar results. Unfortunately, the evidence pertaining to the efficacy of bunion surgery is generally of low quality, and the most recent Cochrane review concluded that inadequate evidence exists to indicate significant benefits of any one surgical technique versus another (Ferrari et al 2000).

Hallux limitus/rigidus

Hallux limitus is a condition in which there is limited range of motion at the first metatarsophalangeal joint of the hallux. If this progresses to complete fusion of the joint, it is termed hallux rigidus. For hallux limitus, treatment involves foot orthoses to facilitate propulsion or manipulation and injection with corticosteroid (Solan et al 2001). For hallux rigidus, footwear modifications or surgery may be necessary. However, in a recent 14-year follow-up study of patients who had chosen not to have surgery, few reported that their condition had worsened, and 75% would still choose not to have surgery if they had to make the decision again. A large proportion of these patients had changed their footwear to that with a more ample toe-box, suggesting that selection of appropriate footwear may be a sufficient treatment in many people (Smith et al 2000). Indeed, a recent retrospective analysis of 772 patients with hallux limitus reported that 55% were successfully treated with conservative measures, including change of footwear, foot orthoses and corticosteroid injection (Grady et al 2002).

Lesser toe deformity

Long-term wearing of ill-fitting footwear, in association with faulty foot mechanics and intrinsic muscle atrophy, can lead to the development of clawing, hammering and retraction of the lesser toes (Coughlin 1984). Hammertoes and clawtoes are one of the most common foot complaints in older people, and can lead to the development of corns on the dorsum of the interphalangeal joints and calluses under the metatarsal heads.

There is also evidence to suggest that toe deformity may impair balance in older people (Menz and Lord 2001b). Treatment involves footwear modification, various splinting devices, and management of secondary lesions. Severe cases often require surgery to realign and stabilize the affected metatarsophalangeal or interphalangeal joints and/or lengthen the long flexor or extensor tendons.

Functional foot problems

The term 'functional foot problems' refers to those related to abnormal mechanics of the foot when walking. A myriad of such conditions may be responsible for pain in the heel, midfoot and forefoot, and differentiating between these conditions requires detailed diagnostic approaches by foot care specialists. The following section will briefly outline the most commonly observed functional foot problems, grouped together according to the region of the foot they affect.

Heel problems

Pain in the region of the heel is one of the most common presentations to foot specialist clinics. Although sound epidemiological data are not available, it has been estimated that the prevalence of heel pain in older people lies between 12.5 and 15% (Black et al 1993). There are a range of causes of heel pain, including proximal plantar fasciitis (also referred to as heel spur syndrome or enthesopathy), nerve entrapment, calcaneal stress fracture and plantar calcaneal bursitis. A number of systemic conditions can also lead to heel pain, including Paget's disease, rheumatoid arthritis, psoriatic arthritis, gout, Reiter's syndrome and ankylosing spondylitis (Barrett and O'Malley 1999).

Older people may be more likely to develop heel pain due to the effects of ageing on the structure and function of the plantar heel pad, a specialized soft tissue structure under the calcaneus consisting of closely packed fat cells that is responsible for shock attenuation when walking. Older people have thicker, but more compressible heel pads that dissipate more energy than younger people (Hsu et al 1998), which may result in greater impact being applied to the musculoskeletal and neural structures in the heel region. The impaired ability of the heel pad to attenuate shock is even more pronounced in the presence of diabetes mellitus (Hsu et al 2000). The other likely contributor to heel pain in older people is excess body weight, as many patients with heel pain have a higher body mass index than controls (Rano et al 2001).

A wide range of treatments have been reported for plantar heel pain, including stretching the calf muscles, foot orthoses/insoles, heel cups, tension night splints, corticosteroid injection, therapeutic ultrasound, non-steroidal anti-inflammatory drugs, galvanic currents, shoe modifications, acupuncture, laser therapy, extracorporeal shock-wave therapy and surgery (Young et al 2001). However, the quality of evidence for each of these interventions is generally poor, and the most recent Cochrane review on the topic concluded that although there is some evidence for the effectiveness of cortisone administered via iontophoresis, the efficacy of other frequently employed treatments has not been fully established in comparative studies (Crawford et al 2002b).

Midfoot problems

Pain in the midfoot can result from a range of conditions. The most commonly diagnosed conditions responsible for pain in this area are plantar fasciitis and osteoarthritis of the talonavicular joint. Less common causes include tarsal tunnel syndrome and tibialis posterior dysfunction. Tarsal tunnel syndrome is a well-known but rare entrapment neuropathy involving the posterior tibial nerve in the tarsal tunnel, a fibro-osseous channel extending from the medial aspect of the ankle to the midfoot. Tarsal tunnel syndrome can result from a range of conditions such as ganglia, sarcoma, talocalcaneal coalition, and the presence of an accessory flexor digitorum longus muscle (Lau and Daniels 1999). Treatment involves surgical decompression of the neurovascular bundle and/or resection of the osseous coalition or accessory muscle.

Tibialis posterior dysfunction is a condition in which the tibialis posterior muscle, which plays a role in maintaining the medial arch of the foot, weakens and may partially rupture, leading to a progressive and disabling flatfoot deformity (Landorf 1995). While the exact cause is unknown, tendon degeneration due to reduced blood supply has been implicated (Frey et al 1990), and the condition is more common in people with obesity, hypertension, diabetes or previous trauma (Holmes and Mann 1992). Treatment options include foot orthoses, tendon reconstruction or surgical fixation of joints in the rearfoot.

Forefoot problems

'Metatarsalgia' is a commonly used, non-specific term to describe pain in the forefoot; however, it is not in itself a clinical entity. Common causes of pain in the forefoot already discussed include hyperkeratosis, hallux valgus, hallux limitus/rigidus and lesser digital deformity. Other common causes in older people include interdigital neuritis and metatarsal stress/insufficiency fracture (Van Wyngarden 1997).

Interdigital neuritis (also referred to as Morton's neuroma) is the term given to plantar digital neuritis affecting the 3rd/4th interdigital space (Youngswick 1994). The pain associated with this condition frequently has a 'pins and needles' quality and radiates towards the toes. While the aetiology is uncertain, this condition is thought to result from the pinching of a plantar digital nerve caused by excessively narrow footwear or abnormal foot mechanics. Treatment involves footwear advice and/or modification, padding to redistribute weight-bearing pressure away from the affected area, or surgical excision (Wu 1996).

Stress fractures are most commonly caused by healthy bones being exposed to intense and/or repetitive loads for which the bone is not prepared, such as a rapid increase in training intensity in a competitive athlete. Insufficiency stress fractures, however, result from normal loads to bones weakened by genetic, metabolic, nutritional or endocrine processes. As bone mineral density decreases with age, older people develop an increased risk of insufficiency fracture, and this increased risk is particularly pronounced in older women with osteoporosis. Insufficiency fractures can occur in the bones of the foot, particularly the metatarsals (Freeman and Randall 2001, Kaye 1988, Varenna et al 1997). Treatment involves pressure redistribution and management of osteoporosis.

Can foot problems be prevented?

Given that many foot problems in older people can be at least partially attributed to inappropriate footwear, it is likely that changing footwear habits could prevent a great deal of discomfort and disability. As stated previously, the prevalence of ill-fitting footwear in older people is very high – between 50 and 80% – and there is solid evidence to indicate that older people who wear ill-fitting shoes are more likely to suffer from foot problems (Burns et al 2002, Chung 1983, Frey et al 1993, 2000, King 1978). However, no studies have adequately evaluated whether changing to more suitable footwear actually reduces rates of foot problems, and convincing older people to change their footwear is a difficult task. Fashion exerts a very powerful influence over footwear selection (Joyce 2000, Seale 1995), so much so that advising older people on suitable footwear has been called 'an exercise in eternal futility' (Rossi 1993). Further work needs to be done to develop effective strategies to influence shoe-wearing behaviour, and to assess the efficacy of such interventions on pain and disability.

In addition to changing footwear, regular podiatric treatment may assist in the prevention of foot problems. Debridement of hyperkeratotic lesions results in immediate relief of pain (Redmond et al 1999), increases the bearable pressure threshold of the foot (Prud'homme and Curran 1999), and decreases the pressures borne by the metatarsal heads when walking (Pitei et al 1999). Pressure redistributing insoles have also been shown to be effective in reducing the size of plantar calluses in people with diabetes (Colagiuri et al 1995), which may prevent damage to subcutaneous tissues. Older people themselves can also prevent or at least slow the development of lesions by the regular application of emollient creams to prevent skin dryness (Ademola et al 2002, Hopp and Sundberg 1974, Jennings et al 1998, 2002, Uy et al 1999).

Strength and flexibility training can markedly improve mobility in older people (see Chapter seven, this volume). However, the role of strengthening foot muscles and maintaining range of motion in foot joints has received very little attention. As stated previously, normal ageing has been shown to influence the contractile properties of lower limb muscles, and a recent study has indicated that older people exhibit 29% less strength in toe plantarflexor muscles compared with young controls (Endo et al 2002). Given the importance of the toes in standing and walking, maintaining the strength of intrinsic foot muscles may offer some functional benefits. A controlled trial by Kobayashi et al (1999) reported that a tri-weekly, 8-week programme of toe grasping exercises (including gathering a towel and picking up beanbags with the toes) resulted in significant reductions in postural sway measures in older people, indicating that toe strength plays an important role in the maintenance of balance. Strength training may also play a role in slowing the progression of conditions such as hallux valgus and lesser digital deformity.

As ageing is also associated with reduced range of motion in subtalar and ankle joints (James and Parker 1989, Nigg et al 1992), and reduced range of motion in the foot can impair balance (Fogel et al 1982, Johansson et al 1982), exercises to maintain range of motion in lower limb joints may hold some promise as a preventative strategy. While no studies have evaluated such an intervention in older people, a preliminary investigation in subjects with diabetes revealed that a programme of passive mobilization exercises resulted in significant increases in range of motion of the ankle, subtalar, first ray and first metatarsophalangeal joints, with many subjects in the treatment group reporting a subjective improvement in gait (Dijs et al 2000). Maintaining mobility in foot joints may improve the lower limb's ability to absorb shock, thereby reducing the likelihood of conditions such as heel pain and metatarsalgia.

Although these small clinical studies indicate that some interventions may be effective, few large-scale studies have been undertaken to adequately evaluate the effect of podiatric intervention on preventing foot problems in older people. The only significant studies of the effects of podiatric intervention have been performed in the context of preventing ulceration and amputation in people with diabetes. These studies have generally found that patients receiving podiatry treatment report less severe foot pain, exhibit some improvements in functional ability and self-care behaviour, and may be less likely to develop ulcers (Rijken et al 1999, Ronnemaa et al 1997). It is likely that similar beneficial effects would be observed with regard to podiatry treatment of older people. However, large-scale studies are yet to be undertaken.

Can treatment of foot problems improve mobility and quality of life?

Given that no large-scale studies of podiatry interventions in older people have been undertaken, any improvement in mobility and quality of life associated with podiatry treatments remains largely speculative. No studies have utilized objective tests of mobility (sit-to-stand, walking speed, etc.) to evaluate podiatry treatments, and only very recently have health-related quality of life instruments been reported in the foot and ankle literature (Wrobel 2000). The Foot Function Index (Budiman-Mak et al 1991), a self-administered index consisting of three domains (activity limitation, pain and disability), has been found to respond positively to foot orthotic interventions in people with hyperkeratotic lesions (Caselli et al 1997) and people with rheumatoid arthritis (Conrad et al 1996, Woodburn et al 2002), while another foot-specific health-related quality of life scale – the Foot Health Status Questionnaire (FHSQ) – has recently been developed, incorporating aspects of the Short Form 36 (SF-36) general health questionnaire (Bennett et al 1998). Significant improvements in the pain, physical function, general foot health, and footwear-related quality of life components of the FHSQ have been reported following foot surgery (Bennett et al 2001) and following orthotic treatment for heel pain (Landorf and Keenan 2002). These preliminary findings are generally positive, and indicate that podiatry treatments may have beneficial effects on mobility and quality of life. However, further research needs to be undertaken in large samples of older people.

Conclusion

Foot problems are an important yet commonly overlooked contributor to impaired physical functioning and reduced quality of life in older people. Many foot problems can be managed effectively with conservative interventions, and although the evidence is sparse, it is likely that maintaining the skin integrity, range of motion and muscle strength of the foot will assist older people to remain active. All older people should undergo regular foot screening to ensure they do not needlessly endure disabling foot pain.

References

Ademola J, Frazier C, Kim S J, Theaux C, Saudez X 2002 Clinical evaluation of 40% urea and 12% ammonium lactate in the treatment of xerosis. American Journal of Clinical Dermatology 3:217–222

Australian Institute of Health and Welfare 2002 Podiatry Labour Force 1999. AIHW cat no. HWL 23. AIHW (National Health Labour Force Series No. 23), Canberra

Barrett S L, O'Malley R 1999 Plantar fasciitis and other causes of heel pain. American Family Physician 59:2200–2206

Bartolomei F J 1995 Onychauxis. Surgical and nonsurgical treatment. Clinics in Podiatric Medicine and Surgery 12:215–220

Beard J D 2000 ABC of arterial and venous disease: chronic lower limb ischaemia. British Medical Journal 320:854–857

Bedinghaus J, Niedfeldt M 2001 Over-the-counter foot remedies. American Family Physician 64:791–796

Bennett P J, Patterson C, Wearing S, Baglioni T 1998 Development and validation of a questionnaire designed to measure foot-health status. Journal of the American Podiatric Medical Association 88:419–428

Bennett P J, Patterson C, Dunne M P 2001 Health-related quality of life following podiatric surgery. Journal of the American Podiatric Medical Association 91:164–173

Benvenutti F, Ferrucci L, Guralnik J, Gangemi S, Baroni A 1995 Foot pain and disability in older persons: an epidemiologic survey. Journal of the American Geriatrics Society 43:479–484

Black J R, Bernard J M, Williams L A 1993 Heel pain in the older patient. Clinics in Podiatric Medicine and Surgery 10:113–119

Blake A, Morgan K, Bendall M, et al 1988 Falls by elderly people at home – prevalence and associated factors. Age and Ageing 17:365–372

Budiman-Mak E, Conrad K J, Roach K E 1991 The foot function index: a measure of foot pain and disability. Journal of Clinical Epidemiology 44:561–570

Burns S L, Leese G P, McMurdo M E T 2002 Older people and ill-fitting shoes. Postgraduate Medical Journal 78:344–346

Caselli M, Levitz S, Clark N, et al 1997 Comparison of Viscoped and Poron for painful submetatarsal hyperkeratotic lesions. Journal of the American Podiatric Medical Association 87:6–10

Chantelau E, Gede A 2002 Foot dimensions of elderly people with and without diabetes mellitus – a data basis for shoe design. Gerontology 48:241–244

Chung S 1983 Foot care. A health care maintenance program. Journal of Gerontological Nursing 9:213–227

Cohen P R, Scher R K 1992 Geriatric nail disorders: diagnosis and treatment. Journal of the American Academy of Dermatology 26:521–531

Colagiuri S, Marsden L, Naidu V, Taylor L 1995 The use of orthotic devices to correct plantar callus in people with diabetes. Diabetes Research and Clinical Practice 28:29–34

Conrad K J, Budiman-Mak E, Roach K E, Hedeker D 1996 Impacts of foot orthoses on rheumatoid arthritics. Journal of Clinical Epidemiology 49:1–7

Coughlin M J 1984 Mallet toes, hammer toes, claw toes and corns. Postgraduate Medicine 75:191–198

Crawford V L S, Ashford R L, McPeake B, Stout R W 1995 Conservative podiatric medicine and disability in elderly people. Journal of the American Podiatric Medical Association 85:255–259

Crawford F, Young P, Godfrey C, et al 2002a Oral treatments for toenail onychomycosis: a systematic review. Archives of Dermatology 138:811–816

Crawford F, Atkins D, Edwards J 2002b Interventions for treating plantar heel pain. The Foot 11:228–250

Davies C T M, White M J 1983 Contractile properties of elderly human triceps surae. Gerontology 29:19–25

Dijs H M, Roofthooft J M A, Driessens M F, et al 2000 Effect of physical therapy on limited joint mobility in the diabetic foot. Journal of the American Podiatric Medical Association 90:126–132

Dolinis J, Harrison J E 1997 Factors associated with falling in older Adelaide residents. Australian and New Zealand. Journal of Public Health 21:462–468

Ebrahim S B J, Sainsbury R, Watson S 1981 Foot problems of the elderly: a hospital survey. British Medical Journal 283:949–950

Elewski B 1997 The effect of toenail onychomycosis on patient quality of life. International Journal of Dermatology 36:754–756

Endo M, Ashton-Miller J, Alexander N 2002 Effects of age and gender on toe flexor muscle strength. Journal of Gerontology 57A:392–397

Ferrari J, Higgins J P T, Williams R L 2000 Interventions for treating hallux valgus (abductovalgus) and bunions. Cochrane Database of Systematic Reviews 2: CD000964

Fogel G R, Katoh Y, Rand J A, Chao E Y S 1982 Talo-navicular arthrodesis for isolated arthrosis. Foot and Ankle 3:105–113

Foster A, Edmonds M, Das A, Watkins P 1989 Corn cures can damage your feet: an important lesson for diabetic patients. Diabetic Medicine 6:818–819

Freeman D B 2002 Corns and calluses resulting from mechanical hyperkeratosis. American Family Physician 65:2277–2280

Freeman D, Randall D B 2001 Stress fracture of the foot secondary to osteoporosis: an atypical presentation. Journal of the American Podiatric Medical Association 91:99–101

Frey C C 1990 Vascularity of the posterior tibial tendon. Journal of Bone and Joint Surgery 72A:884–888

Frey C, Thompson F, Smith J, Sanders M, Horstman H 1993 American Orthopedic Foot and Ankle Society women's shoe survey. Foot and Ankle 14:78–81

Frey C C 2000 Foot health and shoewear for women. Clinical Orthopaedics and Related Research 372:32–44

Gabell A, Simons M A, Nayak U S L 1985 Falls in the healthy elderly: predisposing causes. Ergonomics 28:965–975

George D 1993 Management of hyperkeratotic lesions in the elderly patient. Clinics in Podiatric Medicine and Surgery 10:69–77

Gilchrest B A 1996 A review of skin ageing and its medical therapy. British Journal of Dermatology 135:867–875

Glogau R G 1997 Physiologic and structural changes associated with aging skin. Dermatologic Clinics 15:555–559

Gorecki G A 1978 Shoe related foot problems and public health. Journal of the American Podiatry Association 4:245–247

Gorter K J, Kuyvenhoven M M, deMelker R A 2000 Nontraumatic foot complaints in older people. A population-based survey of risk factors, mobility, and well-being. Journal of the American Podiatric Medical Association 90:397–402

Grady J F, Axe T M, Zager E J, Sheldon L A 2002 A retrospective analysis of 772 patients with hallux limitus. Journal of the American Podiatric Medical Association 92:102–108

Greenberg L 1994 Foot care data from two recent nationwide surveys – a comparative analysis. Journal of the American Podiatric Medical Association 84:365–370

Harris J 1999 Do crinkly toenails really matter? British Medical Journal 319:1197

Hart R, Bell-Syer S, Crawford F, et al 1999 Systematic review of topical treatments for fungal infections of the skin and nails of the feet. British Medical Journal 319:79–82

Holmes G B, Mann R A 1992 Possible epidemiological factors associated with rupture of the posterior tibial tendon. Foot and Ankle 13:70–79

Hopp R A, Sundberg S 1974 The effects of soaking and lotion on dryness of the skin in the feet of the elderly patient. Journal of the American Podiatry Association 64:747–760

Hsu T C, Wang C L, Tsai W C, Kuo J K, Tang F T 1998 Comparison of the mechanical properties of the heel pad between young and elderly adults. Archives of Physical Medicine and Rehabilitation 79:1101–1104

Hsu T C, Wang C L, Shau Y W, et al 2000 Altered heel-pad mechanical properties in patients with type two diabetes mellitus. Diabetic Medicine 17:854–859

Hughes J, Clark P, Klenerman L 1990 The importance of the toes in walking. Journal of Bone and Joint Surgery 72B:245–251

Hung L, Ho Y, Leung P 1985 Survey of foot deformities among 166 geriatric inpatients. Foot and Ankle 5:156–164

Idusuyi O, Kitaoka H, Patzer G 1998 Oblique metatarsal osteotomy for intractable plantar keratosis: 10-year follow-up. Foot and Ankle International 19:351–355

James B, Parker A W 1989 Active and passive mobility of lower limb joints in elderly men and women. American Journal of Physical Medicine and Rehabilitation 68:162–167

Jenkins G 2002 Molecular mechanisms of skin ageing. Mechanisms of Ageing and Development 123:801–810

Jennekens F G I, Tomlinson B E, Walton J N 1971 Histochemical aspects of five limb muscles in old age. Journal of the Neurological Sciences 14:259–276

Jennings M B, Alfieri D, Ward K, Lesczczynski C 1998 Comparison of salicylic acid and urea versus ammonium lactate for the treatment of foot xerosis. A randomized, double-blind, clinical study. Journal of the American Podiatric Medical Association 88:332–336

Jennings M B, Logan L, Alfieri D M, et al 2002 A comparative study of lactic acid 10% and ammonium lactate 12% lotion in the treatment of foot xerosis. Journal of the American Podiatric Medical Association 92:143–148

Johansson J E, Harrison J, Greenwood F A H 1982 Subtalar arthrodesis for adult traumatic arthritis. Foot and Ankle 2:294–298

Joyce P 2000 Women and their shoes: attitudes, influences and behaviour. British Journal of Podiatry 3:111–115

Kaye R A 1988 Insufficiency stress fractures of the foot and ankle in postmenopausal women. Foot and Ankle International 19:221–224

Kilmartin T E, Wallace W A 1993 The aetiology of hallux valgus: a critical review of the literature. The Foot 3:157–167

King P A 1978 Foot assessment of the elderly. Journal of Gerontological Nursing 4:49–52

Kitaoka H, Ahn T, Luo Z, An K 1997 Stability of the arch of the foot. Foot and Ankle. International 18:644–648

Kobayashi R, Hosoda M, Minematsu A, et al 1999 Effects of toe grasp training for the aged on spontaneous postural sway. Journal of Physical Therapy Science 11:31–34

Koski K, Luukinen H, Laippala P, Kivela S-L 1996 Physiological factors and medications as predictors of injurious falls by elderly people: a prospective population-based study. Age and Ageing 25:29–38

Landorf K B 1995 Tibialis posterior dysfunction – early identification is the key to success. Australian Podiatrist 29:9–14

Landorf K B, Keenan A M 2002 An evaluation of two foot-specific, health-related quality-of-life measuring instruments. Foot and Ankle International 23:538–546

Lau J T, Daniels T R 1999 Tarsal tunnel syndrome: a review of the literature. Foot and Ankle International 20:201–209

Leveille S G, Guralnik J M, Ferrucci L, et al 1998 Foot pain and disability in older women. American Journal of Epidemiology 148:657–665

Leveille S G, Bean J, Bandeen-Roche K, et al 2002 Musculoskeletal pain and risk of falls in older disabled women living in the community. Journal of the American Geriatrics Society 50:671–678

London N, Nash R 2000 ABC of arterial and venous disease. Varicose veins. British Medical Journal 320:1391–1394

McDonagh M J N, White M J, Davies C T M 1984 Different effects of ageing on the mechanical properties of human arm and leg muscles. Gerontology 30:49–54

Menz H B, Lord S R 1999 Foot problems, functional impairment and falls in older people. Journal of the American Podiatric Medical Association 89:458–461

Menz H B, Lord S R 2001a The contribution of foot problems to mobility impairment and falls in community-dwelling older people. Journal of the American Geriatrics Society 49:1651–1656

Menz H B, Lord S R 2001b Foot pain impairs balance and functional ability in community-dwelling older people. Journal of the American Podiatric Medical Association 91:222–229

Mohrenschlager M, Wicke-Wittenius K, Brockow K, Bruckbauer H, Ring J 2001 Onychogryphosis in elderly persons: an indicator of long-standing poor nursing care? Report of one case and review of the literature. Cutis 68:233–235

Muehlman C, Rahimi F 1990 Aging integumentary system. Podiatric review. Journal of the American Podiatric Medical Association 80:577–582

Munro B J, Steele J R 1998 Foot-care awareness – a survey of persons aged 65 years and older. Journal of the American Podiatric Medical Association 88:242–248

Nigg B, Fisher V, Allinger T, Ronsky J, Engsberg J 1992 Range of motion of the foot as a function of age. Foot and Ankle 13:336–343

Pitei D, Foster A, Edmonds M 1999 The effect of regular callus removal on foot pressures. Journal of Foot and Ankle Surgery 38:251–255

Prud'homme P, Curran M 1999 A preliminary study of the use of the algometer to investigate whether or not patients benefit when podiatrists enucleate corns. The Foot 9:65–69

Rano J A, Fallat L M, Savoy-Moore R T 2001 Correlation of heel pain with body mass index and other characteristics of heel pain. Journal of Foot and Ankle Surgery 40:351–356

Redmond A, Allen N, Vernon W 1999 Effect of scalpel debridement on the pain associated with plantar hyperkeratosis. Journal of the American Podiatric Medical Association 89:515–519

Rijken P M, Dekker J, Lankhorst GJ, et al 1999 Podiatric care for diabetic patients with foot problems: an observational study. International Journal of Rehabilitation Research 22:181–188

Ronnemaa T, Hamalainen H, Toikka T, Liukkonen I 1997 Evaluation of the impact of podiatrist care in the primary prevention of foot problems in diabetic subjects. Diabetes Care 20:1833–1837

Rosenberg G 1958 Effect of age on peripheral vibratory perception. Journal of the American Geriatrics Society 6:471–481

Rossi W A 1980 The frustration of 'sensible' shoes. Journal of the American Podiatry Association 70:257–258

Rossi W A 1993 The sex life of the foot and shoe. Krieger Publishing Company, Florida.

Rounding C, Hulm S 2001 Surgical treatments for ingrowing toenails. The Foot 11:166–182

Saltzman C L, Nawoczenski D A 1995 Complexities of foot architecture as a base of support. Journal of Orthopedic and Sports Physical Therapy 21:354–360

Scher R 1994 Onychomycosis is more than a cosmetic problem. British Journal of Dermatology 130:15

Scherer W P, Kinmon K 2000 Dermatophyte test medium culture versus mycology laboratory analysis for suspected onychomycosis. A study of 100 cases in a geriatric population. Journal of the American Podiatric Medical Association 90:450–459

Scherer W P, McCreary J P, Hayes W W 2001 The diagnosis of onychomycosis in a geriatric population: a study of 450 cases in South Florida. Journal of the American Podiatric Medical Association 91:456–464

Seale K 1995 Women and their shoes: unrealistic expectations? AAOS Instructional Course Lectures 44:379–384

Singh D, Bentley G, Trevino S 1996 Callosities, corns, and calluses. British Medical Journal 213:1403–1406

Smith R, Katchis S, Ayson L 2000 Outcomes in hallux rigidus patients treated nonoperatively: a long-term follow-up study. Foot and Ankle International 21:906–913

Solan M, Calder J, Bendall S 2001 Manipulation and injection for hallux rigidus. Is it worthwhile? Journal of Bone and Joint Surgery 83B:706–708

Spittell J, Spittell P 1992 Chronic pernio: another cause of blue toes. International Angiology 11:46–50

Stevens J C, Choo K K 1996 Spatial acuity of the body surface over the life span. Somatosensory and Motor Research 13:153–166

Tanaka T, Noriyasu S, Ino S, Ifukube T, Nakata M 1996 Objective method to determine the contribution of the great toe to standing balance and preliminary observations of age-related effects. IEEE Transactions on Rehabilitation Engineering 4:84–90

Thomas S E, Dykes P J, Marks R 1985 Plantar hyperkeratosis: a study of callosities and normal plantar skin. Journal of Investigative Dermatology 85:394–397

Tinetti M E, Speechley M, Ginter S F 1988 Risk factors for falls among elderly persons living in the community. New England Journal of Medicine 319:1701–1707

Torkki M, Malmivaara A, Seitsalo S, et al 2001 Surgery vs orthosis vs watchful waiting for hallux valgus: a randomized controlled trial. JAMA 285:2474–2480

Uy J J, Joyce A M, Nelson J P, West B, Montague J R 1999 Ammonium lactate 12% lotion versus a liposome-based moisturizing lotion for plantar xerosis. A double-blind comparison study. Journal of the American Podiatric Medical Association 89:502–505

Vandervoort A A, McComas A J 1986 Contractile changes in opposing muscles of the human ankle joint with aging. Journal of Applied Physiology 61:361–367

Vandervoort A A, Chesworth B M, Cunningham D A, et al 1992 Age and sex effects on mobility of the human ankle. Journal of Gerontology 47:17–21

Van Wyngarden T M 1997 The painful foot, Part I: common forefoot deformities. American Family Physician 55:1866–1876

Varenna M, Binelli L, Zucchi F, et al 1997 Is the metatarsal fracture in postmenopausal women an osteoporotic fracture? A cross-sectional study on 113 cases. Osteoporosis International 7:558–563

Wild D, Nayak U, Isaacs B 1980 Characteristics of old people who fell at home. Journal of Clinical and Experimental Gerontology 2:271–287

Williamson J, Stokoe I, Gray S 1964 Old people at home – their unreported needs. Lancet i:1117–1120

Woodburn J, Helliwell P 1996 Relation between heel position and the distribution of forefoot plantar pressures and skin callosities in rheumatoid arthritis. Annals of the Rheumatic Diseases 55:806–810

Woodburn J, Stableford Z, Helliwell P 2000 Preliminary investigation of debridement of plantar callosities in rheumatoid arthritis. Rheumatology 39:652–654

Woodburn J, Barker S, Helliwell P 2002 A randomized controlled trial of foot orthoses in rheumatoid arthritis. Journal of Rheumatology 29:1377–1383

Wrobel J S 2000 Outcomes research in podiatric medicine. Journal of the American Podiatric Medical Association 90:403–410

Wu K K 1996 Morton's interdigital neuroma: a clinical review of its etiology, treatment, and results. Journal of Foot and Ankle Surgery 35:112–119

Young C C, Rutherford D S, Niedfeldt M W 2001 Treatment of plantar fasciitis. American Family Physician 63:477–478

Youngswick F D 1994 Intermetatarsal neuroma. Clinics in Podiatric Medicine and Surgery 11:579–592

Zuber T J 2002 Ingrown toenail removal. American Family Physician 65:2547–2252

12

Physical activity and falls prevention

Keith Hill and Kate Murray

CHAPTER CONTENTS

Epidemiology of falls among older people 247

Extrinsic and intrinsic risk factors for falls and fractures 249

The importance of musculoskeletal risk factors in falls prevention 250

Physical activity options to reduce falls risk for older people 251

Physical activity to reduce falls risk in older people – the evidence 251

Physical activity to reduce falls fracture risk in older people 255

Which dimensions of physical activity are most important in reducing falls risk? 255

Criteria for developing a physical activity programme to reduce falls 256

Incorporating balance and strength training into a physical activity programme 258

Lifestyle modification 259

Participation and sustainability 259

Physical activity in other settings 260

Summary 261

References 261

Epidemiology of falls among older people

Falls and associated injuries are common and costly, both to older people themselves, and to the wider community. Approximately one in three people aged over 65 years living in the community fall each year, and this rate increases with advancing age (Campbell et al 1981). In the USA in 1986, 8313 deaths were recorded from falls-related incidents for people aged over 65 years (Nevitt 1990). Additionally, Sattin et al (1990) reported that 7% of people aged over 75 years present to an emergency department after a fall each year, with approximately 40% of these cases being admitted to hospital for an average 14 days stay. The rate of injurious falls increases exponentially with increasing age (Sattin et al 1990). The overall costs associated with falls for people aged over 65 years have been shown to rise with increasing frequency and severity of falls (Rizzo et al 1998), and have been estimated at $US12.6 billion (Runge 1993). The costs associated with injurious falls are projected to escalate with the ageing of the population in the USA, Canada and other Western countries, unless falls and fall injury prevention programmes are successfully implemented (Wiktorowicz et al 2001).

Fractures are one of the most serious injuries associated with falls, and occur if the forces applied to the bone exceed the strength of the bone. Thus the severity of the fall and the strength of bone both play an important role in determining whether a fracture occurs. Osteoporosis is a major factor associated with risk of fracture, weakening both bone density and structural quality. It has been described as a 'silent thief' (Access Economics 2001), with 10% of Australians having osteoporosis. Osteoporosis increases with age, and the prevalence is three times greater in women than men (Access Economics 2001).

Fractures account for 77% of principal diagnoses associated with falls-related hospitalizations (Cripps and Jarman 2001), with over half of these being hip or femoral fractures. In a 1-year prospective study, healthcare costs for a hip fracture patient were more than double that of age- and residence-matched control subjects ($US13 470, compared with $US6170) (Haentjens et al 2001). One in five hip fracture patients experienced a subsequent fracture in a 16-month follow-up period (Colón-Emeric et al 2000). Not only is the management of fractures costly in terms of surgery, hospitalization and therapy, in many cases functional recovery to pre-fracture levels is not achieved (Magaziner et al 2000). Therefore, falls and falls injury prevention programmes need to target both the prevention of falls, and the prevention/management of osteoporosis.

While the costs associated with injurious falls are high, injurious falls requiring medical attention only account for approximately 10% of falls among older people (Hill et al 2002a, Tinetti et al 1995). Even minor falls which do not cause injury can cause loss of confidence in mobility (Tinetti et al 1994a), resulting in reduced activity levels, secondary deconditioning, and an increased risk of further falls. It is important for the signs of reduced confidence to be recognized after a fall, and for targeted treatment strategies to be implemented as soon as possible after the fall. Tools such as the Falls Efficacy Scale (Tinetti et al 1990) and the Modified Falls Efficacy Scale (Hill et al 1996) are useful in identifying specific activities affected by loss of confidence, which can then be addressed by a programme which often incorporates both an exercise and psychological support component (Tennstedt et al 1998, Yardley et al 1998).

Extrinsic and intrinsic risk factors for falls and fractures

Risk factors for falls can be considered to be either extrinsic (related to the environment, or high risk activity being undertaken) or intrinsic (related to the ageing process, and the influence of pathology on the systems involved in balance) (Lord et al 2001). Examples of both extrinsic and intrinsic falls risk factors are listed in Table 12.1. In the majority of cases, falls are multifactorial in nature, often involving a combination of extrinsic and intrinsic risk factors. Of note, older people more commonly attribute falls to extrinsic factors (Weinberg and Strain 1995), even when intrinsic factors may be contributing at least as much to the fall. Older people who experience a fall should undergo a medical review in order to identify and treat any contributory intrinsic factors, as well as addressing the extrinsic risks (Campbell 1997, Hill et al 2002b, Schwarz 1995).

Although low levels of activity have been noted in many studies as a risk factor for falls (Campbell et al 1989, Lord et al 1993), one study suggested that very high levels of physical activity might also be a risk factor for falls and injurious falls (O'Laughlin et al 1993). A potential explanation might be that older people who are more active are more frequently exposed to a greater range of potential environmental falls hazards than less active older people. Clearly, consideration needs to be given to matching exposure to risk to the individual's physical abilities. Most commonly, physical activity programmes which have achieved increased physical activity have not increased risk of falling among participating individuals (see section on 'Physical activity to reduce falls risk in older people – the evidence').

Table 12.1 Falls risk factors

Intrinsic falls risk factors	Extrinsic falls risk factors
■ Increased age	■ Uneven surfaces
■ History of previous fall/s	■ Slippery surfaces
■ History of injuries associated with fall/s	■ Poor lighting
■ Low activity levels	■ Inadequate footwear
■ Impaired balance	■ Loose mats/cords on floor
■ Reduced leg muscle strength	■ Stairs/curbs
■ Impaired walking/use of a gait aid	■ Sun glare/reflective surfaces
■ Polypharmacy	■ High risk activities such as reaching to a high shelf by standing on the edge of a chair
■ Specific high risk medications such as psychotropic drugs and sedatives	
■ Incontinence	
■ Impaired vision	
■ Dizziness	
■ Functional impairments	
■ Decreased reaction time	
■ Postural hypotension	
■ Cognitive problems, including dementia	
■ Chronic medical conditions such as stroke, Parkinson's disease and arthritis	

Some of the falls risk factors are also risk factors for fractures. These include increased age, previous falls and injuries, impaired balance, reduced muscle strength, and low activity level (Deal 1997). Additional risk factors for fractures include osteoporosis, osteomalacia (low vitamin D levels), low calcium intake, and low body weight (Deal 1997, Gregg et al 2000). Situational falls risk factors have also been described with respect to serious injury following a fall (Tinetti et al 1995). These include time and location of fall, for example landing on a hard or a soft surface; height from which the fall occurred, which will influence forces at the point of impact; and body position and direction of impact at the time of the fall.

Injury rates have been reported to be higher in more healthy/physically active older people. Speechley and Tinetti (1991) classified a large community sample into 'frail', 'transitional', or 'vigorous' groups based on a range of measures. While falls rates were lower for the 'vigorous' group, the proportion of falls causing serious injuries was more than double in the 'vigorous' group relative to the 'frail' group. In another sample of healthy women over 65 years of age, 9% experienced fractures due to falls in a 12-month follow-up period (Hill et al 1999). Serious injuries and fractures may be more common in active older people because the majority of falls occur during walking-related activities, and gait speed is significantly greater in healthy older people than in frailer older people. Increased walking speed at the time of a fall results in greater forces at the point of impact, and may cause more serious injuries such as fractures.

The importance of musculoskeletal risk factors in falls prevention

A number of the intrinsic falls risk factors are potentially amenable to remediation with physical activity. These include:

- impaired balance
- leg muscle weakness
- slow reaction time, reduced coordination
- reduced leg muscle flexibility, especially reduced calf length
- impaired or unsteady gait.

A systematic review of the range of physical activity options investigated as part of a series of linked falls prevention programmes – the FICSIT studies – established that those which incorporated some level of balance retraining appeared to be most effective in reducing falls risk (Province et al 1995). In addition, Tinetti et al (1996) investigated the effectiveness of a multifactorial intervention strategy which incorporated a physiotherapy-directed home exercise programme, a medication review, and a home environmental hazard review (Tinetti et al 1994b). A change in balance score of one was shown to be associated with an 11% reduction in falls rate (Tinetti et al 1996), indicating the substantial influence of balance performance on falls risk.

A degree of specificity of training is evident with various forms of physical activity. Some of the more specific health benefits relate to the physical demands placed on the neuromusculoskeletal system in the physical activity programme. For example, studies have shown that balance training can improve balance performance in older people, but may have little effect on muscle strength (Buchner et al 1997a). This highlights the need to train for the specific outcome desired. Additionally, there are a range of generic health benefits across many forms of physical activity. Some of the generic health benefits include improved morale, reduced depression, improved sleep and improved general health rating (Bravo et al 1996, Ellingson and Conn 2000, Singh et al 1997). As discussed previously, balance training seems to be the most important component of a physical activity programme if the goal is to achieve reduced falls among older people. However, older people with specific falls risk factors, for example reduced strength, are also likely to reduce their falls risk by training the problematic risk factor.

Physical activity options to reduce falls risk for older people

A range of physical activity options are available for older people that potentially could reduce risk of falls or fractures. Broadly these can be considered as either structured or incidental physical activities. Structured physical activities are those that occur as part of a formal programme. These are commonly performed as part of a class setting (Day et al 2002), or could also include home exercise programmes (Campbell et al 1997). Examples include strength training classes at a gymnasium (Buchner et al 1997b), combined group exercise programmes at community halls (Day et al 2002, Lord et al 1996), and tai chi classes (Wolf et al 1996). Incidental physical activities are components of routine lifestyle that have a physical component. Examples include walking to shops instead of driving, and using stairs instead of elevators. The majority of the falls prevention research literature has investigated structured physical activity programmes, although health promotion programmes advocate that a mix of both structured and incidental activity can contribute to improved health at the population level (Christmas and Andersen 2000).

Physical activity to reduce falls risk in older people – the evidence

Structured physical activity programmes are often used to prevent falls (Department of Human Services 2001, Gardner et al 2000). Various types of physical activity have been shown to reduce intrinsic risk factors for falling among older people with varying levels of frailty (Fiatarone et al 1994, Lord et al 1996, Morey et al 1996). However, relatively few randomized controlled trials have investigated the effectiveness of physical activity programmes on reducing falls rates (Gillespie et al 2001). The research evidence identifying effectiveness of different forms of physical activity in reducing falls among older people can be summarized as follows.

Balance training programmes

Balance training programmes are those where the emphasis of training is on improving postural stability and reducing falls. They have been shown to improve balance performance in older people (Ledin et al 1990, Rose and Clark 2000, Wolfson et al 1996). However, rarely has this approach been investigated in isolation using a randomized controlled trial design, with falls as an outcome. In one such study, Wolf et al (1996) used balance training on a force platform as one of three interventions in a falls prevention study. The platform training group improved balance performance, but this did not result in reduced falls. The use of force platform training in isolation, and its lack of transferability to balance requirements in everyday activities may have contributed to the lack of effect on falls. There have been several combined exercise approaches which have incorporated balance training and been shown to be effective in reducing falls among older people (see below).

Strength training programmes

There is evidence from randomized controlled trials that graduated strength training programmes can improve muscle strength in frail older people (Fiatarone et al 1990, 1994) and in less frail older people (Bravo et al 1996, Singh et al 1997). Randomized controlled trials have also demonstrated the effectiveness of strength training programmes in improving mobility and function in community-dwelling older people (Chandler et al 1998, Skelton et al 1995). However, there have been no strength training programmes implemented in isolation that have used falls rates as an outcome measure. There have been several combined exercise approaches which have included strength training with one or more other forms of exercise that have been shown to reduce falls (see below) (see also Chapter 7).

Cardiovascular fitness programmes

Cardiovascular training programmes aim to improve general fitness, and have an associated effect on general activity level. These programmes often include walking, bicycle riding (stationary or free wheeled), aerobic exercise programmes, or swimming/aquarobics programmes. Activities which incorporate a moderate amount of walking, such as golf or lawn bowls, may also be included in this category. In order to achieve a beneficial health effect, performance during the cardiovascular activity should aim to increase the exercising heart rate to 50–75% of the maximum heart rate (American Council on Exercise 1998, Awerbuch 2001), or to exercise between levels 12 to 14 on the Borg Rating of Perceived Exertion scale (American Council on Exercise 1998). Sedentary older people planning on commencing a cardiovascular programme are recommended to have a medical review prior to commencing the programme (see Chapter 14).

Cardiovascular physical activity programmes have been shown to improve cardiovascular health outcomes (e.g. lowered resting heart rate, quicker return to resting heart rate after activity ceases, improved VO_{2max}) in older people (King et al 1998). Randomized controlled trials have demonstrated significant improvements in cardiovascular measures among older people undertaking walking programmes (Hamdorf and Penhall 1999) and bicycle ergometry programmes (Posner et al 1992). The comparative effectiveness of three forms of group-based endurance training techniques (stationary bike, walking, and aerobic movement) was evaluated in a randomized controlled trial of sedentary, community-dwelling older people with mild balance deficits (Buchner et al 1997a). Only the walking programme significantly improved at least one outcome measure in each of the areas of muscle strength, endurance, balance, gait and health status. Walking is a particularly important form of cardiovascular training to consider, as it is an easily performed, low cost activity, requiring no specialized equipment or training. However, one of the few randomized controlled trials to evaluate the effectiveness of a brisk walking programme on falls identified an increased number of falls in the intervention group (Ebrahim et al 1997). Positive outcomes from the study included maintenance of bone mineral density at the femoral neck in the walking group. Participants were women who had had at least one upper limb fracture in the previous 2 years, and hence would be considered at increased risk of further falls. These results highlight the importance of ensuring a physical activity programme is targeted appropriately and safely, particularly for those with increased falls risk. Further research is needed to clarify the specific health benefits, including effect on falls and falls injury, associated with walking programmes.

Combined balance, strength, cardiovascular programmes

Many physical activity approaches incorporate a combination of two or more of balance, flexibility, coordination, strength and cardiovascular fitness activities.

Home programmes

Home programmes are usually undertaken following an assessment, with a programme developed which is tailored to the individual in terms of the specific exercises, frequency and intensity. Individualized home exercise programmes have been used as part of multiple intervention programmes that have resulted in reduced falls among older people, although it was not possible to separate the direct effect of the exercise component relative to other components in these studies (Tinetti et al 1994b).

Campbell and colleagues (Campbell 1997, Campbell et al 1997, 1999) conducted a randomized controlled trial evaluating the effectiveness of a home-based, physiotherapy-directed programme incorporating balance and strengthening exercises and a walking programme. Participants were women aged greater than 80 years. Recommended exercise frequency was three times weekly for 6 months, with four visits by the physiotherapist in this period to monitor and modify the exercises, and facilitate ongoing participation. The exercise group achieved significant improvements in balance and strength, and also a significantly lower rate of falls compared to the control group. A 12-month follow-up revealed that 42% of the intervention group had continued their exercises, whereas the control subjects had become less active and reported an increased fear of falling. Two years after the programme, the rate of falls remained significantly lower in the exercise group compared with the control group (Campbell et al 1999). Interestingly, this benefit was sustained without further home visits from the physiotherapist beyond the initial 12-month period. Two subsequent studies conducted by the same research group have also achieved a significant reduction in falls, using trained nurses to implement the home programme (Robertson et al 2001a, 2001b). If health professionals other than physiotherapists are to be involved in developing and implementing balance programmes, emphasis needs to be focused on effective training. The challenge in these programmes is to sufficiently challenge balance to achieve therapeutic benefit in a safe manner.

Group/supervised programmes

Community-based group exercise programmes are also a commonly adopted approach to maintaining or improving physical status. Typically, these programmes incorporate a combination of balance, strength, flexibility and endurance activities. Improved strength and balance, and reduced falls rates have been reported for this type of programme (Day et al 2002). Lord et al (1995) also found improved balance, strength and reaction time among older women participating in a group programme, and a strong trend for reduced falls rates among the subgroup who had high attendance rates at the classes.

Buchner et al (1997b) compared the outcomes of strength training using weight machines, endurance training using stationary bicycles, and combined strength and endurance training, in a group setting. Sessions were of 1 hour duration, three times each week, for 6 months, with post-study planning to promote continued exercise either in existing community classes or unsupervised settings. The control group maintained usual activities. At 6-month follow-up, strength gains were maximal in the strength training group and aerobic capacity had increased only in the endurance training and combined training groups. There were no significant improvements on any measures of gait or balance, but exercise across all three intervention groups was found to have a protective effect on the risk of falling.

Another randomized controlled trial investigated the effectiveness of a combined programme of supervised progressive strength training, followed by functional and balance training, performed three times a week for 12 weeks (Hauer et al 2001). Participants in the programme had an average age of 82 years, had been discharged from a geriatric hospital, and had a history of injurious falls requiring medical treatment. Seventy-four percent of participants had fall-related fractures and 12% were cognitively impaired. Falls were reduced by 25% in the intervention group compared with the control group by the end of the 6-month programme. Physical activity prior to hospital admission was typically low in the study population and more than doubled with the training. There were no training-related medical problems in the study group, and the adherence rate was excellent (85%).

Tai chi is another form of physical activity gaining increased popularity in Western countries. Tai chi chuan is a gentle form of tai chi considered appropriate for older people (Wolf et al 1997a). There are a number of different types of tai chi, which are commonly described in relation to the number of movements (forms). Most commonly, the 24-form Beijing style has been reported (Shih 1997). However, a number of abbreviated versions of tai chi have also been described for older people. An abbreviated 10-form version of tai chi was compared with individualized balance training on a force platform, or a social-information control group, in a randomized controlled trial (Wolf et al 1996, 1997b). Tai chi was found to reduce the risk of multiple falls by 48% when compared with control subjects over the 4-month follow-up period. No significant change was observed in falls rates for the other two groups. Other benefits of the tai chi programme included reduced fear of falling, lower systolic blood pressure after a 12-minute walk, increased confidence in balance and movement, and improvement in daily activities (Kutner et al 1997, Wolf et al 1996). In view of specificity of training, these results cannot be generalized to other types of tai chi. Further investigations of a more comprehensive set of forms, such as the Beijing 24-form, in reducing falls among older people are warranted.

Physical activity to reduce falls fracture risk in older people

Cross sectional and longitudinal studies have identified that low levels of physical activity are associated with significantly increased risk of hip fracture among older people (Gregg et al 2000, Høidrup et al 2001, Norton et al 2001). Intervention programmes aiming to prevent injurious falls should address both falls-related factors such as muscle strength and balance, as well as maintenance of bone mass (Luukinen et al 1997).

In order to target maintenance of bone mass, a physical activity programme needs to incorporate weight-bearing activities. A meta-analysis of ten studies evaluating the effect of aerobic exercise on lumbar spine bone mineral density identified differences between people who performed weight-bearing exercises compared with controls, as a result of loss of bone mineral density in the control group relative to the exercise group (Kelley 1998). Programmes such as exercise to music classes which incorporate varying types of weight-bearing movements appear to be effective in maintaining or improving bone mineral density in postmenopausal women (Bassey 2001, Welsh and Rutherford 1996). Brisk walking programmes (Brooke-Wavell et al 1997), weight-bearing exercises including walking, stepping on and off blocks, aerobic dance activities (Bravo et al 1996), and a weight-bearing programme in combination with calcium supplementation (McMurdo et al 1997) have also been shown to result in stabilized bone mineral density. Only the study by McMurdo et al (1997) investigated falls, finding fewer falls among the group undertaking exercise and calcium supplementation, compared with the control group who received calcium supplementation only. The difference was, however, statistically significant only between 12 and 18 months post training. The effectiveness of these programmes on falls-related injury rates in older people is yet to be determined.

Which dimensions of physical activity are most important in reducing falls risk?

Physical activity programmes can vary substantially in terms of the:

- type of physical activity
- frequency of participation in the physical activity
- duration of the physical activity per session
- intensity of the physical activity training programme.

Studies successfully resulting in falls reduction have generally incorporated a component of balance training, and have often also used combinations of strength and cardiovascular fitness training (Campbell et al 1997, Day et al 2002, Wolf et al 1996). The comparative effectiveness of each of these components, used individually or in combination, in reducing falls rates remains unclear. For example, it is not known whether a specific dosage of tai chi is twice as effective in reducing falls rates as a walking programme. Knowledge of the comparative health benefits of different types of physical activity would be valuable to facilitate decision-making by older people about participation in physical activity, as well as being useful for policy and programme planners.

The minimum dosage of physical activity required to achieve the benefits of reduced falls rates is also yet to be determined. In those studies which have identified significant reduction in falls rates, frequencies of 1–3 times weekly, and durations of 15–60 minutes have commonly been reported (Carter et al 2001, Gardner et al 2000). Further investigation is required to evaluate whether a higher frequency or intensity of physical activity and a longer period of activity can result in greater improvements in falls rates. On review, it would appear that factors associated with some of the inconclusive results in this area include inadequate physical activity intensity and low participant compliance (Gardner et al 2000). On the basis of the studies published to date, it is not possible to provide an optimum rationale for exercise prescription to prevent falls.

Criteria for developing a physical activity programme to reduce falls

A number of important issues need to be considered in the development and implementation of physical activity programmes, to maximize the likelihood that the programme will reduce falls.

1. The physical demands of the programme need to be appropriate for the health status of those in the programme. This is particularly important in terms of the balance requirements, because if the balance requirements exceed capabilities, then a fall may occur. Those running the programme need to ensure that the content, dosage and schedule are matched to each individual. Older people who are commencing any new form of physical activity programme should also have a general health review and clearance from their doctor prior to commencing the programme.
2. There may need to be different levels and types of programmes for older people to cater for different physical abilities. Gardner and colleagues (2000) found that one reason why some exercise falls prevention programmes did not reduce falls was inadequate intensity of the physical activity.
3. Each programme needs to incorporate balance training, which may consist of specific dynamic balance retraining activities, or be a component of combination movements such as tai chi chuan.

4. The programme should have a 'warm-up' component, which pre-
   pares the body for the type of physical activity to be undertaken, and
   a 'warm-down' component to finish the physical activity programme.
   The 'warm-down' component consists of gentle exercise, flexibility
   and relaxation, to minimize post-exercise muscle soreness.
5. The programme needs to be increased in difficulty over time, to
   accommodate improvements in physical performance associated
   with the programme.

There are a number of other factors that may influence decisions about
which specific types of physical activity programmes to use. These
include:

1. Identifying pre-existing physical disabilities that impact upon falls
   risk, such as reduced muscle strength. Programmes targeting the
   specific risk factor affecting an individual are more likely to have a
   beneficial effect on that risk factor, and falls risk.
2. Personal preferences for group classes, individual, or home-based
   activities. Each of these approaches has been used successfully to
   reduce falls in older people (Campbell 1997, Day et al 2002). Individual
   or home-based programmes tend to require greater self-motivation
   to maintain compliance (Christmas and Andersen 2000). One of the
   strong support mechanisms arising from group-based physical activity
   programmes is the opportunity for social interaction, peer support, and
   networking before and after the physical activity component. This support can have a positive influence over ongoing participation in activity programmes.
3. Acknowledging that personal motivation to participate and sustain
   involvement in a physical activity programme affects outcome
   (Christmas and Andersen 2000). According to the stages of change
   model (Prochaska et al 1994), individuals may be at one of five stages
   of being prepared to undertake specific health-promoting behaviours
   such as physical activity. These are:
   ■ pre-contemplation: period when the health behaviour is not even
     being considered
   ■ contemplation: period when the individual is seriously consid-
     ering participating in the health-promoting behaviour in the next
     6 months
   ■ preparation: period when the individual is seriously considering
     commencing the health-promoting behaviour in the next month
   ■ action: the period when the individual has commenced the health-
     promoting behaviour
   ■ maintenance: the period involving sustaining participation in the
     health-promoting behaviour long term (greater than 6 months)
     (Prochaska et al 1994).
   Those who are at early stages of preparation for change are likely to
   benefit more from motivation by external facilitators such as occurs
   in group programmes, as well as social networking during the group
   programme.

Incorporating balance and strength training into a physical activity programme

Balance is a complex function which requires a well-functioning integrated system incorporating sensory (vision, somatosensory and vestibular), central integration of afferent information, and efficient efferent (neuromotor) responses (Lord et al 2001). Balance tasks can be considered static where there is no overt body movement, or dynamic, where there is movement of the body's centre of mass, or limbs, around the base of support. An example of a static balance task is standing on one leg, while examples of dynamic balance tasks include reaching, stepping or turning. Greatest benefit appears to be associated with practice of dynamic balance activities rather than static activities. Functional balance also requires the allocation of cognitive and attentional resources to the balance task, often while performing one or more unrelated activities, such as when talking and looking in shop windows whilst walking. Reduced ability to perform dual tasks, one of which incorporates balance, is associated with increased falls risk (Condron and Hill 2002, Shumway-Cook et al 1997) (see Chapter 13).

Physical activity programmes can incorporate a range of different types of balance activities that may improve balance performance and reduce falls risk. These include:

- standing balance tasks with varying width/area of base of support (feet apart, feet together, heel to toe stance, or single limb stance)
- tasks incorporating arm or head movements into other balance activities (turning head side to side while performing heels to toes balancing movement)
- balance tasks with concurrent dual task activity (walking and talking, or throwing a ball in the air while balancing on a narrow beam)
- changing the sensory demands of the activity, for example eyes closed, or standing on foam
- walking quickly, with sudden changes in direction
- practice of mobility activities at differing speeds, on various terrains.

In order for improvements in balance to occur, a physical activity programme needs to challenge individual abilities. The specific components of the programme depend upon the abilities of participants, the type of programme being undertaken, and may be incorporated into a home-based or group programme. For older people with a history of falls or impaired balance, a comprehensive assessment by a physiotherapist is recommended to identify the appropriate type and intensity of balance training. According to Gardner et al (2001) balance activities that are closely related to lifestyle and function and can be incorporated into exercise programmes include sit-to-stand, walking and turning around, with the challenge of each task being able to be graded from 'easy' to 'most difficult' to match individual ability. Skelton and Dinan (1999) also report a progressive series of exercises, including balance and strength training.

Strength training programmes are becoming more acceptable to older people as a realistic and practical exercise option to improve general health and function. Strength training programmes for older people usually involve working with either machines or free weights, or resistance band training (Awerbuch 2001). Programmes often involve identifying the individual's one repetition maximum (1 RM, the maximal weight able to be controlled and lifted with a specific muscle group), and the programme commences with individuals lifting 70–80% of 1 RM. Each targeted muscle group is worked in a 'set', which is the number of repetitions of the exercise, usually 8–15, and progression involves gradually increasing the number of sets for each muscle group up to two or three within a session, then progressing the weight being lifted (American Council on Exercise 1998). Strength training is recommended up to 3 days a week, with a rest day in-between to allow for muscle recuperation and development (Gardner et al 2001). Use of body weight in functional activities such as standing up from a chair, and going up and down steps can also have a strength training effect (Sherrington and Lord 1997).

Key muscles to target are the ankle dorsiflexors, quadriceps, hip abductors and extensors, trunk stabilizing muscles, the abdominals and trunk extensors, because they are important for a range of important functional activities such as safe and efficient transferring, getting up from the floor, standing from a chair and walking. These movements are performed more poorly by fallers than by non-fallers (Nevitt et al 1989, Tinetti et al 1988).

Lifestyle modification

With more than 40% of individuals over the age of 65 not participating in any leisure activities involving physical exertion (Resnick and Spellbring 2000), strategies that encourage lifestyle modification in order to include more physical activity are vital. Gardner et al (2001) recommended that walking be included as an essential element of falls prevention exercise programmes. Guidelines suggest a total of 30 minutes walking every day, which may be achieved by strategies such as getting off the bus one stop too early, or using the stairs rather than the elevator.

For older people who are already generally active, increasing the volume of aerobic activity can be achieved using brisk walking, swimming, playing golf, and water aerobics. While the specific falls prevention benefits of these types of activities have not been formally investigated, they are likely to have beneficial health effects on general fitness, balance, walking and muscle strength.

Participation and sustainability

To achieve long-term effectiveness of physical activity programmes aimed at reducing falls, consideration needs to be given to engaging initial participation, and maintaining long-term participation and sustainability. Whether or not an older person participates in a particular physical activity programme can be influenced by factors such as:

- how the programme is promoted
- whether the target group identifies with the health problem being targeted by the programme (Managing Innovation 2000)

- pre-existing medical problems
- medical advice to participate in the programme
- perception of ability to undertake the physical activity programme
- suitability of the venue
- ease of access/availability of transport
- cost (Gardner et al 2000, King et al 1998).

Sustainability refers to factors that increase the likelihood of continued participation with a programme or its message in the longer term, and may include:

- perceived benefit of the programme, which may be facilitated by intermittent review of participants on key physical measures
- enjoyment in participating
- social and other benefits
- the ability of the programme to respond to changing needs (Resnick and Spellbring 2000).

The effectiveness of an exercise programme in reducing falls rates has been shown to be greater for those who are high compliers than for people who fail to adhere (Lord et al 1995). Campbell et al (1999) reported that 42% of those performing a home-based strength and balance training programme continued with the programme at a 1-year follow-up. They hypothesized that the individual nature of the programme may have enhanced compliance and suggested 6-monthly reviews to maintain enthusiasm. Those participants who were more physically active at baseline, those with a previous fall and those who remained confident about not falling were more likely to continue exercising. In a supervised centre-based programme, however, Hauer and colleagues (2001) reported an excellent adherence rate (85%) in a previously sedentary group of older women. It was concluded that the use of specific training equipment, coupled with the motivating effect of the group setting was more acceptable to some individuals than home-based programmes. Another study by Williams and Lord (1995) showed that impaired balance and strength, and use of psychoactive medications were associated with reduced compliance in a group programme for older women. These are generally indicators of increased frailty and falls risk, and indeed older people with these problems need to be among those targeted with appropriate physical activity options. Similarly, Campbell et al (1997) found that older people who were more frail and at greater risk of falling were most difficult to involve and sustain in a home-based programme. Alternative strategies to increase ongoing participation by more frail older people, or consideration of alternative intervention types, need to be further explored.

Physical activity in other settings

Older people living in the community have been the focus of the majority of the falls prevention research investigating effectiveness of physical activity programmes (Gillespie et al 2001). Falls are an even more common problem for frail older people living in residential aged care settings (Norton and Butler 1997). Although studies have identified improvement in falls risk factors such as muscle weakness and impaired balance using both individual and group physical activity programmes in residential aged care settings (Fiatarone et al 1994, Harada et al 1995), none have identified significant reduction in falls rates.

Summary

There is growing evidence that a range of physical activity programmes reduce the risk of falling in older people. Programmes need to be targeted to different groups within the community, from well older people through to more frail older people. Strategies to maximize uptake and facilitate long-term participation are important to ensure that these research findings are translated into practice, and to reduce the unacceptably high current rate of falls amongst older people.

References

Access Economics Pty Ltd 2001 The burden of brittle bones: costing osteoporosis in Australia. Canberra. Prepared for Osteoporosis Australia

American Council on Exercise 1998 Exercise for older adults: ACE's guide for fitness professionals. (Cotton R, ed). American Council on Exercise, San Diego

Awerbuch M 2001 Live Stronger Live Longer: an exercise and lifestyle program for over 40s. McGraw-Hill, Sydney

Bassey E J 2001 Exercise for prevention of osteoporotic fracture. Age and Ageing 30 (Suppl):29–31

Bravo G, Gauthier P, Roy P, et al 1996 Impact of a 12-month exercise program on the physical and psychological health of osteopenic women. Journal of the American Geriatrics Society 44:756–762

Brooke-Wavell K, Jones P, Hardman A 1997 Brisk walking reduces calcaneal bone loss in postmenopausal women. Clinical Science 92:75–80

Buchner D M, Cress M E, de Lateur B J, et al 1997a A comparison of the effects of three types of endurance training on balance and other fall risk factors in older adults. Aging (Milano) 9(1–2):112–119

Buchner D M, Cress M E, de Lateur B J, et al 1997b The effect of strength and endurance training on gait, balance, falls risk, and health service use in community-living older adults. Journal of Gerontology 52:M218–224

Campbell A 1997 Preventing falls by dealing with the causes. Medical Journal of Australia 167:407–408

Campbell A, Robertson M, Gardner M, et al 1997 Randomised controlled trial of a general practice programme of home based exercise to prevent falls in elderly women. British Medical Journal 315:1065–1069

Campbell A J, Robertson M, Gardner M, et al 1999 Falls prevention over 2 years: a randomised controlled trial in women 80 years and older. Age and Ageing 28:513–518

Campbell J, Reinken J, Allan B, et al 1981 Falls in old age: a study of frequency and related clinical factors. Age and Ageing 10:264–270

Campbell J, Borrie M, Spears G 1989 Risk factors for falls in a community-based prospective study of people 70 years and older. Journal of Gerontology 44:M112–117

Carter N, Kannus P, Khan K 2001 Exercise in the prevention of falls in older people: a systematic literature review examining the rationale and the evidence. Sports Medicine 31:427–438

Chandler J, Duncan P, Kochersberger G, et al 1998 Is lower extremity strength gain associated with improvement in physical performance and disability in frail, community-dwelling elders? Archives of Physical Medicine and Rehabilitation 79:24–30

Christmas C, Andersen R 2000 Exercise and older patients: guidelines for the clinician. Journal of the American Geriatrics Society 48:318–324

Colón-Emeric C S, Sloane R, Hawkes W G, et al 2000 The risk of subsequent fractures in community-dwelling men and male veterans with hip fracture. American Journal of Medicine 109(4):324–326

Condron J, Hill K 2002 Reliability and validity of a dual task force platform assessment of balance performance: effect of age, balance impairment and cognitive task. Journal of the American Geriatrics Society 50:157–162

Cripps R, Jarman J 2001 Falls by the elderly in Australia: trends and data for 1998. Injury Research and Statistics Series. Australian Institute of Health and Welfare, Adelaide.

Day L, Fildes B, Gordon I, et al 2002 A randomised factorial trial of falls prevention among community-dwelling older people. British Medical Journal 325:128

Deal C L 1997 Osteoporosis: prevention, diagnosis, and management. American Journal of Medicine 102:35–39

Department of Human Services: Public Health Division 2001 Evidence-based health promotion: resources for planning #3 – Falls prevention. Melbourne.

Ebrahim S, Thompson P, Baskaran V, et al 1997 Randomised placebo-controlled trial of brisk walking in the prevention of postmenopausal osteoporosis. Age and Ageing 26:253–260

Ellingson T, Conn V S 2000 Exercise and quality of life in elderly individuals. Journal of Gerontological Nursing 26(3):17–25

Fiatarone M, Marks E, Ryan N, et al 1990 High-intensity strength training in nonagenarians. Effects on skeletal muscle. JAMA 263:3029–3034

Fiatarone M, O'Neill E, Doyle Ryan N, et al 1994 Exercise training and nutritional supplementation for physical frailty in the oldest old. New England Journal of Medicine 330:1769–1775

Gardner M M, Robertson M C, Campbell A J 2000 Exercise in preventing falls and fall related injuries in older people: a review of randomised controlled trials. British Journal of Sports Medicine 34(1):7–17

Gardner M, Buchner D, Robertson M, et al 2001 Practical implementation of an exercise-based falls prevention programme. Age and Ageing 30:77–83

Gillespie L D, Gillespie W J, Robertson M C, et al 2001 Interventions for preventing falls in elderly people (Cochrane Review). Cochrane Database of Systematic Reviews 3:CD000340

Gregg E, Pereira M, Caspersen C 2000 Physical activity, falls, and fractures among older adults: a review of the epidemiologic evidence. Journal of the American Geriatrics Society 48:883–893

Haentjens P, Autier P, Barette M, et al 2001 The economic cost of hip fractures among elderly women. A one-year, prospective, observational cohort study with matched-pair analysis. Belgian Hip Fracture Study Group. Journal of Bone and Joint Surgery: America 83A(4):493–500

Hamdorf P, Penhall R 1999 Walking with its training effects on the fitness and activity patterns of 79–91 year old females. Journal of Medicine 29:22–28

Harada N, Chiu V, Fowler E, et al 1995 Physical therapy to improve functioning in older people in residential care facilities. Physical Therapy 75:830–839

Hauer K, Rost B, Rutschle K, et al 2001 Exercise training for rehabilitation and secondary prevention of falls in geriatric patients with a history of injurious falls. Journal of the American Geriatrics Society 49(1):10–20

Hill K, Schwarz J, Kalogeropoulos A, et al 1996 Fear of falling revisited. Archives of Physical Medicine and Rehabilitation 77:1025–1029

Hill K, Schwarz J, Flicker L, et al 1999 Falls among healthy community dwelling older women: a prospective study of frequency, circumstances, consequences and prediction accuracy. Journal of Public Health 23:41–48

Hill K, Kerse N, Lentini F, et al 2002a Falls: a comparison of trends in community, hospital and mortality data in older Australians. Aging (Milano) 14:18–27

Hill K, Schwarz J, Sims J 2002b Falls. In: Ratnaike R (ed) Practical guide to geriatric medicine. McGraw-Hill, Sydney

Høidrup S, Sorensen T I, Stroger U, et al 2001 Leisure-time physical activity levels and changes in relation to risk of hip fracture in men and women. American Journal of Epidemiology 154(1):60–68

Kelley G 1998 Aerobic exercise and lumbar spine bone mineral density in postmenopausal women: a meta-analysis. Journal of the American Geriatrics Society 46:143–152

King A, Rejeski W, Buchner D 1998 Physical activity interventions targeting older adults. A critical review and recommendations. American Journal of Preventive Medicine 15(4):316–333

Kutner N, Barnhart H, Wolf S L, et al 1997 Self-report benefits of tai chi practice by older adults. Journal of Gerontology 52(5):P242–246

Ledin T, Kronhed A C, Moller C, et al 1990 Effects of balance training in elderly evaluated by clinical tests and dynamic posturography. Journal of Vestibular Research 1(2):129–138

Lord S, Ward J, Williams P, et al 1993 An epidemiological study of falls in older community-dwelling women: the Randwick falls and fractures study. Australian Journal of Public Health 17:240–245

Lord S, Ward J, Williams P, et al 1995 The effect of a 12-month exercise trial on balance, strength, and falls in older women: a randomised controlled trial. Journal of the American Geriatrics Society 43:1198–1206

Lord S, Ward J, Williams P 1996 Exercise effect on dynamic stability in older women: a randomised controlled trial. Archives of Physical Medicine and Rehabilitation 77:232–236

Lord S, Sherrington C, Menz H 2001 Falls in older people: risk factors and strategies for prevention. Cambridge University Press, Cambridge

Luukinen H, Koski K, Laippala P, et al 1997 Factors predicting fractures during falling impacts among home-dwelling older adults. Journal of the American Geriatrics Society 45:1302–1309

Magaziner J, Hawkes W, Hebel J R, et al 2000 Recovery from hip fracture in eight areas of function. Journal of Gerontology 55(9):M498–507

Managing Innovation 2000 A study into the information needs and perceptions of older Australians concerning falls and their prevention. Managing Innovation (Marketing Consultancy Network Inc) for the Commonwealth Department of Health and Aged Care, Canberra

McMurdo M, Mole P, Paterson C 1997 Controlled trial of weight bearing exercise in older women in relation to bone density and falls. British Medical Journal 314:569

Morey M, Pieper C, Sullivan R, et al 1996 Five-year performance trends for older exercisers: a hierarchical model of endurance, strength, and flexibility. Journal of the American Geriatrics Society 44:1226–1231

Nevitt M 1990 Falls in older persons: risk factors and prevention. In: Berg R, Cassels J (eds) The second fifty years: promoting health and preventing disability. National Academy Press, Washington, DC

Nevitt M, Cummings S, Kidd S, et al 1989 Risk factors for recurrent non-syncopal falls. JAMA 261:2663–2668

Norton R, Butler M 1997 Prevention of falls and falls related injuries among institutionalised older people. National Advisory Committee on Health and Disability, Wellington, New Zealand

Norton R, Galgali G, Campbell A J, et al 2001 Is physical activity protective against hip fracture in frail older people? Age and Ageing 30(3):262–264

O'Loughlin J, Robitaille Y, Boivin J, et al 1993 Incidence of and risk factors for falls and injurious falls among the community dwelling elderly. American Journal of Epidemiology 137:342–354

Posner J, Gorman K, Windsor-Landsberg L, et al 1992 Low to moderate intensity endurance training in healthy older adults: physiological response after four months. Journal of the American Geriatrics Society 40:1–7

Prochaska J, Velicer W, Rossi J, et al 1994 Stages of change and decisional balance for 12 problem behaviours. Health Psychology 13:39–46

Province M, Hadley E, Hornbrook M, et al 1995 The effects of exercise on falls in elderly patients: a preplanned meta-analysis of the FICSIT trials. JAMA 273:1341–1347

Resnick B, Spellbring A 2000 Understanding what motivates older adults to exercise. Journal of Gerontological Nursing 26:34–42

Rizzo J, Friedkin R, Williams C, et al 1998 Health care utilization and costs in a Medicare population by fall status. Medical Care 36:1174–1188

Robertson M C, Devlin N, Gardner M, et al 2001a Effectiveness and economic evaluation of a nurse delievered home exercise programme to prevent falls. 1: randomised controlled trial. British Medical Journal 322:697

Robertson M C, Gardner M M, Devlin N, et al 2001b Effectiveness and economic evaluation of a nurse delivered home exercise programme to prevent falls. 2: controlled trial in multiple centres. British Medical Journal 322:701–704

Rose D, Clark C 2000 Can the control of bodily orientation be significantly improved in a group of older adults with a history of falls? Journal of the American Geriatrics Society 48:275–282

Runge J 1993 The cost of injury. Emergency Medicine Clinics of North America 11:241–253

Sattin R, Lambert Huber D, DeVito C, et al 1990 The incidence of fall injury events among the elderly in a defined population. American Journal of Epidemiology 131:1028–1037

Schwarz J 1995 Falls in the elderly: management and prevention in general practice. Modern Medicine in Australia 38:89–95

Sherrington C, Lord S 1997 Home exercise to improve strength and walking velocity after hip fracture: a randomised controlled trial. Archives of Physical Medicine and Rehabilitation 78:208–212

Shih J 1997 Basic Beijing twenty-four forms of tai chi exercise and average velocity of sway. Perceptual and Motor Skills 84:287–290

Shumway-Cook A, Woollacott M, Kerns K, et al 1997 The effects of two types of cognitive tasks on postural stability in older adults with and without a history of falls. Journal of Gerontology 52A:M232–240

Singh N A, Clements K M, Fiatarone M A 1997 A randomized controlled trial of progressive resistance training in depressed elders. Journal of Gerontology 52(1):M27–35

Skelton D, Dinan S 1999 Exercise for falls management: rationale for an exercise programme aimed at reducing postural stability. Physiotherapy Theory and Practice 15:105–120

Skelton D, Young A, Greig C, et al 1995 Effects of resistance training on strength, power, and selected functional abilities of women aged 75 and older. Journal of the American Geriatrics Society 43:1081–1087

Speechley M, Tinetti M 1991 Falls and injuries in frail and vigorous community elderly persons. Journal of the American Geriatrics Society 39:46–52

Tennstedt S, Howland J, Lachman M, et al 1998 A randomised, controlled trial of a group intervention to reduce fear of falling and associated activity restriction in older adults. Journal of Gerontology 53B(6):P384–392

Tinetti M, Speechley M, Ginter S 1988 Risk factors for falls among elderly persons living in the community. New England Journal of Medicine 319:1701–1707

Tinetti M, Richman D, Powell L 1990 Falls efficacy as a measure of fear of falling. Journal of Gerontology 45:P239–243

Tinetti M, deLeon C, Doucette J, et al 1994a Fear of falling and fall-related efficacy in relationship to functioning among community-living elders. Journal of Gerontology 49:M140–147

Tinetti M, Baker D, McAvay G, et al 1994b A multifactorial intervention to reduce the risk of falling among elderly people living in the community. New England Journal of Medicine 331:821–827

Tinetti M, Doucette J, Claus E 1995 The contribution of predisposing and situational risk factors to serious fall injuries. Journal of the American Geriatrics Society 43:1207–1213

Tinetti M, McAvay G, Claus E 1996 Does multiple risk factor reduction explain the reduction in fall rate in the Yale FICSIT Trial? American Journal of Epidemiology 144:389–399

Weinberg L, Strain L 1995 Community-dwelling older adults' attributions about falls. Archives of Physical Medicine and Rehabilitation 76:955–960

Welsh L, Rutherford O M 1996 Hip bone mineral density is improved by high-impact aerobic exercise in postmenopausal women and men over 50 years. European Journal of Applied Physiology and Occupational Physiology 74(6):511–517

Wiktorowicz M, Goeree R, Papaioannou A, et al 2001 Economic implications of hip fracture: health service use, institutional care and cost in Canada. Osteoporosis International 12:271–278

Williams P, Lord S 1995 Predictors of adherence to a structured exercise program for older women. Psychology and Aging 10:617–624

Wolf S, Barnhart H, Kutner N, et al 1996 Reducing frailty and falls in older persons: an investigation of tai chi and computerised balance training. Journal of the American Geriatrics Society 44:489–497

Wolf S, Coogler C, Tingsen X 1997a Exploring the basis for tai chi chuan as a therapeutic exercise approach. Archives of Physical Medicine and Rehabilitation 78:886–892

Wolf S, Barnhart H, Ellison G, et al 1997b The effect of tai chi quan and computerised balance training on postural stability in older subjects. Physical Therapy 77:371–381

Wolfson L, Whipple R, Derby C, et al 1996 Balance and strength training in older adults: intervention gains and tai chi maintenance. Journal of the American Geriatrics Society 44(5)S:498–506

Yardley L 1998 Fear of imbalance and falling. Reviews of Clinical Gerontology 8:23–29

13

Effects of dual task interference on postural control, movement and physical activity in healthy older people and those with movement disorders

Sandra G Brauer and Meg E Morris

CHAPTER CONTENTS

Introduction 267

Balance, movement and physical activity require attention 268

Factors influencing dual task interference 269

Dual task interference in healthy older adults 272

Dual task interference in older people with balance impairment 275

Dual task interference in older people with movement disorders 278

Clinical assessment of dual task interference 281

Clinical interventions to reduce dual task interference in older people 282

References 284

Introduction

Many activities of daily life involve performing several tasks at once, such as talking and walking, or maintaining standing balance whilst dressing. Although most people are able to perform several tasks at the same time, some individuals experience difficulty, particularly if one is a 'postural task' that requires them to maintain balance and upright stance. The term 'dual task interference' refers to the deterioration in performance that occurs when two tasks are performed simultaneously. Severe dual task interference is more common in older adults than younger people, and in those with balance impairments, movement disorders or a history of falls. Because more than one-quarter of adults aged over 65 years fall each year (Campbell et al 1989), a major focus of this chapter will be on how dual task interference compromises postural control and gait in older people. In addition, theories as to why dual task interference occurs will be outlined and evidence of dual task interference in healthy older adults and those with impairments or disabilities will be presented. The chapter will finish by summarizing clinical measures of dual task interference and rehabilitation strategies used to optimize performance.

Balance, movement and physical activity require attention

Traditionally, the control of balance and gait has been viewed as an 'automatic' process, requiring minimal cognitive processing for effective and efficient function. However, more recent studies have shown that even simple balance and gait tasks require attention. Attention has been given several definitions, and in this context we consider it to be the information processing required to complete a task. Depending on the task, it can involve filtering information, selecting information, or focussing, shifting, dividing or sustaining attention (Groth-Marnat 1997).

A dual task paradigm can be used to investigate the changes in performance that occur when performing multiple tasks, and to determine the attentional requirements of tasks such as balance maintenance. In this paradigm, the person performs a primary task alone, a secondary task alone and then both the primary and secondary task together. A comparison is then made between performances for the dual and single task conditions. If performance of the secondary task deteriorates when it is performed concurrently with the primary task, then the primary task is considered to be attention-demanding. Dual task methodology has the underlying assumptions that: (i) a limited central processing capacity exists; (ii) performing a task requires part of the limited processing capacity; and (iii) if two tasks share processing capacity, the performance in one or both tasks can be disturbed when the processing capacity is exceeded (Kahneman 1973).

Several theories explain why there may be a deterioration in performance when a person performs more than one task at a time. These relate to either structural limitations or capacity limitations. The term 'structural limitation' refers to an anatomical limitation whereby only one signal can pass through an area of the neurological system at a time. A 'capacity limitation' is where the finite size of information processing space available is exceeded. Simultaneous multiple tasks can be performed if there is adequate processing capacity. If the capacity is saturated, performance in one or all of the tasks deteriorates, and the system may have to prioritize between the tasks.

Structural and capacity limitations can act as 'rate-limiting factors', by creating a bottleneck to the rate or the number of processes that can be performed simultaneously (Kahneman 1973). An example of a structural limitation acting as a rate-limiting factor is where visual afferent input pathways may be needed for both a secondary task that requires a response to a visual cue, and maintain postural stability. Thus, the limitation in performance may be due to the competition between the tasks to use the same pathways or structures. This explanation has been used to help explain interference between different rhythmic movements, such as gait and fast finger tapping (Ebersbach et al 1995). In Ebersbach's study, structural interference was considered to occur at the level of sub-cortical networks that organize and regulate competing rhythmic outputs. Considering that postural control is such a complex behaviour involving input and activity in many sensory, planning and motor areas, it is conceivable that interference while performing some concurrent tasks could be at least in part due to structural limitations.

While structural limitation theory can explain some performance constraints, it does not explain situations where dual task interference occurs despite the use of different inputs and outputs that do not use the same anatomical structures. One example is talking whilst walking. Whereas human speech is controlled mainly by the frontal and temporal cortices of the brain, locomotion is regulated by brainstem, spinal, cerebellar and basal ganglia nuclei, with a small amount of cortical input (Morris et al 1995). Several studies investigating dual task interference in young and balance-impaired adults have concluded that interference is due to a limited capacity (Dault et al 2001a, 2001b, O'Shea et al 2002, Yardley et al 2001). Furthermore, with increased age, attentional capacity is reduced (Crossley and Hiscock 1992, Jensen and Goldstein 1991). The processing requirements of some tasks may also increase with age or pathology. For example, more resources may be required to perceive sensory stimuli if the thresholds are raised due to age-related decline in function. Considering that with age there is a reduction in capacity and a possible increase in attention required for task completion, it is not surprising that some older people experience difficulty performing dual tasks.

Factors influencing dual task interference

Several factors have been shown to influence dual task interference. These relate to the tasks performed and the individual. Task-related factors include task complexity, task type, task response mode and the timing of task performance. Individual factors include chronological age, health status and physiological arousal.

Task-related interference

The attentional capacity used by a task is considered to be proportional to the postural demands placed on the system. Thus, a more challenging task may use more attentional resources and thus demonstrate interference with a secondary task earlier or to a greater degree than a less challenging postural task. Lajoie and colleagues (1993) illustrated this when they found that reaction time on a secondary task increased from sitting, to standing to walking, implying that cognitive processing requirements increase with increasing task complexity, even in young healthy adults. They also found that reaction time was longest during the single support phase, the most stability-demanding aspect of gait. An increase in attentional demand has been demonstrated when stability has been incrementally challenged by reducing the size of the base of support

(Lajoie et al 1996, Teasdale et al 1993), or by adopting more difficult postures or movements (Bourdin et al 1998). Insufficient challenge to the system due to tasks not being complex enough has been used as a common explanation by researchers who did not find any dual task interference (Barin et al 1997). In young adults, the tasks have to be sufficiently demanding or complex for a dual task interference to arise. Several studies have found that young adults can maintain a quiet stance position when simultaneously performing a reaction time task with no interference to either task (Barin et al 1997, Maylor and Wing 1996, Redfern et al 1999a, Shumway-Cook and Woollacott 2000, Shumway-Cook et al 1997, Teasdale et al 1993).

Another way to increase the postural challenge is to modify the sensory inputs available. Teasdale and colleagues (1993) found that reducing visual and somatosensory cues increased the attention demand of standing in both young and older adults. Similarly, Redfern et al (1999a) found that reaction time for the secondary task was greatest in the condition of conflicting sensory information (standing on a sway-referenced platform with a scene) in young adults. Alternatively, performance on the primary balance task has also been shown to deteriorate with reduction in sensory cues, particularly in elderly or balance-impaired individuals (Shumway-Cook and Woollacott 2000, Shumway-Cook et al 1997).

The type of secondary task has been shown to influence the degree of dual task interference. This may be due to structural interference if the secondary task competes for similar cognitive resources to the postural task, or capacity issues if the task has a greater attentional demand. Kerr and colleagues (1985) investigated the influence of two different cognitive tasks – a spatial and a non-spatial task on the ability to maintain a tandem stance position. The type of secondary task was found to influence balance when elderly subjects performed stability-demanding tasks. Performing a spatial memory task (placing numbers in an imagined matrix) interfered with postural stability more than a non-spatial memory task (remembering sentences). Maylor and Wing (1996) also investigated the influence of several different cognitive tasks on standing postural stability in young and older adults and found a reduction in postural stability in older adults when performing two of the five cognitive tasks (Brooks spatial memory task and backward digit recall). The Brooks spatial memory task is recognized as having a visuo-spatial component, and recent studies (Li and Lewandowsky 1995) have also suggested that the backward digit recall can also use this type of cognitive processing. Despite these early studies concluding that spatial cognitive tasks influence postural stability more than non-spatial, later studies indicate that the issue is not simple.

Shumway-Cook and colleagues (1997) reported a greater interference between postural and cognitive task performance with a non-spatial rather than a spatial task. Elderly fallers demonstrated a reduction in balance (as measured by an increased centre of pressure (COP) displacement) in both task conditions, whereas young and non-falling elderly adults demonstrated a reduction in balance only while simultaneously performing the non-spatial task. Another study found that in younger adults, the source of the input for the secondary task (visual versus auditory) made no difference to the performance of the primary postural (stance) or secondary cognitive (reaction time) tasks (Redfern et al 1999a). Further studies are required to investigate this issue while performing tasks that are more stability-demanding and with greater sophistication in the measurement of the postural task. It is likely that the degree of dual task interference will vary depending on the individual tasks and the groups studied, as it is difficult to examine the impact of task type while ensuring task complexity is controlled.

Most paradigms investigating dual task interference have used secondary tasks requiring articulation during the postural task such as responding verbally to an auditory signal (Lajoie et al 1993, Teasdale et al 1993), counting aloud (Shumway-Cook and Woollacott 2000), identifying spatial locations (Andersson et al 1998), or holding a conversation (Lundin-Olsson et al 1997). The articulation itself may be enough to cause interference in the postural task as Yardley and colleagues found articulation resulted in an increased quiet stance sway path, but a silent mental task did not (Yardley et al 1999). This supports others studies where minimal interference was found when performing a silent mental task (Kerr et al 1985, Maki and McIlroy 1996, Maylor and Wing 1996). Thus, another factor to consider is the mode of responding to a second task. It appears that talking results in greater interference with postural control than silent mental tasks.

The timing of the secondary task may influence the degree of interference. Most balance recovery tasks appear to be most attention demanding between 150 and 500 ms after the stimulus, after the immediate response is made and when the person is regaining the pre-stimulus position or movement (Brauer et al 2001, Maki et al 2001, Norrie et al 2002, Rankin et al 2000). Similarly, interference with human locomotion appears to be sensitive to the timing of the introduction of a secondary stimulus (Chen et al 1996). Thus, the characteristics of both the primary and secondary tasks have a strong influence over the degree of dual task interference exhibited. Notwithstanding, several factors relating to the individual also have been demonstrated to have a major impact on dual task interference.

Individual factors and dual task interference

Individual factors shown to impact on dual task interference when one task is a postural one include cognitive impairment, physiological arousal, prioritization between tasks, age, balance impairment and the presence of movement disorders such as hypokinesia or dystonia. For example, older people with cognitive impairment show greater dual task interference than non-cognitively impaired individuals (Camicioli et al 1997). Physiological arousal, possibly due to anxiety, has also been shown to influence quiet stance when concurrently performing a mental arithmetic task (Maki and McIlroy 1996). It appears that increased arousal or stress should be considered as a contributor to dual task interference with postural control, rather than just the cognitive load placed by competing tasks.

The degree of interference to either the postural or secondary task is likely to be influenced by the individual's prioritization of the tasks. Preferential attention may be instructed (e.g. maintain balance as best as possible while talking) or may arise out of the tasks themselves. For example, greater priority may be given to a postural task that poses a greater (perceived or real) threat to stability than to the concomitant secondary task. Three factors that individuals cannot control that have been shown to have a major influence on dual task interference are age, balance impairment and movement disorders. Evidence of these factors will now be presented when examining the effect of a second task on balance maintenance, reactive balance ability and gait.

Dual task interference in healthy older adults

Several studies have shown that performing a secondary cognitive task has a greater impact on postural stability in old people than in young adults (Brown et al 1999, Maylor and Wing 1996, Melzer et al 2001, Teasdale et al 1993). This may be due to capacity-related factors such as a reduction in attentional capacity with advancing age, and postural stability requiring a greater proportion of the attentional resources in older adults. Increased cognitive processing may be required by older adults due to decreased afferent sensitivity (e.g. visual acuity, joint position sense), decreased automaticity in sensory integration, altered postural response strategies, and changes in muscle activation. Muscle activation changes with advanced age can include a delayed onset of postural muscles such as gluteus medius when performing rapid movements (Brauer and Burns 2002), increased co-contraction of opposing muscle groups such as gastrocnemius and tibialis anterior when balancing, and a change in the patterning of postural muscle activity. An example of pattern changes with age is found when reactions to underfoot balance perturbations are studied. Young adults respond first with distal muscles (gastrocnemius for backward perturbations), then thigh and then trunk (Woollacott 1986). Older adults reverse this pattern so the first muscles active are the trunk muscles, then thigh muscles then distal muscles (Woollacott 1986). Interference will be discussed in the categories of balance maintenance, reactive balance control and gait.

Balance maintenance

Healthy older adults generally demonstrate dual task interference even when the task is simply to maintain a bilateral stance position (Dault et al 2001a, Maylor and Wing 1996, Melzer et al 2001, Redfern et al 1999b, Shumway-Cook et al 1997). The interference is frequently shown as an increase in centre of pressure (COP) motion in comparison to a single task condition, and in comparison to young adults. Movement of the COP can be measured when a person stands on a force platform, as seen in Figure 13.1, which senses the downward and shearing forces they impart on the plate. The COP reflects the control of the body's centre of mass, and so the more adjustments a person needs to make to maintain their balance, the greater their COP motion. This is illustrated in Figure 13.2, where

Figure 13.1 Measuring centre of pressure motion in stance using a force platform.

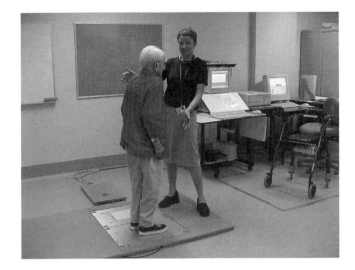

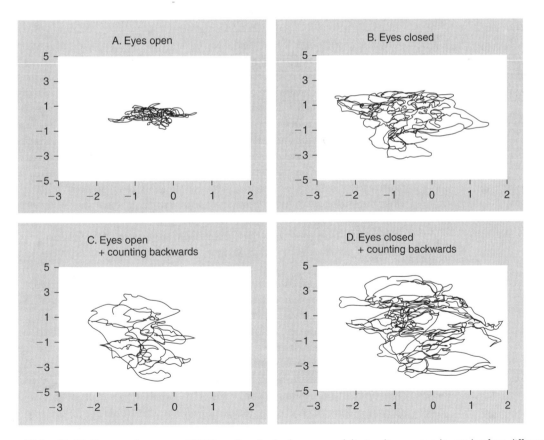

Figure 13.2 (A–D) Centre of pressure (COP) motion (cm) of a young adult standing on one leg under four different conditions.

13.2A shows COP motion of a healthy young adult standing on one leg. When the balance task becomes more difficult by closing the eyes (13.2B), or adding a second task (13.2C and 13.2D), the COP motion increases in distance and area.

Infrequently, dual task interference is only apparent with a marked alteration in sensory cues such as provided by a sway-referenced surface, no visual input or optokinetic stimulation (Shumway-Cook and Woollacott 2000). A sway-referenced surface is available with some commercially produced computerized balance assessment equipment whereby the standing surface moves the same amount and in the same direction as the person swaying. The term 'optokinetic stimulation' refers to visual stimuli such as rapidly moving lines that stimulate the vestibular system to perceive that the person is moving. Conversely, greater interference in the secondary task has also been reported in older adults in comparison to young adults, particularly when stability is challenged (Marsh and Geel 2000, Teasdale et al 1993). This deterioration is likely to occur sometime after 60 years of age, as most studies of healthy elders investigate persons aged over 65 years, and a study of dual task ability across decades found no change in adults aged between 20 and 60 years (Barin et al 1997).

Reactive balance

In healthy older adults, the immediate response to recover balance following a perturbation is not affected by the performance of a secondary task (Brauer et al 2001, 2002, Brown et al 1999, Rankin et al 2000, Redfern et al 2002, Stelmach et al 1990). One likely explanation is that healthy elders may prioritize balance recovery over the secondary task. In support, studies have found dual task interference with the secondary task when there was no impact on balance recovery (Brown et al 1999, Redfern et al 2002). In addition, the cortical control or processing required to initiate the postural response may be minimal, and thus another task does not interfere with this more automatic aspect of balance recovery. Studies investigating the impact of the timing of a second task suggest that minimal interference occurs with reactive control until at least after 150 ms following the perturbation (Maki et al 2001, Norrie et al 2002). These two experiments investigated whether a continuous second task deteriorates while reacting to a sudden lower limb displacement. They used a tracking task where subjects used a hand-held joystick to keep a marker within two lines that formed a winding track on the computer screen in front of them, whilst standing on a force-plate. The plate was suddenly moved and subjects had to regain their balance. Although they recovered well from the balance perturbation, they moved out of the lines on the hand tracking task at least 150 ms after the disturbance to their feet. Nevertheless this was well after they had reacted to regain balance.

Dual task interference with balance is apparent in healthy elders in the ongoing recovery of balance. This has been demonstrated as taking a longer time to recover standing balance (Stelmach et al 1990), a reduction in EMG magnitude of muscles important in balance recovery (Rankin et al 2000) and taking a longer time to initiate the recovery step (Brown et al 1999). This dual task interference may have dire consequences if the initial response is not sufficient to regain stability.

Human locomotion

Gait appears to have a larger attentional cost in healthy older people than young adults, as greater interference in the secondary task is generally reported under dual task conditions than single (Eichhorn et al 1998, Lindenberger et al 2000). Whether a second task interferes with the gait of healthy elders is still contentious. A reduction in gait speed and increase in double support time has been found in healthy elders under dual task conditions (O'Shea et al 2002). Other studies have found no interference with gait with an added task (Eichhorn et al 1998, Lindenberger et al 2000), even in persons aged over 80 years (Camicioli et al 1997). Like young adults, the second tasks need to be of sufficient challenge before interference is likely.

When the gait task is made more challenging, dual task interference is evident in healthy elders. When asked to step over a virtual object (a band of light), obstacle contact was more frequent when subjects had to simultaneously respond verbally to a visual signal (Chen et al 1996). There were larger errors in older adults than in young adults. Obstacle contact in healthy elders under dual task conditions has been predicted by clinical cognitive tests of attention maintenance, selective attention, and the ability to flexibly and efficiently problem solve (Persad et al 1995). The ability to switch response sets due to task demands has been associated with frontal lobe function and a decline in frontal lobe function has been demonstrated with age (Lezak et al 1994). The importance of the frontal lobe to dual task performance is highlighted by a case study of a 36-year-old man with multiple sclerosis whose balance and gait was deteriorating. He had reported falls when talking and walking together (Sandyk 1997). As part of his usual treatment for multiple sclerosis, he was given two transcranial treatments with AC pulsed electromagnetic fields to the frontal lobes. After these two sessions his dual task performance during gait and balance was dramatically improved and he showed improvement in the Thurstone's Word-Fluency Test, a neuropsychological test of frontal lobe dysfunction.

Dual task interference in older people with balance impairment

Persons with balance impairment demonstrate greater dual task interference than unimpaired people. This includes elderly people who are frail or who have fallen, and those with neurological disorders such as Parkinson's disease, Alzheimer's disease and Lewy body dementia. While not all have a reduction in attentional capacity, balance and gait are likely to be more attentionally demanding in these populations due to the compensations required by their pathology. For example, walking with a standard walker is more attentionally demanding than gait with a rolling walker or no aids (Wright and Kemp 1992).

Two studies have been able to prospectively predict elderly fallers from their dual task interference with gait. Elders living in residential care who had to stop walking when engaging in a conversation were predicted to fall in the following year (Lundin-Olsson et al 1997). In a seminal study, Lundin-Olsson and colleagues investigated elderly nursing home residents and found that those who had to stop walking to engage

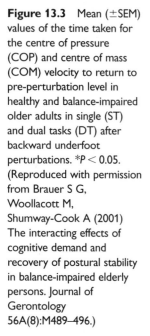

Figure 13.3 Mean (±SEM) values of the time taken for the centre of pressure (COP) and centre of mass (COM) velocity to return to pre-perturbation level in healthy and balance-impaired older adults in single (ST) and dual tasks (DT) after backward underfoot perturbations. *P < 0.05. (Reproduced with permission from Brauer S G, Woollacott M, Shumway-Cook A (2001) The interacting effects of cognitive demand and recovery of postural stability in balance-impaired elderly persons. Journal of Gerontology 56A(8):M489–496.)

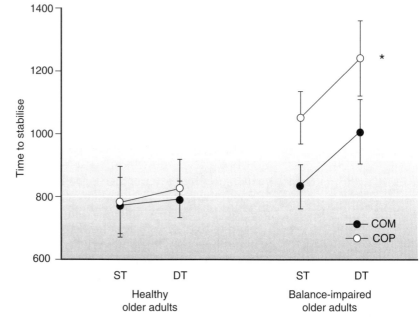

in a conversation were most likely to fall within the following year. More recently, community-dwelling elders who fell over in a 1-year follow-up period were predicted by a slower time to complete more complex walking while talking tasks (Verghese et al 2002).

It follows that older people with a history of falls or postural instability have greater dual task interference in balance and gait tasks than healthy elders. With a reduction in sensory cues, they show a greater COP excursion than healthy elders under dual task conditions (Shumway-Cook and Woollacott 2000, Shumway-Cook et al 1997), implying greater instability when maintaining a position. Elderly fallers actually fell when attempting dual task balance tasks with sensory system manipulation, with all unable to complete the two most difficult tasks under sway-referenced conditions (Shumway-Cook and Woollacott 2000).

When perturbed by an underfoot force plate movement, balance-impaired elders take a longer time for their centre of mass and COP to regain a stable position (Brauer et al 2001), and show a greater amplitude of COP motion (Condron and Hill 2002) when responding by keeping their feet in place. Figures 13.3 and 13.4 illustrate that balance-impaired elders take a longer time to restabilize their body with an added task than do healthy elders. Balance-impaired elders are more likely to need to take a step to recover balance when performing a concurrent cognitive task, than when recovering balance alone (Brauer et al 2001). Similar to healthy elders, muscle activity and body segment motion was monitored throughout these studies and dual task conditions had no effect on their response. Thus dual tasking may show greatest interference in balance-impaired elders when using sensory inputs to realize where one is in

Figure 13.4 Time for the centre of pressure (COP) to stabilize in a representative healthy and balance-impaired older adult when regaining balance after a backward underfoot perturbation while also responding to auditory tones via a headset. (Reproduced with permission from Brauer S G, Woollacott M, Shumway-Cook A (2001) The interacting effects of cognitive demand and recovery of postural stability in balance-impaired elderly persons. Journal of Gerontology 56A(8):M489–496.)

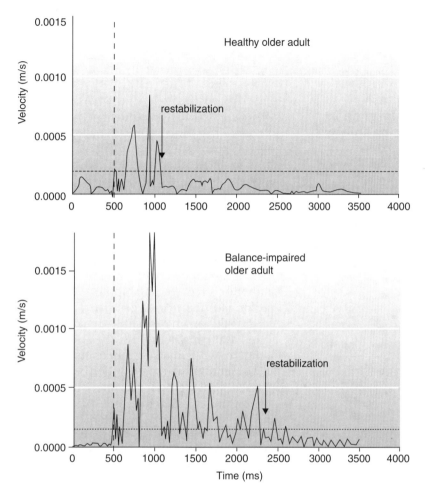

space and provide ongoing responses, rather than when recovering with an automatic postural strategy.

Increased COP excursion under dual task conditions suggests that balance-impaired elders are unable to prioritize or allocate attention to the postural task first. A study of reactive balance ability demonstrated clearly that balance-impaired individuals performed the balance recovery first, then the secondary cognitive task (Brauer et al 2002). Allocation of attention to tasks is dependent on factors such as threat of injury, instructions to subjects, goal of the tasks and the nature of all tasks (Shumway-Cook et al 1997).

Several balance-impaired populations have demonstrated dual task interference with gait. Frail elders have shown a reduction in speed, increase in lateral deviations and number of stops (Beauchet et al 2002). Stroke survivors and spinal cord injured persons both reduced gait velocity and increased double support time when concurrently answering questions (Bowen et al 2001, Lajoie and Baarbeau 1999). Finally, several studies have shown persons with Parkinson's disease to demonstrate dual task interference with gait, but the reasons for this interference are compounded by the nature of their pathology (Morris et al 1996, 2001).

Dual task interference in older people with movement disorders

In addition to age-related changes in motor performance in healthy individuals, movement disorders and cognitive impairment can exacerbate dual task interference in those with conditions such as Parkinson's disease, Huntington's disease and Alzheimer's disease. People with basal ganglia dysfunction are particularly at risk of severe dual task interference due to the role of this part of the brain in the regulation of movement automaticity. Iansek et al (1995) and Seitz and Roland (1992) have described how the motor cortical regions of the frontal cortices play a key role in enabling a person to perform a motor skill during the early stages of motor learning. Once the skill has been practised to the level that it is well-learned, it is relegated to the basal ganglia for control. Thus whilst the basal ganglia enable the motor skill to be executed 'automatically' with the correct speed, amplitude and force for the context in which it is performed, the frontal cortical regions of the brain are free to control other tasks 'on line', such as speaking, walking, balancing or arithmetic.

In basal ganglia disease, the ability to perform more than one task at a time can become severely compromised due to the loss capacity for movement automaticity. In both Parkinson's disease and Huntington's disease, well-learned, complex motor skills such as walking, dressing, writing and speaking become exceedingly slow due to the need to control movement using attentional processes (Morris 2000, Churchyard et al 2001). Visual guidance and conscious attention to every step of a motor sequence often takes the place of quick, 'subconscious', basal-ganglia regulated performance. Dual task performance becomes increasingly compromised with disease progression, presumably due to both structural and information capacity limitations. Using the dual task interference models presented at the beginning of this chapter, it could be proposed that a structural anatomical limitation may occur because only a limited number of signals can pass through the frontal motor control regions at a given time. In addition, a capacity limitation is likely to occur due to the finite information processing space of the frontal cortices. As shown by Brown and Marsden (1991), people with Parkinson's disease have diminished attentional resources as well as difficulty shifting attention between multiple tasks. Thus, whereas people with Parkinson's disease can perform a simple movement (such as throwing a ball or waving) quickly and easily because there are no structural or capacity limitations for single-component actions, the performance of simultaneous tasks is markedly compromised (Benecke et al 1986, Brown and Marsden 1991, Dalrymple-Alford et al 1994, Elble 1998, Horstink et al 1990).

When people with advanced basal ganglia disease are required to perform two tasks at the same time, the one that runs through the frontal cortical regions and is under conscious control can usually be performed relatively normally, whereas the task controlled by the defective basal ganglia is under-scaled in speed, amplitude and force (Morris et al 2001). In severe cases, such as when a person has severe akinesia, it may not be possible for the person to actually perform the secondary task at all (Camicioli et al 1997). Camicioli et al measured akinetic Parkinsonian patients with motor freezing, who were required to maintain verbal fluency whilst walking. Compared with non-freezers with Parkinson's disease and control subjects, footstep size was markedly reduced and gait speed was abnormally slow in the dual task condition. As pointed out by O'Shea et al (2002) only the secondary task (gait) was measured. This makes it difficult to determine the extent to which the fluency task interfered with gait, as compliance with the fluency task could not be confirmed.

In an earlier series of gait studies, Morris et al (1996) showed that dual task interference in people with Parkinson's disease was directly proportional to the complexity of the secondary task. When people were required to recite a simple sentence ('Where is the child?') over and over whilst walking, their gait speed and stride length reduced only marginally. As the sentence complexity increased, the speed and amplitude of footsteps diminished. For the most difficult condition (reciting the days of the week backwards) these variables were often less than half the values for healthy older people, resulting in marked shuffling, tiny steps and reduced ground clearance. This is particularly dangerous, because reduced ground clearance during gait increases the risk of tripping on obstacles and falling.

Several other investigations have verified that the complexity of the primary task is a key determinant of dual task interference in people with Parkinson's disease. Bond and Morris (2000) showed that people with Parkinson's disease had slight reductions in gait speed and stride length and increased double limb support duration when instructed to carry a wooden tray whilst walking. When required to carry the same tray with two plastic wine glasses on top, they exhibited marked reductions in speed and stride length, which were much greater than the performance deficits measured in age-matched control subjects. An investigation on people with Huntington's disease by Churchyard et al (2001) reiterated this theme. When people with Huntington's disease were required to recite numbers backwards or attend to metronome beats whilst walking, their gait speed and stride length showed marked deterioration. Morris et al (2000) reported similar findings in relation to postural control. People with Parkinson's disease performed poorly on a series of standing balance tasks when required to direct their attention towards reciting the days of the week backwards. Those who were frequent fallers showed the greatest dual task interference, suggesting the need for patient education about the increased risk of falls in multi-task situations. Using a multiple tasks test (comprising one cognitive task and seven motor tasks performed in different combinations), Bloem et al (1991a) showed that the number of healthy older people and those with Parkinson's disease who made movement errors increased as the secondary tasks became more complex. Predictably, those with Parkinson's disease made the most errors.

Whether the type of secondary task is a major determinant of the severity of dual task interference in people with Parkinson's disease requires further investigation. In a preliminary study, O'Shea et al (2002) found that both a motor task (transferring coins from one pocket to another) and a cognitive task of a similar level of difficulty (digit recital) compromised gait in people with Parkinson's disease. These investigators concluded that the complexity and difficulty of secondary tasks have more powerful effects on gait impairment than whether the secondary task is motor or cognitive in type. These findings await replication.

An interesting finding of the Parkinson's disease literature is that some 'secondary tasks' act as movement facilitators rather than inhibitors or distracters. For example, Morris et al (1994) found that when elderly people with gait hypokinesia were instructed to focus their attention on stepping over white strips of cardboard placed on the floor at their criterion step length, the 'visual cues' enabled them to walk with normal footstep size and speed. In contrast, when they were required to step in time to a metronome set at the correct stepping frequency for their age, the step length and speed diminished. The reasons why the secondary visual cue task facilitated movement whereas the secondary auditory cue task compromised movement in people with hypokinesia is not completely clear. One hypothesis is that the fundamental deficit in gait hypokinesia is one of stride amplitude regulation, and the visual cues enabled people to use the frontal cortices and visual system to bypass the defective basal ganglia in order to control stride size. Auditory cues do not enable a person to directly control stride size as they provide no information on movement amplitude. Of note, the visual cues were not mandatory for normalizing footstep size in people with Parkinson's disease. As long as people were cognitively intact, they could learn to focus conscious attention on walking with long strides (Morris et al 1996). This cognitive strategy only produces transient performance effects – as soon as the person's attention is diverted to another activity the step speed and size revert back to their usual low levels (Morris et al 1996).

Severe dual task interference is not only associated with basal ganglia lesions. It can occur in any neurological condition that requires a person to compensate for their motor deficit using frontal attentional mechanisms. Due to frontal lobe capacity limitations combined with their motor, sensory or cognitive disorders, people with cerebellar disorders (Bronstein et al 1990), brainstem lesions, spinal or peripheral nerve lesions (Lajoie et al 1994) can experience disproportionate levels of movement slowing when required to attend to a secondary task. Thus people with Alzheimer's disease, acquired brain injury, stroke, multiple sclerosis, motor neurone disease or cerebral palsy frequently report difficulty in simultaneous task performance. Those with Alzheimers's disease are particularly at risk, because cognitive impairment compromises their ability to adequately compensate for movement slowness using the frontal cortical regions (Camicioli et al 1997, Lundin-Olsson et al 1997).

Clinical assessment of dual task interference

Several clinical tools have been developed to assess dual task interference during gait, but no clinical tools have yet been published to assess interference with balance. All tests have been developed and validated for the elderly population. Lundin-Olsson and colleagues (Lundin-Olsson et al 1997) investigated the effect of performing dual tasks on balance, mobility and falls in frail older adults residing in an institutional setting. If a patient demonstrated dual task interference with gait whereby they stopped walking when talking, they were likely to fall in the following year. This was termed the 'stops walking while talking' test. While this first dual task test of interference is quick and simple, it does not measure the degree of interference between tasks.

The same researchers addressed this issue by developing the motor timed up and go test. The timed up and go test (TUG) involves timing how quickly a person can rise from sitting, walk 3 metres, turn, walk 3 metres back again and sit down (Podsiadlo and Richardson 1991). This was modified to add a manual task of carrying a glass of water simultaneously with the walking (Lundin-Olsson et al 1998). Frail residents who had a time difference of >4.5 seconds between the motor TUG and the TUG were more prone to falls during the following six months (Lundin-Olsson et al 1998).

Because different types of secondary tasks have a varying impact on balance and gait in older people (Kerr et al 1985, Maylor and Wing 1996, Shumway-Cook et al 1997), Shumway-Cook and colleagues added a cognitive task to the motor TUG and assessed the dual task TUG test (DTTUG) (Shumway-Cook et al 2000). It consisted of performing the TUG, the motor TUG and adding the condition of performing the TUG while counting backwards by three's from a random number selected by the assessor. The addition of either a cognitive or manual task increased the time taken to perform the TUG in all older subjects. Cut-off points of 13.5, 14.5, and 15 seconds for the TUG, motor TUG and TUG with the cognitive task respectively were able to correctly predict approximately 90% of elders into faller and non-faller groups. While the DTTUG tests were no better than a simple TUG test at predicting who had fallen in the past, they are reliable, quantitative measures that may be useful in identifying situations where dual task interference may occur.

The multiple tasks test is a further extension of the above tests, developed to measure the ability to perform multiple tasks concurrently (Bloem et al 2001a, 2001b). It involves timing the speed to walk a path while incrementally adding tasks, so the final condition involves performing eight tasks together. The tasks manipulate a variety of elements (motor, cognitive, sensory), with the tasks chosen by clinicians and patients as those difficult to perform or related to falls in the elderly. The test has been validated in healthy elders and in persons with Parkinson's disease (Bloem et al 2001a, 2001b). While the full test is time-consuming, a smaller subsection has been validated and may be useful to objectively assess dual task interference, particularly in older people with a higher level of function.

The walking while talking test measures the time taken to walk 20 feet, turn and return (40 feet total) at the person's normal walking pace while simultaneously performing a simple and complex added task (Verghese et al 2002). The simple task involves reciting the letters of the alphabet aloud, and the complex task involves reciting alternate letters of the alphabet (a, c, e ...). Older persons who had fallen took a longer time to complete both elements of the test, and several cut-off scores were presented that predicted elderly people to be fallers or non-fallers. As expected, the complex task was better than the simple task in differentiating fallers from non-fallers.

Finally, neuropsychological evaluation of attention is recommended, particularly in persons likely to have problems, such as frail older adults. There is no single test of attention. Frequently used clinical tests where attention is a primary component include the trail making tests (Reitan 1958) and the PASAT (paced auditory serial addition test) (Gronwall 1977). Both have demonstrated reliability, validity and sensitivity in several populations (Leclercq and Zimmermann 2002). Assessment of general cognitive status may also be helpful using the Mini Mental State Examination (MMSE), which is a quick screening tool (Folstein et al 1975).

Clinical interventions to reduce dual task interference in older people

Clinical interventions to reduce dual task interference can be divided into rehabilitation, to improve the ability to perform multiple tasks, or compensatory strategies, if the underlying difficulty cannot be overcome. For both of these approaches, raising awareness about the problem of dual task interference with the person, their caregiver and support team is an initial step. Easy changes can make a difference, including altering the environment (ensure good lighting, reduce obstacles) and simplifying the way in which daily activities are performed (e.g. sit down to talk on the telephone or get dressed; avoid talking whilst walking; carry objects in a backpack rather than in the hands). This approach is important for safety, to reduce the chance of a trip or fall resulting from inability to multi-task. Assessment by a skilled clinician can reveal under what situations the older person has most interference with balance or gait, and when to be particularly vigilant about safety.

There is very little published regarding the rehabilitation of dual task interference with balance or gait. Most work has been published on balance re-education in amputees. With usual rehabilitation, balancing on a sound limb and prosthesis becomes less attention-demanding (Geurts et al 1991) and attention can be successfully directed to a second task (Geurts and Mulder 1994). This suggests that in persons where postural ability has potential to improve, so can their dual task ability.

As outlined earlier, dual task interference increases with increasing complexity of both the postural task (e.g. walking more demanding than standing) and the second task (e.g. holding a tray with glasses interferes more with walking than holding a tray alone). So, increasing the difficulty of both tasks could be a logical way to progress treatment.

Table 13.1	Clinical guidelines
Well elderly	■ May have problems with multi-tasking when there is a sensory system conflict; e.g. when walking in poor lighting, at night, on uneven surfaces or with poor footwear ■ Should not have dual task interference with usual daily activities ■ If dual task interference arises, use as a 'red flag' for the clinician to further investigate balance and walking ■ Good test = dual task timed up and go test
Mild motor disability	■ Are likely to frequently experience slowing or difficulty with dual task performance ■ Already a high risk for falls ■ Dual task interference is likely to occur when performing difficult postural tasks; e.g. walking up stairs or along a narrow pathway ■ Have the potential to learn new ways of moving or to improve dual task ability ■ Need to be frequently assessed by a trained clinician ■ Good tests = dual task timed up and go test or multiple tasks test
Mild cognitive disability	■ High risk for falls ■ May not be able to learn to improve dual task ability – so advise caregivers of risky situations; adapt environment to reduce risk of overbalancing; avoid multi-tasking ■ Neuropsychological assessment of attention and executive function advised ■ Good test = clinical tests of cognitive function advised; include trail-making A and B tests, Mini-Mental State Examination
Frail elderly	■ Likely to experience dual task interference even with simple tasks, such as walking and talking ■ Very high risk for falls ■ Dual task interference with gait more likely in those using a walker, stick, other aids ■ Intervention aimed to reduce environmental risks, train staff/ caregivers in how to optimize balance and gait function ■ Need to be aware of dual task situations where other problems could arise; e.g. skin tear when getting out of bed and not paying attention ■ Need to be aware of effects of medication on task performance ■ Good test = talking while walking test

Similarly, intervention could progress from performing dual tasks to multiple tasks, as in the multiple tasks test, so that the person ends up walking, talking, and carrying an object all under changed sensory conditions such as in dim light.

The studies reviewed earlier in this chapter demonstrated that the type of secondary task may differentially influence postural tasks, so it is important to assess and include a variety of different types of secondary tasks in rehabilitation. The type of task can vary from a cognitive one (e.g. maths: counting backwards, language: thinking of names beginning with a certain letter) to a motor task (e.g. carrying a tray), to a visuo-spatial task (e.g. reciting the way from their bed to the dining room). Clinical experience has shown that a range of tasks is required as elders vary widely as to what combinations are most interfering.

Prioritization is also important in maintaining safety when performing more than one task. This may be asserted initially with conscious cognitive control, where attention is diverted away from the postural task for short and then increasing lengths of time, or during more critical phases of balance recovery. Alternatively, changing the prioritization toward the postural task is required when compensating for dual task interference that is not improving or when safety is the primary concern.

Dual task interference is most likely to occur in older adults, adults with balance impairment or those with cognitive deficits. This represents a substantial proportion of the rehabilitating population. Further research is required to provide evidence that dual task interference can be reduced with intervention, and to provide an evidence-based framework from which to approach therapy.

References

Andersson G, Yardley L, et al 1998 A dual-task study of interference between mental activity and control of balance. American Journal of Otology 19(5):632–637

Barin K, Jefferson G D, et al 1997 Effect of aging on human postural control during cognitive tasks. ISA Transactions 388–393

Beauchet O, Dubost V, et al 2002 Study of the influence of a specific cognitive task on spatial-temporal walking parameters in frail elderly patients. Presse Medicale 31(24):1117–1122

Benecke R, Rothwell J C, et al 1986 Performance of simultaneous movements in patients with Parkinson's disease. Brain 109:739–757

Bloem B, Valkenburg V, et al 2001a The Multiple Tasks Test: strategies in Parkinson's disease. Experimental Brain Research 137:478–486

Bloem B, Valkenburg V, et al 2001b The Multiple Tasks Test: development and normal strategies. Gait and Posture 14(3):191–202

Bond J, Morris M E 2000 Effects of goal-directed secondary task performance on gait in subjects with Parkinson disease. Archives of Physical Medicine and Rehabilitation 81:110–116

Bourdin C, Teasdale N, et al 1998 High postural constraints affect the organization of reaching and grasping movements. Experimental Brain Research 122(3):253–259

Bowen A, Wenman R, et al 2001 Dual-task effects of talking while walking on velocity and balance following a stroke. Age and Ageing 30:319–323

Brauer S G, Burns Y 2002 The influence of preparedness on rapid stepping in young and older adults. Clinical Rehabilitation 16(7):741–748

Brauer S G, Woollacott M, et al 2001 The interacting effects of cognitive demand and recovery of postural stability in balance-impaired elderly persons. Journal of Gerontology 56(8):M489–496

Brauer S G, Woollacott M, et al 2002 The influence of a concurrent cognitive task on the compensatory stepping response to a perturbation in balance-impaired and healthy elders. Gait and Posture 15(1):83–93

Bronstein A M, Hood J D, et al 1990 Visual control of balance in cerebellar and parkinsonian syndromes. Brain 113:767–779

Brown L A, Shumway-Cook A, et al 1999 Attentional demands and postural recovery: the effects of aging. Journal of Gerontology 54(A4):M165–171

Brown R G, Marsden C D 1991 Dual task performance and processing resources in normal subjects and patients with Parkinson's disease. Brain 114:215–231

Camicioli R, Howieson D, et al 1997 Talking while walking: the effect of a dual task in aging and Alzheimer's disease. Neurology 48:955–958

Campbell J, Borrie M, et al 1989 Risk factors for falls in a community-based prospective study of people 70 years and older. Journal of Gerontology 44:M112–117

Chen H C, Schultz A B, et al 1996 Stepping over obstacles: dividing attention impairs performance of old more than young. Journal of Gerontology 51A(3):M116–122

Churchyard A, Morris M E, et al 2001 Gait dysfunction in Huntington's disease: parkinsonism and a disorder of timing. Advances in Neurology 87:375–385

Condron J, Hill K 2002 Reliability and validity of a dual task force platform assessment of balance performance: effect of age, balance impairment and cognitive task. Journal of the American Geriatrics Society 50:157–162

Crossley M, Hiscock M 1992 Age-related differences in concurrent task performance of normal adults: evidence for a decline in processing resources. Psychology and Aging 7(4):499–506

Dalrymple-Alford J C, Kalders A S, et al 1994 A central executive deficit in patients with Parkinson's disease. Journal of Neurology, Neurosurgery and Psychiatry 57:360–367

Dault M, Frank J, et al 2001a Influence of a visuospatial, verbal and central executive working memory task on postural control. Gait and Posture 14:110–116

Dault M, Geurts A, et al 2001b Postural control and cognitive task performance in healthy participants while balancing on different support surface configurations. Gait and Posture 14:248–255

Ebersbach G, Dimitrijevic M, et al 1995 Influence of concurrent tasks on gait: a dual task approach. Perceptual and Motor Skills 81:107–113

Eichhorn J, Orner J, et al 1998 Ageing effects on dual task methodology using walking and verbal reaction time. Issues on Aging 21:8–12

Elble R J 1998 Gait and freezing in Parkinson disease. In: Proceedings 5th international conference of Parkinson's disease and movement disorders. Seminar 4.2, 1998, New York, USA

Folstein M F, Folstein S E, et al 1975 'Mini-Mental State' A practical method for grading the cognitive state of patients for the clinician. Journal of Psychiatric Research 12:189–198

Geurts A C H, Mulder T W 1994 Attention demands in balance recovery following lower limb amputation. Journal of Motor Behaviour 26(2):162–170

Geurts A C H, Mulder T W, et al 1991 Dual-task assessment of reorganisation of postural control in persons with lower limb amputation. Archives of Physical Medicine and Rehabilitation 72:1059–1064

Gronwall D 1977 Paced Auditory Serial Addition Task: a measure of recovery from concussion. Perceptual and Motor Skills 44:367–373

Groth-Marnat G 1997 Handbook of psychological assessment, 3rd edn. Wiley, New York

Horstink M W I M, Berger H, et al 1990 Bimanual simultaneous motor performance and impaired ability to shift attention in Parkinson's disease. Journal of Neurology, Neurosurgery and Psychiatry 53:685–690

Iansek R, Bradshaw J, et al 1995 Interaction of the basal ganglia and supplementary motor area in the elaboration of movement. In: Glencross D, Piek J (eds) Motor control and sensorimotor integration. Elsevier Science, Amsterdam, p 37–59

Jensen G, Goldstein L 1991 A microcomputerized task assessment of cognitive change in normal elderly and young adults. Experimental Ageing Research 17(2):119–121

Kahneman D 1973 Attention and Effort. Prentice Hall, Englewood Cliffs, NJ

Kerr B, Condon S M, et al 1985 Cognitive spatial processing and the regulation of posture. Journal of Experimental Psychology 11(5):617–622

Lajoie Y, Baarbeau H 1999 Attentional requirements of walking in spinal cord injured patients compared to normal subjects. Gait and Posture 9:S25

Lajoie Y, Teasdale N, et al 1993 Attentional demands for static and dynamic equilibrium. Experimental Brain Research 97:139–144

Lajoie Y, Teasdale N, et al 1994 Gait of a deafferented subject without large myelinated sensory fibres below the neck. Neurology 47:109–115

Lajoie Y, Teasdale N, et al 1996 Attentional demands for walking: age-related changes. In: Ferrandez A-M, Teasdale N (eds) Changes in sensory motor behavior in aging. Elsevier Science, Amsterdam, p 235–256

Leclercq M, Zimmermann P 2002 Applied neuropsychology of attention: theory, diagnosis and rehabilitation. London, New York. Psychology Press, Hove

Lezak M, Legall D, et al 1994 Assessment of executive function after frontal lobe damage. Revue de Neuropsychologie 4(3):327–343

Li S, Lewandowsky S 1995 Forward and backward recall – different retrieval processes. Journal of Experimental Psychology and Learning 21(4):837–847

Lindenberger U, Marsiske M, et al 2000 Memorizing while walking: increase in dual-task costs from young adulthood to old age. Psychology and Aging 15(3):417–436

Lundin-Olsson L, Nyberg L, et al 1997 Stops walking when talking. Lancet 349:617

Lundin-Olsson L, Nyberg L, et al 1998 Attention, frailty and falls: the effect of a manual task on basic mobility. Journal of the American Geriatrics Society 46:758–761

Maki B, McIlroy W 1996 Influence of arousal and attention on the control of postural sway. Journal of Vestibular Research 6:53–59

Maki B, Zecevic A, et al 2001 Cognitive demands of executing postural reactions: does aging impede attention switching? NeuroReport 12(16):3583–3587

Marsh A, Geel S 2000 The effect of age on the attentional demands of postural control. Gait and Posture 12:105–113

Maylor E A, Wing A M 1996 Age differences in postural stability are increased by cognitive demands. Journal of Gerontology 51B(3):P143–154

Melzer I, Benjuya N, et al 2001 Age-related changes of postural control: effect of cognitive tasks. Journal of Gerontology 47(4):189–194

Morris M E 2000 Movement disorders in people with Parkinson's disease: a model for physical therapy. Physical Therapy 80:578–597

Morris M E, Iansek R, et al 1994 The pathogenesis of gait hypokinesia in Parkinson's disease. Brain 117:1161–1182

Morris M E, Iansek R, et al 1995 Motor control considerations for gait rehabilitation in Parkinson's disease. In: Glencross D, Piek J (eds) Motor control and sensorimotor integration. Elsevier Science, Amsterdam, p 61–93

Morris M E, Iansek R, et al 1996 Stride length regulation in Parkinson's disease: normalization strategies and underlying mechanisms. Brain 119:551–568

Morris M E, Iansek R, et al 2000 Postural instability in Parkinson's disease: a comparison with and without a concurrent task. Gait and Posture 12(3):205–216

Morris M E, Huxham F, et al 2001 Gait disorders and gait rehabilitation in Parkinson's disease. Advances in Neurology 87:347–361

Norrie R, Maki B, et al 2002 The time course of attention shifts following perturbation of upright stance. Experimental Brain Research 146:315–321

O'Shea S, Morris M E, et al 2002 Dual task interference during gait in people with Parkinson's disease: effects of motor versus cognitive secondary tasks. Physical Therapy 82(9):888–897

Persad C, Giordani B, et al 1995 Neuropsychological predictors of complex obstacle aviodance in healthy older adults. Journal of Gerontology 50B(5):P272–277

Podsiadlo D, Richardson S 1991 The timed up and go: a test of basic functional mobility for frail elderly persons. Journal of the American Geriatrics Society 39:142–148

Rankin J, Woollacott M H, et al 2000 Cognitive influence on postural stability: a neuromuscular analysis in young and older adults. Journal of Gerontology 55A(3):M112–119

Redfern M, Jennings J, et al 1999a The influence of attention on postural control in stance. Gait and Posture 9:S11

Redfern M, Jennings J, et al 1999b Attention influences sensory integration for postural control in older adults. Gait and Posture 14:211–217

Redfern M, Muller M, et al 2002 Attentional dynamics in postural control during perturbations in young and older adults. Journal of Gerontology 57A(8):B298–303

Reitan R 1958 Validity of the Trail Making Test as an indicator of organic brain damage. Perceptual and Motor Skills 8:271–276

Sandyk R 1997 Treatment with electromagnetic field improves dual task performance (talking while walking) in multiple sclerosis. International Journal of Neurosciences 92(1–2):95–102

Seitz R J, Roland P E 1992 Learning of sequential finger movements in man: a combined kinematic and positron emission tomography (PET) study. European Journal of Neurosciences 4:154–165

Shumway-Cook A, Woollacott M 2000 Attentional demands and postural control: the effect of sensory context. Journal of Gerontology 55A(1):M10–16

Shumway-Cook A, Woollacot M, et al 1997 The effects of two types of cognitive tasks on postural stability in older adults with and without a history of falls. Journal of Gerontology 52A(4): M232–240

Shumway-Cook A, Brauer S G, et al 2000 Predicting the probability for falls in community-dwelling older adults using the timed up and go test. Physical Therapy 80(9):896–903

Stelmach G E, Zalaznik H N, et al 1990 The influence of ageing and attentional demands on recovery from postural instability. Aging 2(2):155–161

Teasdale N, Bard C, et al 1993 On the cognitive penetrability of postural control. Experimental Ageing Research 19:1–13

Verghese J, Buschke H, et al 2002 Validity of divided attention tasks in predicting falls in older individuals: a preliminary study. Journal of the American Geriatrics Society 50(9):1572–1576

Woollacott M H 1986 Gait and postural control in the ageing adult. Elsevier Science, Amsterdam

Wright D, Kemp T 1992 The dual-task methodology and assessing the attentional demands of ambulation with walking devices. Physical Therapy 72:306–309

Yardley L, Gardner M, et al 2001 Interference between postural control and mental task performance in patients with vestibular disorder and healthy controls. Journal of Neurology, Neurosurgery and Psychiatry 71(1):48–52

Yardley L, Gardner M, et al 1999 Effect of articulatory and mental tasks on postural control. NeuroReport 10(2):215–219

14

Precautions and contraindications for exercise in elderly people with cardiorespiratory or musculoskeletal conditions

Helen McBurney and Jill Cook

CHAPTER CONTENTS

Cardiovascular conditions 289

Musculoskeletal conditions 292

Medication 296

Environment 297

Summary 299

References 300

Regular physical activity is now recognized as a major component of a healthy lifestyle. People can benefit from physical activity at all ages and exercise is regarded as a 'best buy' in public health (Morris 1994, Pate et al 1995, Roos 1997). Physical inactivity is relatively more common in elderly people than for other age groups and can lead to a loss of function and independence in older age (Mazzeo and Tanaka 2001). Activity need not be vigorous to achieve health and fitness benefits. It appears that the greatest health benefits occur when the least active individuals become moderately active (Haskell 1994). Therefore to enhance health in elderly people, it is more important to promote an increase in activity volume (as described by duration and frequency) in sedentary individuals, rather than to increase intensity above a moderate level relative to the individual's capacity. A frequent community misconception is that if moderate activity is good then more or harder activity must be even better. It is well recognized that health benefits can be achieved from exercise that is performed more regularly and for longer durations but at lower intensities than exercises typically prescribed to achieve fitness (ACSM 2000, Haskell 1994, Mazzeo and Tanaka 2001).

The health of older people results from a combination of ongoing exposure to risk factors and ageing processes. Environmental factors rather than genetic factors are the main source of disease-specific variation in the later stages of life (AIHW 2002, p. 228). Individuals of the same age differ in their physiological status and it may be difficult to differentiate differences due to deconditioning, age-related decline or disease processes (ACSM 2000, p. 225). Just as exercise has benefits regardless of age, it appears that there are no direct contraindications or precautions regarding activity that are directly related to the attainment of any specific chronological age (Mazzeo and Tanaka 2001).

Contraindications, precautions or special considerations regarding activity relate to particular diseases or impairments acquired over the lifespan and to the exercise environment. Older people may have more than one chronic condition that limits their ability to exercise, for example ischaemic heart disease, chronic pulmonary disease or peripheral vascular disease. Modification of activity on an individual basis may therefore be necessary. Pre-participation assessment of the previously sedentary older person may be initiated with the use of a simple questionnaire such as the Physical Activity Readiness Questionnaire (PAR-Q) (ACSM 2000, p. 23). This will provide quick and ready identification of those who require further screening of their health status prior to exercise participation.

Cardiovascular conditions

Cardiovascular disease is the most prevalent disease group in older adults in the USA, UK, Canada and Australia. It accounts for 37% of all disability-adjusted life years (AIHW 2002, p. 228). Within the cardiovascular group, ischaemic heart disease is the most common condition in both males and females. This pattern is prevalent throughout the developed world. It appears, however, that the cardiovascular responses of older adults are similar to those of young adults and that the same beneficial cardiovascular adaptations to exercise occur in response to training (ACSM 1998).

Ischaemic heart disease

The increased myocardial demands of vigorous exercise may precipitate cardiovascular events in individuals with known or subclinical heart disease. Cardiovascular complications of activity are more frequently associated with clinical signs of: previous myocardial infarction, an ejection fraction lower than 30%, unstable angina pectoris, angina at rest and cardiac arrhythmias. Other causes may be chronotropic impairment caused by medication or inotropic impairment such as exercise hypotension. The lack of adequate warm-up or cool-down activities and the use of excessively too vigorous activity can potentiate further events.

The lower the exercise intensity, the less likely it is that exercise-related cardiovascular complications will occur. Swain and Franklin (2002) were not able to identify a lower threshold of intensity for aerobic training in individuals with known cardiac disease and yet noted that

Table 14.1 Contraindications to exercise for people with cardiac conditions

Angina	At rest or unstable
Exertional hypertension	Exercise systolic blood pressure >240 mmHg and/or exercise diastolic blood pressure >110 mmHg
Exertional hypotension	Failure of blood pressure to increase appropriately with exertion
Signs of cardiac failure	Pale, cold, sweaty, short of breath, pulmonary crackles inappropriate for level of exertion and environmental conditions
Arrhythmias	On exertion or exacerbated by exertion

Table 14.2 Precautions for exercise in people with cardiac conditions

Angina	Exercise intensity just below that where angina is precipitated
Known silent ischaemia	Exercise intensity just below that where ischaemia is precipitated
Cardiac failure	Activity at a level where symptoms are not increased
Atrial fibrillation	With controlled ventricular response rate. Adequate warm-up. Activity at a level where additional symptoms such as breathlessness are minimal

benefits were achieved at intensities as low as 42% of oxygen uptake reserve.

Prior to commencing a new exercise programme of moderate intensity, individuals with known cardiac disease should be assessed in a controlled and monitored exercise environment using a standardized exercise test protocol for the signs of high risk as summarized in Table 14.1.

If a low or moderate level activity programme is undertaken in older people with known or suspected ischaemic heart disease, attention to the precautions summarized in Table 14.2 will enhance the safety of the programme.

Recommendations for exercise in individuals with cardiovascular conditions can be readily found in books and papers such as those of the American College of Sports Medicine (ACSM 1997, 1998, 2000). In general it is recommended that individuals undertake low to moderate intensity activity for at least half an hour on a daily basis. Twice a week this should include some specific strength training activities. Flexibility exercises should be include in warm-up and cool-down sessions. Tudor-Locke et al (2002) found that whilst walking for exercise was frequently reported in community-dwelling older adults, participation in structured exercise classes was the only source of regular resistance and flexibility training.

Monitoring activity

With the current trend towards encouraging older individuals to continue with regular exercise, it is likely that physical activity will become a routine part of daily life. Physical activity levels can be increased or maintained with such things as a daily walk, gardening, using stairs, cycling or vigorous housework. The intensity of activity should be monitored and it is appropriate that the individual learns at least one way to do this. Monitoring of activity by rating perceived exertion is simple and has the advantage that as fitness increases, the individual achieves more within the same activity intensity perception. The Borg Rating of Perceived Exertion Scales are easy to use and have been found to be reliable as indicators of intensity of effort when the individual has sufficient training to be well calibrated to the scale (Williams and Eston 1989). Moderate intensity activity would be rated between 12 and 14 on the categorical scale or between three and four on the category ratio scale (Borg 1982). These scales account for specificity of training as familiar activities are rated by individuals at lower levels of perceived effort than unfamiliar activity or exercise that might otherwise be expected to be of a similar intensity.

Neurological disorders that compromise cardiopulmonary function

When disorders of movement or balance are the result of damage to the nervous system, such as in stroke, Parkinson's disease or motor neuron disease, cardiopulmonary function can sometimes be compromised. Poor control of movement or muscle weakness can make physical activity more difficult and require a higher level of oxygen consumption than for unimpaired individuals of the same age. In neurological conditions where there is an extended period of inactivity, the older person can find that ordinary activities such as dressing and walking require high heart rates and a matching feeling of effort (Russo 1990). Strategies to improve cardiovascular fitness should therefore be a part of the rehabilitation programme. Activities that require a high level of effort may need to be interspersed throughout one session rather than repeated in a short time frame, or broken down into less physically taxing parts, with each part to be performed and practised separately. If the person has a chest infection or difficulty activating respiratory muscles effectively for breathing, then standard cardiopulmonary treatments apply.

Peripheral vascular disease

Individuals with lower limb peripheral vascular disease may experience claudication with associated pain during physical activity as a result of poor oxygen supply to working muscles. Exercise has been advocated to improve peripheral muscle function within the limits of the available oxygen supply (Gardner and Poehlman 1995). Weight-bearing exercise has the most beneficial effect but may be poorly tolerated initially. If this is the case, non-weight-bearing activity such as exercise bicycling is an appropriate alternative.

Multiple chronic conditions

Elderly people frequently have more than one chronic condition that limits their ability to exercise. In considering how best to encourage regular physical activity it is necessary to take into account the limitations imposed by each condition, to consider which of these if any may be reversible with activity and to prescribe activity at an intensity, frequency and duration that it is possible for the person to complete within the limits of their capacity.

A common query relates to the exercise capacity of an individual who has suffered a stroke in conjunction with a cardiac event. Cardiac symptoms such as angina or breathlessness might impose the main limitations on exercise intensity whilst the stroke might be the cause of major impairments in movement or postural control. In this situation it is common for the client to attend rehabilitation for their neurological condition initially. In such a setting they might be asked to perform activities that require a high level of effort and are repeated frequently, such as rising from a chair or stair-climbing. In order to minimize the occurrence of hypertension or angina, early rehabilitation of this individual might require some low level aerobic training, practice at easier levels of the task such as starting from a high chair, or practice at sections of the task and frequent rests. This is before moving on to practise the functional activity or to incorporate activities into daily life in order to increase societal participation.

Musculoskeletal conditions

As discussed by Dodd and colleagues in Chapter 7, advanced age is associated with loss of muscle strength (number of fibres), bone mass, cardiovascular function (heart output and heart rate), respiratory function (lung volume) and metabolic rate (increasing the likelihood of weight gain). As a result, exercise can become more difficult and activity levels may decrease unless the individual takes active steps to maintain fitness. Staying fit and strong can limit the level of impairment and activity limitation that occurs, keep muscles strong and reduce bone mass loss (Pescatello et al 1999). Fitness can also assist recovery from musculoskeletal injuries. Recovery after injury, especially hip fracture, is better when pre-injury fitness levels are high (Horan and Clague 1999).

Many activities can be undertaken by older people to maintain physical abilities and health. Weight-bearing and non-weight-bearing exercises can benefit the musculoskeletal system, although skeletal benefits are only obtained from progressive resistance strength training exercises, or weight-bearing activities such as intense walking/running or stair-climbing (Berard et al 1997). Walking does not appear to increase the risk of injury, and the length of time walked or frequency does not increase the chance of injury (Hootman et al 2001). Vigorous walking is a good exercise because people with a wide range of fitness levels can perform this activity without increased risk of injury (Ready et al 1999). Women may be more susceptible to injury in a walking or jogging programme than men (Ready et al 1999).

Musculoskeletal risks of exercise

Exercise can be associated with injuries in people of all age groups, and active older people are also exposed to this risk. Musculoskeletal injuries can be divided into those that are 'acute' or those that result from 'overuse'. Acute injuries are more commonly associated with high velocity physical activities such as running and impact sports such as jumping (e.g. basketball). It is also possible for some older individuals to sustain an acute injury with low velocity activity. Overuse injuries can occur in any sport or activity and are usually associated with change in activity or an increase in the intensity of exercise.

Common musculoskeletal injuries in active older people

Tendon injury

As tendons age they become stiffer and less elastic. This places them at risk of developing pathology and pain, most commonly in the Achilles and the lateral elbow. These injuries are nearly always due to overuse, and they respond best to progressive eccentric exercise programmes (Khan et al 2000). Tendon ruptures are common in older people, and the rotator cuff and Achilles are the most common tendon ruptures in this age group. Due to hormonal influences, women have some protection against tendon rupture until they are postmenopausal (Maffulli et al 1999). In contrast, men are at risk of tendon rupture throughout the life-span (Maffulli et al 1999). Management after Achilles tendon rupture is dependent on fitness levels, age and individual factors such as smoking and vascular status. Conservative management may be undertaken if there is any compromise to wound healing. Conservative management is reported to have a higher risk of re-rupture (Moller et al 2001), but is also reported to have a reasonable outcome if successful.

The rotator cuff is exposed to sustained workload throughout life and can tear with a small force in the older person. Thus tears commonly occur after a fall on an outstretched hand. Playing golf loads the rotator cuff of the non-dominant shoulder and individuals with pre-existing disease in the shoulder may be better choosing another activity (Lindsay et al 2000). Rotator cuff tears can also be managed conservatively or surgically. Surgery can include primary repair or arthroscopic debridement. Both surgical and conservative treatments offer a good chance of recovery (Vad et al 2002).

Joint degeneration

As discussed in detail in Chapter 10, arthritis commonly affects the knees and hips of older adults and can be a primary presentation or secondary to injury earlier in life. In many people arthritis remains pain-free and symptoms in a joint that result from exercise can resolve even with underlying arthritic changes. Maintaining muscle strength around the joint may offer protection to the joint and minimize further damage (Fransen et al 2001).

Exercise does not adversely affect joint pain in most older people with OA. For example, low impact exercises such as strength training and riding an exercise bike did not aggravate joint pain in elderly people with arthritis (Coleman et al 1996). The benefits of exercise were preserved, and people with joint disease gained similar strength as individuals without arthritis (Coleman et al 1996). Golf places high loads on the lead hip with rotational torque and care should be taken in those with pre-existing hip joint disease (Lindsay et al 2000).

Back pain

The discs and joints of the spine are exposed to repeated use during life and often have signs and symptoms of degeneration in older people. The discs become more fibrous and less hydrated, which impairs their load-bearing capacity. Disc degeneration may be associated with changes in the facet joints and neural structures. In combination, these changes result in decreased spinal movement in older people. In turn this can be associated with muscle weakness. Specific exercise routines may offer some protection from further injury and pain (Hodges and Richardson 1996). Notwithstanding, high compressive loads on the spine occur during the golf swing and as such, golf should not be undertaken by individuals with osteoporosis (Lindsay et al 2000).

Fractures

As bone density decreases and the propensity to fall increases, the incidence of fractures in older people also increases. Common fractures occur to the humerus (surgical neck), distal radius, femoral fractures (neck), thoracic vertebrae and patella (Horan and Clague 1999). Chapter 9 in this volume provides a comprehensive account of the pathogenesis and management of fractures in older people.

Management of musculoskeletal injuries in older people

Do older people have more limited recovery than younger athletes who sustain musculoskeletal injuries? For more severe injuries that require hospital care, the length of stay in hospital is longer for elderly people than for young adults (Gomberg et al 1999). Nevertheless full recovery eventually occurs in most older individuals. Very old people with a neck of femur fracture are at risk of poor outcome, given that 12–20% die within 12 months of fracture (Khan et al 2001).

Immediate management of an acute injury

For more minor injuries, there appears to be no evidence that the older person will recover less than younger individuals, although lower pre-trauma levels of strength, bone density and fitness affect outcome. Traditionally, rest, ice, compression and elevation (RICE) are the preferred treatment options after acute injury. This is empirically based treatment, and little evidence supports any of the parts of the RICE approach. Ice application may or may not cause vasoconstriction, and tissue temperatures may not lower sufficiently to effect changes in blood flow in the presence of subcutaneous fat (MacAuley 2002). In the absence of research to indicate best practice acute management, clinically used guidelines must be used. Thus RICE for acute injuries is still considered to be appropriate management. Assessment by a medical practitioner for the correct diagnosis and the prescription of anti-inflammatory and pain-relieving medication is also strongly advised. Time frames for application of the RICE regime are also empirically based; 24–72 hours is suggested in most textbooks; clinical assessment of injury severity appears to guide the time needed for acute management.

Subacute management

Early mobilization after injury is also considered to be essential for good tissue repair (Maffulli and King 1992) and is especially critical in older people, to restore and preserve function. Exercise should be guided by symptoms (during and after exercise), and the area protected as necessary with appropriate orthoses or taping. Early professional advice about correct management of injury and exercise levels may prevent the onset of secondary conditions and loss of function.

Management of overuse injuries

Overuse injuries are again managed on clinical grounds, with load management, anti-inflammatory medication and exercise. Strength and flexibility exercises are important, and reduction of load to levels that do not exacerbate the pain are also a management strategy. Application of ice after exercise is encouraged, and taping and use of orthoses may be beneficial during exercise for pain relief, load reduction or biomechanical correction.

Prevention of musculoskeletal injuries during exercise

Instituting some simple strategies may prevent overuse injuries associated with exercise. These can be listed as follows:

1. It is considered important to include a warm-up and cool-down period. Warm-up will have cardiovascular effects (decreased vascular resistance), muscular effects (increased blood flow, decreased muscular stiffness) and joint range effects (increased connective tissue compliance). Warm-up may include stretching of any main muscles that will be subject to higher loads. Recent studies have shown reduction in injury rates when stretching was used as part of the warm-up (e.g. McKay et al 2001).
2. Progress increases in exercise slowly. Although many people aim for large gains in fitness or strength in short time frames, this can result in overuse injuries. Muscles and connective tissues require time to adapt to the level of exercise, and progressing before adaptation may cause symptoms (Ready et al 1999). The amount to progress exercise may be difficult to know, especially in individuals that do not have a strong exercise history. The Borg scale and recommended heart rate provide some guidelines for exercise progression.
3. Choose the exercise that suits the individual and their fitness, exercise history and current injury and disease. Bike and lower impact exercises may be best for those with joint disease; however, these activities have their own injury risks. Cycling in older people can be associated with accidents due to loss of balance and pedal problems (Kingma et al 1997).
4. Choose appropriate footwear and maintain it in good condition. Injuries such as plantar fasciitis and metatarsalgia are common in this age group (Matheson et al 1989, Ready et al 1999).
5. Previous injury is a risk factor for further injury (McKay et al 2001, Ready et al 1999), so protect any areas that have been previously injured and use braces, tape or other support where appropriate.

Medication

Therapists need to be aware of medications taken by their clients as well as the side effects and implications for activity. This knowledge can increase the safety of an exercise session and allow more individual consideration of activity prescription. Elderly people consume a high proportion of all prescribed medication and may take multiple medications at the behest of differing prescribers, particularly where they have more than one chronic condition and consult different medical staff for each specific problem. This 'polypharmacy' can increase the risk of adverse drug reactions or interactions (Bryant et al 2003).

Ageing is further associated with a variety of physiological changes that may alter pharmacokinetics. The absorption, distribution, metabolism and excretion of drugs may be affected. There are a number of categories of medications that will affect the physiological responses of an individual to exercise. Their effects may be heightened or attenuated depending on such changes in elderly people. For example, some long-acting sedatives are cleared from the body more slowly in elderly people and may be associated with side effects such as light-headedness, fatigue, poor coordination, altered balance and confusion (Upfal 2000). Individuals may be less responsive to one drug or class of drugs and more sensitive to others so that dose may need to be altered to achieve desired effects without side effects.

Beta-blockers

Beta-blocking medications are frequently used in the management of cardiac disease to reduce myocardial oxygen demand by decreasing myocardial contractility, heart rate and systolic blood pressure. At high doses or using a variety that is not cardiac selective, their use may potentiate other detrimental effects such as bronchoconstriction in asthma or reducing time to claudication in peripheral vascular disease. Beta-blocking medication will reduce heart rate during exercise by 20–30% (Head 1999). If exercise is of moderate intensity, adequate cardiac output appears to be maintained despite the reduced heart rate. Thermoregulation can also be adversely affected by the use of beta-blocking medication (Eston and Connolly 1996).

Anti-anginals

Anti-anginal medications, in particular the nitrates, cause dilatation of arterial and venous circulation by relaxation of smooth muscle in vessel walls. They reduce the work of the heart by decreasing peripheral resistance and venous return. This can allow an increased exercise capacity by increasing the anginal threshold. Prescribed nitrates can be used prior to exercise to remove or reduce the likelihood of the occurrence of angina. Hypotension may occur in individuals taking such medication if they cease exercise abruptly, so an effective cool-down is important.

Any medications used to lower blood pressure have the potential to induce dizziness or faints in elderly people, particularly in extreme heat or with sudden increases in activity (Upfal 2000).

Environment

Elderly people are at increased risk of slower responses to extremes of temperature or air pollution and are therefore more vulnerable to body stress when ambient conditions are not ideal.

Cold

Physical activity in the cold can be safe provided appropriate clothing is worn. Inhalation of or exposure to cold air may increase stroke volume and cardiac work and activate thermoregulatory reflexes even in mild exposure. This may cause cutaneous systemic vasoconstriction in an effort to conserve body heat. Reflex coronary artery spasm or constriction may also be triggered. The consequent increase in peripheral vascular resistance and arterial pressure with reduced coronary blood flow can precipitate myocardial ischaemia. People with coronary artery disease are likely to experience symptoms at lower activity intensity in the cold. In addition, the vasomotor responses of older persons to cold may be slower and less effective in decreasing skin blood flow. However, when these responses are active the resulting increase in blood pressure may be more pronounced (ACSM 2000). Practical actions for exercise in cold conditions are summarized in Table 14.3.

Heat

High ambient temperature and humidity impede the normal mechanisms used by the body to dissipate heat. Physical activity in heat causes increases in heart rate and myocardial oxygen demand that are disproportionate in relation to increased aerobic needs. Both heat of >24 °C and humidity add to heart rate increases. Early symptoms of heat stress to be noted and acted upon include elevated body temperature and heart rate, dehydration, cramps, syncope and exhaustion (ACSM 2001). Practical actions for exercising during heat are described in Table 14.4.

Table 14.3 Practical actions for exercise in cold conditions

- Wear layers of light clothing, shed and replace as needed
- Change clothing quickly if wet
- Hydrate with warm fluids, preferably caffeine free
- Keep moving
- Cover those parts of the body likely to lose heat because of their large surface area to mass ratio such as hands, feet and head

Table 14.4 Practical actions for exercise in heat

- Maintain adequate hydration
- Reduce dose at >27 °C or >75% relative humidity
- Use the cooler parts of the day
- Use an air-conditioned environment
- Wear light clothing that can 'breathe'
- Remember to use sunscreen

Pollution

Air quality can affect activity capacity and health. Pollution 'dosage' is a consequence of the length of exposure and concentration of pollutant in inspired air. Air pollution may affect the eyes or skin but primarily affects the respiratory tract and is particularly important for individuals whose airways become irritated and react by constricting (Green 1995). Older individuals with asthma or other forms of chronic obstructive respiratory disease are particularly at risk (Seaton et al 1995). Pollutants may be those associated with industry, motor vehicle emissions or may be specific allergens such as pollens. The primary method of preventing the harmful effects of pollution is to avoid exposure. Other methods of dealing with air pollution include starting or increasing the dose of inhaled prophylactic drugs and modifying activity (Ayres 1994). Practical actions for exercise during air pollution are summarized in Table 14.5.

Hydrotherapy

Exercise in water has become increasingly popular with older individuals as it provides health and fitness benefits in a warm and supportive activity medium. Ruoti et al (1994) provide evidence for the effect of non-swimming water exercises in increasing fitness for older adults. On land, gravity and external applied resistance are the forces that muscles must overcome. In the water, buoyancy, turbulence and viscosity are the forces affecting movement of the body (Johnson et al 1977).

In stationary seated individuals immersed in thermoneutral water to the level of the sternal notch, as a result of the hydrostatic pressure, there is a decrease of blood pooling in the limbs and an increase in central venous return. Cardiac output increases by up to 50% due to increased stroke volume while little change occurs in heart rate or in blood pressure. Peripheral resistance is lower due to cutaneous vasodilation as the skin temperature rises. Water at a temperature of 35°C is regarded as thermoneutral as it has no effect on core temperature (Hall et al 1990). If water temperature is increased, blood pressure at rest decreases.

Under exercise conditions, in an upright stance, there is evidence that energy expenditure in the pool is higher than for the equivalent activity on land (Evans et al 1978, Johnson et al 1977). It is suggested that intensity of activity is regulated by pace and by altering resistance (shortening a lever arm or adding/removing resistance equipment). Oxygen consumption is greatest when walking in water at mid-thigh depth. At water levels higher than this, the effect of buoyancy reduces oxygen consumption. Monitoring of exercise intensity using rate of perceived exertion (RPE) scales remains appropriate in water exercise.

Table 14.5 Practical actions for exercise during air pollution

- Select an optimal location for activity; this may be indoors
- Lower the intensity and duration of activity
- Use appropriate respiratory medication if prescribed
- Be aware of daily or seasonal patterns of air quality

Table 14.6 Individual precautions for hydrotherapy

- The thermoregulatory system of the body needs to be efficient to cope with exercise in warm water as evaporation is largely ineffective
- Balance: In the water, input for proprioception is reduced and refraction of light may give a false perception of the bottom of the pool. Turbulence of the water may further upset the recovery reactions of an individual with poor balance
- Where the older person is not comfortable in a water environment their anxiety, fear or insecurity can impede participation
- Cognitive status, particularly concentration and attention, judgement, insight and perceptual abilities, needs to be sufficient to cope with the altered exercise environment. Individual caregivers may be required for participation in water exercise programmes for those with impaired cognition
- Impairment of sight or hearing may reduce the communication abilities in elderly people. This can pose difficulties in a noisy pool environment
- Illnesses of short duration or recent onset that include episodes of dizziness, nausea, faintness or palpitations should be warnings to reduce exercise participation. It is difficult to provide assistance in a water environment and it may be more appropriate to miss a session in these circumstances.

Table 14.7 Contraindications to hydrotherapy

- Incontinence of either urine or faeces
- Epilepsy
- Hypertension
- Infection, particularly open skin lesions and vesicular skin conditions
- Indwelling catheters or other invasive lines
- Severe cognitive impairment or dementia

Precautions and contraindications for water-based exercise are those with respect to the safety of the individual undertaking the exercise and facility safety for all participants in a multi-user environment (Levin 1997). Participants should always be reminded to self-monitor their level of exertion and check for symptoms of cardiac insufficiency. Individual concerns may be associated with ageing changes such as loss of hearing or sight or with specific acute or chronic ill health. Individual precautions are summarized in Table 14.6.

Water-based exercise can provide an effective and enjoyable alternative to land-based programmes for fitness and health in elderly people. Nevertheless, the water exercise facility needs to be as safe as possible for all users. Changing rooms and pool environments need to have non-slip flooring and hand rails with easy entry to the pool. The contraindications to hydrotherapy relate to maintaining a safe and infection-free environment and are presented in Table 14.7.

Summary

The benefits of exercise can be enjoyed by older individuals by using a sensible approach to activity selection and implementation. Simple practical actions can be utilized to lessen the risks of activity in many situations. Exercise at appropriate levels is the simplest and most effective way to improve muscle mass, muscle strength, cardiorespiratory function, balance and movement control. In older athletes or others in whom decreases in these body functions can compromise independence, exercise is strongly recommended.

References

American College of Sports Medicine 1997 The recommended quantity and quality of exercise for maintaining cardiorespiratory and muscular fitness, and flexibility in healthy adults. Medicine and Science in Sports and Exercise 29:975–991

American College of Sports Medicine 1998 Exercise and physical activity for older adults. Medicine and Science in Sports and Exercise 30:992–1008

American College of Sports Medicine 2000 ACSM's guidelines for exercise testing and prescription, 6th edn. Lippincott Williams & Wilkins, Philadelphia

American College of Sports Medicine 2001 ACSM's resource manual for guidelines for exercise testing and prescription, 4th edn. Lippincott Williams & Wilkins, Philadelphia

Australian Institute of Health and Welfare (AIHW) 2002 Australia's health 2002. AIHW, Canberra, p 228

Ayres J 1994 Asthma and the atmosphere. British Medical Journal 309:619–620

Berard A, Bravo G, et al 1997 Meta-analysis of the effectiveness of physical activity for the prevention of bone loss in postmenopausal women. Osteoporosis International 7:331–337

Borg G A 1982 Psychophysical bases of perceived exertion. Medicine and Science in Sports and Exercise 14:377–381

Bryant B, Knights K, et al 2003 Pharmacology for health professionals. Mosby, Sydney

Coleman E, Buchner D, et al 1996 The relationship of joint symptoms with exercise performance in older athletes. Journal of the American Geriatrics Society 44(1):14–21

Eston R, Connolly D 1996 The use of ratings of perceived exertion for exercise prescription in patients receiving beta-blocker therapy. Sports Medicine 21(3):176–190

Evans B W, Cureton K J, et al 1978 Metabolic and circulatory responses to walking and jogging in water. Research Quarterly for Exercise and Sport 49(4):442–449

Fransen M, Crosbie J, et al 2001 Physical therapy is effective for patients with osteoarthritis of the knee: a randomized controlled clinical trial. Journal of Rheumatology 28:156–164

Gardner A W, Poelhman E T 1995 Exercise rehabilitation programs for the treatment of claudication pain: a meta analysis. JAMA 274:975–980

Gomberg B, Gruen G, et al 1999 Outcomes in acute orthopaedic trauma: a review of 130 506 patients by age. Injury 30:431–437

Green M 1995 Air pollution and health. British Medical Journal 311:401–402

Hall J, Bisson D, et al 1990 The physiology of immersion. Physiotherapy 76(6):517–521

Haskell W L 1994 Health consequences of physical activity: understanding and challenges regarding dose–response. Medicine and Science in Sports and Exercise 26:649–660

Head A 1999 Exercise metabolism and beta-blocker therapy: an update. Sports Medicine 27:81–96

Hodges P W, Richardson C A 1996 Inefficient muscular stabilization of the lumbar spine associated with low back pain. Spine 21(22):2640–2650

Hootman J, Macera C, et al 2001 Association among physical activity level, cardiorespiratory fitness and risk of musculoskeletal injury. American Journal of Epidemiology 154(3):251–258

Horan M, Clague J 1999 Injury in the aging: recovery and rehabilitation. British Medical Bulletin 55(4):895–909

Johnson B L, Stromme S B, et al 1977 Comparison of oxygen uptake and heart rate during exercises on land and in water. Physical Therapy 57(3):273–278

Khan K, Cook J, et al 2000 Overuse tendinosis, not tendinitis. Physician and Sports Medicine 28(9):38–48

Khan K, McKay H, et al 2001 Physical activity and bone health. Human Kinetics, Champaign, IL

Kingma J, Duursma N, et al 1997 The aetiology and long-term effects of injuries due to bicycle accidents in persons aged fifty years and older. Perceptual and Motor Skills 85:1035–1041

Levin A 1997 Water fitness for the older adult and frail aged. In: Campion M R (ed) Hydrotherapy: principles and practice. Butterworth-Heinemann, Oxford

Lindsay D, Horton J, et al 2000 A review of injury characteristics, aging factors and prevention programmes for the older golfer. Sports Medicine 30(2):89–103

MacAuley D 2002 What is the role of ice in soft tissue injury management? In: MacAuley D, Best T, Evidence-based Sports Medicine. BMJ Books, London

Maffulli N, King J B 1992 Effects of physical activity on some components of the skeletal system. Sports Medicine 13(6):393–407

Maffulli N, Waterston W, et al 1999 Changing incidence of Achilles tendon rupture in Scotland: a 15 year study. Clinical Journal of Sports Medicine 9(3):157–160

Matheson G, Macintyre J, et al 1989 Musculoskeletal injuries associated with physical activity in older adults. Medicine and Science in Sports and Exercise 21(4):379–385

Mazzeo R S, Tanaka H 2001 Exercise prescription for the elderly: current recommendations. Sports Medicine 31(11):809–818

McKay G D, Goldie P A, et al 2001 Ankle injuries in basketball: injury rate and risk factors. British Journal of Sports Medicine 35:103–108

Moller M, Movin T, et al 2001 Acute rupture of the tendon Achillis. Journal of Bone and Joint Surgery (Br) 83:843–848

Morris J N 1994 Exercise in the prevention of coronary heart disease: today's best buy in public health. Medicine and Science in Sports and Exercise 26:807–814

Pate R R, Pratt M, et al 1995 Physical activity and public health. JAMA 273(5):402–407

Pescatello L 1999 Physical activity, cardiometabolic health and older athletes. Sports Medicine 28(5):315–323

Ready A E, Bergeron G, et al 1999 Incidence and determinants of injuries sustained by older women during a walking program. Journal of Aging and Physical Activity 7:91–104

Roos R J 1997 The Surgeon General's report: a prime resource for exercise advocates. The Physician and Sports Medicine 25:122–127

Ruoti R G, Troup J T, et al 1994 The effects of non swimming water exercises on older adults. Journal of Orthopedic and Sports Physical Therapy 19(3):140–145

Russo P 1990 Cardiovascular responses associated with activity and inactivity. In: Ada L, Canning C (eds) Key issues in neurological physiotherapy. Oxford, Heinemann Medical, p 127–154

Seaton A, MacNee W, et al 1995 Particulate air pollution and acute health effects. Lancet 345:176–178

Swain D P, Franklin B A 2002 Is there a threshold intensity for aerobic training in cardiac patients? Medicine and Science in Sports and Exercise 34(7):1071–1075

Tudor-Locke C, Jones G R, et al 2002 Contribution of structured exercise class participation and informal walking for exercise to daily physical activity in community dwelling older adults. Research Quarterly for Exercise and Sport 73(3):350–356

Upfal J 2000 The Australian drug guide, 5th edn. Bookman, Melbourne

Vad V, Warren R, et al 2002 Negative prognostic factors in managing massive rotator cuff tears. Clinical Journal of Sport Medicine 12(3):151–157

Williams J G, Eston R G 1989 Determination of the intensity dimension in vigorous exercise programmes with particular reference to the rating of perceived exertion. Sports Medicine 8:177–189

15

Exercise training for older people with type 2 diabetes

Scott Bradley

CHAPTER CONTENTS

Introduction 303

Diagnosis of type 2 diabetes 304

Complications of type 2 diabetes 304

Aetiology of type 2 diabetes 305

Prevention of IGT and type 2 diabetes by physical activity 306

Correcting IGT and treating type 2 diabetes with physical activity 308

Mechanism of improved glucose tolerance with physical activity 309

Recommended exercise for individuals with type 2 diabetes 313

Risks and complications of exercise 317

Factors affecting the adoption and maintenance of exercise 319

Summary of exercise guidelines 321

Conclusions 321

References 321

Introduction

Type 2 diabetes, previously referred to as non-insulin-dependent diabetes mellitus or NIDDM, accounts for approximately 85–90% of all cases of diabetes (WHO 1994). Worldwide, it is now recognized as a serious health problem that has evolved with rapid cultural and social changes, ageing populations, increasing urbanization, dietary changes and reduced physical activity (WHO 1994). In 1997 an estimated 120 million people had type 2 diabetes worldwide (Amos et al 1997), with that number predicted to rise to 220 million by 2010 (Amos et al 1997), and soaring to nearly 300 million by 2025 (WHO 1994).

Type 2 diabetes is a metabolic disorder characterized by insulin resistance, relative insulin deficiency and elevated blood glucose concentrations. Insulin is the hormone that stimulates the movement of glucose from the bloodstream into insulin-sensitive tissues such as skeletal muscle and adipose tissue. Insulin resistance is the inability of the body to respond normally to insulin, and therefore blood glucose levels remain elevated. Type 2 diabetes is preceded by the development of impaired glucose tolerance (IGT), during which blood glucose levels are elevated, but not to the same extent as in type 2 diabetes. In this chapter, evidence for the role of exercise in preventing and treating IGT and type 2 diabetes will be presented. Further, the mechanisms by which exercise improves blood glucose control will be discussed. Finally, exercise prescription guidelines, including the efficacy, safety concerns and limitations of exercise in an ageing population with type 2 diabetes, will be provided.

Diagnosis of type 2 diabetes

The World Health Organization criteria for diagnosing type 2 diabetes and IGT are based on fasting, and 2-hour post glucose load blood or plasma glucose concentrations (Alberti and Zimmet 1998). Table 15.1 shows the criteria used for diagnosing type 2 diabetes and IGT using plasma glucose.

Complications of type 2 diabetes

The clinical course and prognosis for people with type 2 diabetes is influenced by the duration of diabetes and degree of metabolic control. People with type 2 diabetes have a substantially reduced life expectancy, with age-specific mortality rates approximately twice that of the non-diabetic population in developed countries (Panzram 1987).

The main complications associated with type 2 diabetes are microvascular and macrovascular disease. Microvascular complications of diabetes include retinopathy, nephropathy and neuropathy. Macrovascular disease complications, such as coronary artery disease (CAD) and

Table 15.1   Criteria for impaired glucose tolerance (IGT) and type 2 diabetes. WHO criteria for the diagnosis of impaired glucose tolerance (IGT) and type 2 diabetes (using fasting and 2-hour post glucose load venous plasma glucose) (Adapted from Alberti and Zimmet 1998)

Category	Venous plasma glucose (mmol/l)		
	Fasting		2 hour
'Normal' glucose tolerance	<6.1	and	<7.8
Impaired glucose tolerance (IGT)	<7.0	and	7.8–11.0
Type 2 diabetes (NIDDM)	≥7.0	and/or	≥11.1

Fasting plasma glucose is typically recorded following at least 8 hours fasting.
The 2-hour glucose is taken 2 hours after ingestion of a 75 g glucose load.
To convert mmol/l to mg/dl, multiply by 18; e.g. 7.8 mmol/l = 140 mg/dl.

peripheral vascular disease (PVD), affect a large number of people with diabetes, and are common causes of morbidity and mortality.

| **Aetiology of type 2 diabetes** | Blood glucose concentration is determined by processes that add glucose to, and remove glucose from, the circulation. In the fasted state, release of glucose from the liver is balanced with uptake of glucose by the body and therefore blood glucose levels are stable. However, after eating, glucose is absorbed from the digestive system and results in a rise in blood glucose. The increase in blood glucose stimulates insulin release from the pancreas, which increases glucose uptake by insulin-sensitive tissues and reduces glucose output from the liver. The increase in glucose clearance by insulin-sensitive peripheral tissues such as skeletal muscle and adipose tissue is more important than the reduction in hepatic glucose output. Normally, skeletal muscle accounts for 70–90% of the glucose uptake of an oral or intravenous glucose challenge (Baron et al 1988, DeFronzo et al 1981, Katz et al 1983), and suggests that changes in skeletal muscle may play an important role in blood glucose regulation. A normal response to insulin prevents excessive and prolonged increases in blood glucose levels. As mentioned above, a major characteristic of type 2 diabetes is insulin resistance, which causes insufficient clearance of blood glucose and/or insufficient inhibition of hepatic glucose output in response to insulin. The initial effects of insulin resistance are hyperinsulinaemia and IGT. That is, insulin resistance results in the need for higher insulin levels in order to regulate blood glucose concentrations. IGT refers to a condition in which the blood glucose level is higher than normal, but not high enough to be classified as type 2 diabetes (Table 15.1). |

Whilst the full aetiology of type 2 diabetes is unknown, there are some well-established risk factors, including inactivity and ageing, for the development of type 2 diabetes. In this chapter, only the association between physical inactivity and type 2 diabetes will be discussed, as it appears much of the risk associated with ageing is due to decreased physical activity, rather than the ageing process itself (Ivy et al 1999). Physical inactivity appears to expose a genetic predisposition to the disease. Two possible mechanisms by which physical inactivity may cause type 2 diabetes in those individuals genetically susceptible have been proposed (Ivy 1997).

The first mechanism proposes that physical inactivity leads to a positive energy balance, increased fat storage and adipocyte (fat cell) hypertrophy (Ivy 1997). As adipocytes enlarge, they develop reduced insulin sensitivity due to a reduced insulin receptor density. This results in reduced plasma free fatty acid (FFA) clearance, and elevated plasma FFAs stimulate hepatic gluconeogenesis (the production of glucose by the liver) (Golay et al 1987, Williamson et al 1969). In addition, elevated FFAs inhibit insulin-stimulated muscle glucose clearance (Boden et al 1991). This results in a compensatory increase in insulin secretion from the pancreas and hyperinsulinaemia in order to control blood glucose concentration. Eventually, the increased necessity for insulin causes pancreatic β cell impairment and reduced plasma insulin levels. This exacerbates the insulin resistant state, reduces FFA clearance, accelerates hepatic glucose output, and results in type 2 diabetes (Ivy 1997).

The second mechanism proposes that physical inactivity exposes a genetic defect in skeletal muscle which results in muscle insulin resistance (Ivy 1997). This leads to increased blood glucose concentration and a compensatory increase in pancreatic β cell insulin secretion and hyperinsulinaemia to control blood glucose. However, the hyperinsulinaemia suppresses fatty acid oxidation and increases triglyceride storage and adipocyte hypertrophy. Next, adipocytes become insulin resistant (as described above) and there is a reduced ability of insulin to clear plasma FFA. This causes an increase in hepatic glucose output and further development of muscle insulin resistance. Eventually the increased reliance on insulin to control blood glucose results in β cell impairment, exacerbating the situation and causing development of type 2 diabetes (Ivy 1997).

Prevention of IGT and type 2 diabetes by physical activity

Epidemiological studies

It is generally agreed that habitual physical activity reduces the chances of developing type 2 diabetes (Ivy et al 1999). For example, there is a high incidence of IGT and type 2 diabetes in urbanized indigenous Australians. Research by O'Dea (1984) showed that when a group of indigenous Australians resumed a traditional hunter-gathering lifestyle which included increased physical activity and a low caloric, low fat diet for only 7 weeks, there were significant improvements in their fasting glucose concentrations, fasting insulin concentrations, and glucose tolerance to an oral glucose challenge (O'Dea 1984). Similarly, in a group of Pima Indians, low levels of current and lifetime leisure physical activity were associated with higher rates of type 2 diabetes (Kriska et al 1993).

In a study that determined the incidence of type 2 diabetes in nearly 6000 male University of Pennsylvania alumni, it was found that the incidence of type 2 diabetes decreased as the reported caloric energy expenditure of physical activity increased (Helmrich et al 1991). In an initial cohort of over 87 000 female nurses, the risk of developing type 2 diabetes within the 8-year follow-up period was 35% less for women who reported engaging in vigorous exercise at least once per week compared with women who exercised less regularly (Manson et al 1991). Similarly, male physicians who reported participation in vigorous exercise at least once per week had a lower incidence of type 2 diabetes than those who did not exercise regularly (Manson et al 1992).

Individuals who had low cardiovascular fitness (i.e. the least fit 20% of the cohort) as measured by maximal incremental treadmill testing at baseline had a 1.9-fold increased risk of IGT and 3.7-fold increased risk of type 2 diabetes compared with those in the high cardiovascular fitness group (the most fit 40% of the cohort) (Wei et al 1999). The protective effects of exercise may be more pronounced in individuals who are at higher risk of developing type 2 diabetes (Lynch et al 1996).

Perhaps the most powerful epidemiology studies are those that involve some degree of intervention. Eriksson and Lindgarde (1991) tested the effectiveness of increased physical activity and improved dietary habits on the prevention of type 2 diabetes. After initially screening nearly 7000 males (aged 47–49 years), over 200 subjects with IGT or early-stage type 2 diabetes were selected to receive treatment including dietary advice and treatment and/or increased physical activity and exercise training. After 5 years, oral glucose tolerance was normalized in over 50% of the IGT subjects, and the incidence of type 2 diabetes was 10.6%. By comparison, oral glucose tolerance had deteriorated 67.1% and the prevalence of type 2 diabetes was 28.6% in the non-intervention IGT group after 5 years (Eriksson and Lindgarde 1991).

Physical activity studies

Although sometimes extreme in study design compared with the more gradual decline in physical activity that typically accompanies ageing, results from bedrest and detraining studies provide support for the importance of physical activity in the prevention of insulin resistance.

Bedrest studies

It has long been known that bedrest is associated with the development of impaired glucose tolerance (Blotner 1945, Deitrick et al 1948, Lutwak and Whedon 1959). Bedrest studies now provide good evidence that a minimal level of physical activity is required to maintain normal glucose tolerance and insulin sensitivity (Dolkas and Greenleaf 1977, Lipman et al 1970, 1972, Misbin et al 1983, Myllynen et al 1987, Stuart et al 1988). After only 3 days of bedrest, insulin-stimulated glucose uptake was reduced by 50% (Lipman et al 1972). Bedrest not only impairs insulin sensitivity and glucose tolerance in previously healthy individuals, but also exacerbates the insulin resistance of individuals with pre-existing glucose intolerance (Misbin et al 1983).

Training cessation

Insulin sensitivity rapidly decreases when trained subjects stop exercising. After only 5 days inactivity in previously trained subjects, the insulin response to maintain normal blood glucose concentration was increased during intravenous glucose infusion (Mikines et al 1989). Following 10 days of detraining, blood glucose concentration was increased in response to an oral glucose load and the maximal rise in plasma insulin concentration was doubled (Heath et al 1983). Following 14 days of detraining, the lower insulin response to an intravenous glucose infusion in the trained state was abolished (King et al 1988).

Effects of ageing

Ageing is associated with the development of insulin resistance, which contributes to the high incidence of IGT and type 2 diabetes in older people (DeFronzo et al 1981, Fink et al 1983, Shimokata et al 1991). Nevertheless insulin resistance may not be due to the ageing process itself. Insulin resistance appears to be determined more by changes in lifestyle and body composition, especially decreased physical activity, accumulation of body fat and decreased lean body mass (Boden et al 1993, Shimokata et al 1991). Skeletal muscle mass decreases by more than 5% per decade beyond 50 years of age (Lynch et al 1999). It has been reported that obesity and poor fitness, rather than age, account for the difference in glucose tolerance between young adults and middle-aged adults (Shimokata et al 1991).

Studies comparing physically active older individuals with sedentary older subjects and younger trained athletes support the notion that the association between ageing and insulin resistance is secondary to changes in physical activity and body composition. Endurance-trained older individuals have lower body fat (Heath et al 1981, Houmard et al 1993, Van Pelt et al 1997) and greater insulin sensitivity than untrained counterparts (Pratley et al 1995, Seals et al 1984, Yamanouchi et al 1992). Master athletes have lower fasting plasma glucose (Pratley et al 1995) and plasma glucose responses to oral glucose challenges that are similar to those of young athletes, and significantly better than sedentary men of similar age (Seals et al 1984).

Correcting IGT and treating type 2 diabetes with physical activity

Exercise training in healthy individuals

Physically active individuals have the same (or slightly lower) plasma glucose responses to an oral glucose challenge than untrained individuals, despite lower insulin levels (Davidson et al 1966, Hartley et al 1972, Heath et al 1983, LeBlanc et al 1981, Lohmann et al 1978, Rodnick et al 1987). Increased insulin sensitivity has been observed for both aerobically-trained (Heath et al 1983, LeBlanc et al 1981, Lohmann et al 1978, Rodnick et al 1987) and strength-trained athletes (Craig et al 1981, Miller et al 1984). These findings suggest that a physically active lifestyle reduces the insulin concentration required to maintain normal plasma glucose. Increased insulin sensitivity with exercise training occurs rapidly in healthy individuals: only 7 days of aerobic training was required to significantly lower the insulin response to an oral glucose challenge (Cononie et al 1994).

Exercise training and impaired glucose tolerance (IGT)

Exercise training appears to be beneficial in individuals with IGT (Ivy et al 1999). Three months to one year of aerobic training by individuals with IGT lowered the plasma glucose response to an oral glucose challenge, even though plasma insulin levels were also reduced (Holloszy et al 1986, Hughes et al 1993). The plasma glucose and insulin responses following training in older people who were previously sedentary were similar to those expected for young individuals without glucose intolerance (Holloszy et al 1986). These studies demonstrate that exercise training can improve glucose tolerance and insulin sensitivity in individuals with IGT.

Exercise training and type 2 diabetes

Whereas early studies failed to demonstrate an improvement in glucose tolerance or insulin sensitivity in individuals with type 2 diabetes following exercise training (Ruderman et al 1979, Saltin et al 1979), more recent experiments have found that both glucose tolerance and insulin sensitivity are improved by exercise training (Dela et al 1995, Holloszy et al 1986, Reitman et al 1984, Schneider et al 1984). One year of aerobic exercise training in individuals with type 2 diabetes improved both glucose tolerance and the insulin response to an oral glucose tolerance test (OGTT), and fasting plasma glucose was also normalized (Holloszy et al 1986). Similarly, only 6–10 weeks of exercise training in individuals with type 2 diabetes lowered fasting plasma glucose and improved oral glucose tolerance even with a reduced insulin response (Reitman et al 1984).

Mechanism of improved glucose tolerance with physical activity

Exercise has both short-term and long-term effects on insulin action (Ivy et al 1999). Firstly, an acute exercise bout has short-lasting insulin-like effects on muscle glucose transport (Holloszy and Narahara 1965, Wallberg-Henriksson and Holloszy 1984). Secondly, an acute exercise bout produces a marked increase in the sensitivity of muscle glucose uptake and muscle glycogen synthesis to insulin (Cartee et al 1989, Garetto et al 1984) that persists until muscle glycogen reaches above normal levels (Cartee et al 1989). Finally, exercise training has been found to result in sustained improvements in insulin action, due to several physiological and cellular adaptations (Ivy et al 1999). These adaptations are discussed below.

Control of hepatic glucose output

Increased hepatic glucose output may contribute to the elevated plasma glucose levels seen in type 2 diabetes (Campbell et al 1988, Vaag et al 1995). Exercise training may reduce the elevated postabsorptive glucose output. Twelve weeks of endurance exercise training reduced hepatic glucose output by over 20% (Segal et al 1991). Further, insulin produced a greater suppression of hepatic glucose output in trained subjects compared with untrained subjects (Rodnick et al 1987). These results indicate that hepatic sensitivity to insulin is improved with training, and thus there is reduced postabsorptive hepatic glucose output. It should be remembered that in the postprandial state when insulin levels are elevated, suppression of hepatic glucose output plays only a minor role in the control of blood glucose, with the difference in blood glucose being mainly due to differences in the response of peripheral tissues to insulin-stimulated glucose uptake (Ivy et al 1999).

Control of body fat

There is an association between excessive body fat and the development of insulin resistance. In particular, the accumulation of abdominal fat accounts for much of the insulin resistance (Kohrt et al 1993). The control of body fat, and especially abdominal fat, may be an important effect of regular physical activity in those with type 2 diabetes. For example, 14 months of moderate aerobic exercise training was associated with a preferential loss of abdominal fat in obese women, and with improved insulin sensitivity (Despres et al 1988).

The mechanism by which central adiposity adversely affects glucose tolerance (and therefore the mechanism by which reductions in abdominal fat improves insulin sensitivity) is not fully understood. It has been speculated that production of tumour necrosis factor-α (TNF-α) from adipocytes in the abdominal region increases (Ivy et al 1999), as it has been found that plasma TNF-α levels are increased in obese individuals with type 2 diabetes (Katsuki et al 1998). Interestingly, infusion of TNF-α causes insulin resistance in rats (Miles et al 1997). It is currently unknown whether exercise training reduces TNF-α levels in the same way as it reduces abdominal adiposity and improves insulin sensitivity. A second proposed mechanism by which abdominal fat may contribute to insulin resistance is by increasing plasma FFAs (Ivy 1997). As previously mentioned, increased FFAs lead to an increase in gluconeogenesis and hepatic glucose output, and can inhibit insulin-stimulated skeletal muscle glucose uptake.

Control of muscle mass

In addition to a decrease in fat mass, it is now apparent that an increase in muscle mass may significantly improve glucose tolerance and insulin action (Ivy et al 1999). Skeletal muscle accounts for 70–90% of the clearance of an oral or intravenous glucose challenge (Baron et al 1988, DeFronzo et al 1981, Katz et al 1983). Therefore, reduced muscle mass could reduce the effectiveness of insulin to clear glucose from the circulation. Conversely, increased muscle mass could increase available insulin-responsive tissue, thereby increasing glucose uptake from the bloodstream and reducing the insulin levels required to maintain normal plasma glucose levels. Miller et al (1984) attributed the reduced insulin response to an OGTT in young men following 10 weeks of resistance training to an increase in muscle mass (Miller et al 1984). Resistance training has also been shown to lower fasting plasma glucose (Fluckey et al 1994) and improve glucose tolerance (Craig et al 1981). It appears that an increase in muscle mass reduces the insulin response necessary to maintain normal blood glucose concentrations.

If individuals are physically inactive, there is a steady decline in muscle mass, particularly past the age of 50 years (Lynch et al 1999, Shimokata et al 1991). Therefore strength training may be important for the maintenance of a normal glucose tolerance. An increase in muscle mass in 50–65 year-old-men following 16 weeks of resistance training was associated with reduced fasting insulin and lower insulin during an OGTT (Miller et al 1994).

Biochemical changes in skeletal muscle

A number of biochemical defects have been identified in insulin-resistant skeletal muscle (Ivy et al 1999). These defects include (1) reduced insulin receptor number and proteins of the insulin signalling cascade (Caro et al 1987), (2) impaired glucose transporter system, (3) reduced activity of enzymes controlling the phosphorylation and disposal of intracellular glucose (Kelley et al 1992, 1996, Lillioja et al 1986, Schalin-Jantti et al 1992), and (4) alterations in plasma membrane phospholipids. Exercise training has been shown to improve all four of these defects (Ivy et al 1999).

Exercise training increases the binding of insulin to rat skeletal muscle (Bonen et al 1986, Dohm et al 1987). However, neither increases in insulin receptor binding nor increases in the number of insulin receptors have been observed in humans following training (Dela et al 1993). The finding that exercise training has no effect on insulin receptor tyrosine kinase activity in human skeletal muscle (Dela et al 1993) suggests that the exercise training induced improvements in insulin action are mediated by events downstream of the insulin receptor kinase activation. This notion has been subsequently been supported. Houmard et al (1999) reported that insulin-stimulated glucose uptake was improved, and skeletal muscle phosphatidylinositol (PI) 3-kinase activity increased following one week of endurance exercise training (Houmard et al 1999). In summary, these results suggest that improvements in insulin-stimulated glucose uptake in healthy individuals following exercise training are due, in part, to changes in the insulin signalling cascade distal to insulin receptor tyrosine kinase activity, and may involve PI 3-kinase.

Exercise training has been shown to increase the concentration of the important skeletal muscle glucose transporter, GLUT4 (Ivy et al 1999). This finding has been demonstrated in young healthy humans (Phillips et al 1996), previously sedentary middle-aged men (Houmard et al 1993), individuals with IGT (Hughes et al 1993) and individuals with type 2 diabetes (Dela et al 1994).

Once glucose is transported into the muscle cell it is phosphorylated to glucose-6-phosphate (G-6-P). The majority of G-6-P formed during insulin-stimulated glucose uptake is rapidly converted to glycogen or oxidized (Ivy and Holloszy 1981, Lillioja et al 1986). In skeletal muscle, the conversion of glucose to G-6-P is catalysed by the enzyme hexokinase and proceeds rapidly, thus maintaining a low intracellular glucose concentration and providing the concentration gradient essential for skeletal muscle glucose transport (Ivy et al 1999). Exercise training increases the activity of hexokinase II (Coggan et al 1993, Holloszy 1975, Mandroukas et al 1984), glycogen synthase (Ebeling et al 1993) and oxidative enzymes (Holloszy 1975, Mandroukas et al 1984), and therefore there is an increased capacity of skeletal muscle to transport, phosphorylate and dispose of glucose following training. These adaptations should contribute to improved insulin sensitivity that results from defects in the glucose disposal pathways (Ivy et al 1999).

The lipid composition of skeletal muscle may be an important predictor of insulin action (Borkman et al 1993, Pan et al 1995, Storlien et al 1991, Vessby et al 1994). Insulin sensitivity is associated with phospholipids that contain unsaturated fatty acids (Borkman et al 1993, Pan et al 1995) and negatively related with phospholipids that contain saturated fatty acids (Vessby et al 1994). Exercise training has been shown to alter the composition of the phospholipids in skeletal muscle in a manner that would improve insulin action (Andersson et al 1998).

Muscle fibre type

Investigations in rats show that type I (slow oxidative) skeletal muscle fibres have higher insulin sensitivity than type IIa (fast oxidative/glycolytic) and IIb (fast glycolytic) fibres (James et al 1985, Richter et al 1982). This difference has been attributed to the higher insulin receptor density (Bonen et al 1986) and GLUT4 protein concentration (Henriksen et al 1990, Kern et al 1990) in type I fibres compared with type IIa and IIb fibres. Skeletal muscle from obese insulin-resistant individuals (Holm and Krotkiewski 1988, Krotkiewski et al 1983, Lillioja et al 1987) and individuals with type 2 diabetes (Lillioja et al 1987, Marin et al 1994) have a low percentage of type I fibres and an increased percentage of type II fibres, particularly type IIb fibres.

The potential conversion of type II fibres to type I fibres with exercise training remains controversial, and if it does occur it would require a considerable period of consistent training (Ivy et al 1999). On the other hand, the conversion of type IIb to type IIa fibres may occur after only a few weeks training (Coggan et al 1993, Krotkiewski and Bjorntorp 1986, Saltin et al 1977). An increase in the percentage of type IIa fibres (at the expense of type IIb fibres) should increase muscle insulin sensitivity.

Capillary density

Individuals with type 2 diabetes have reduced skeletal muscle capillary density compared with subjects without diabetes (Lillioja et al 1987, Marin et al 1994). Exercise training increases skeletal muscle capillary density (Coggan et al 1993, Mandroukas et al 1984, Saltin et al 1977). Increased capillary density should enhance glucose and insulin delivery to the skeletal muscle fibres, and further improve insulin action and blood glucose clearance. For example, the improvement in oral glucose tolerance was significantly related to the increase in muscle capillary density in obese women following 3 months of exercise training (Mandroukas et al 1984).

Control of muscle blood flow

Insulin not only increases skeletal muscle glucose transport, but also increases muscle blood flow. As muscle glucose uptake depends on muscle blood flow, it is clear that increasing glucose delivery by increasing blood flow may independently enhance the effects of insulin on muscle glucose uptake. The insulin-dependent increase in blood flow may account for up to 50% of the increase in glucose uptake (Baron et al 1990, Edelman et al 1990).

Studies indicate that exercise-trained individuals have greater basal and insulin-stimulated muscle blood flow compared with untrained subjects (Dela et al 1992, Ebeling et al 1993, Hardin et al 1995). Hardin et al (1995) reported that leg blood flow was approximately 30% higher in endurance-trained athletes than in untrained subjects following maximal insulin stimulation (Hardin et al 1995). Enhanced insulin-stimulated muscle blood flow has also been demonstrated following exercise training in individuals with type 2 diabetes (Dela et al 1995). These results indicate that exercise training can enhance insulin-mediated blood flow in both normal and insulin-resistant muscle, and contributes to the improved muscle glucose uptake response to insulin.

It is clear that acute exercise as well as exercise training induce significant improvements in insulin sensitivity and blood glucose control in individuals with type 2 diabetes. The improvement in glycaemic control is attributable, at least partially, to reduced hepatic glucose production, increased skeletal muscle mass, reduced body fat and increased insulin sensitivity and glucose uptake within individual muscles.

Recommended exercise for individuals with type 2 diabetes

For older people with type 2 diabetes who do not have significant diabetic complications or other co-morbidities, physical activity programmes that follow the guidelines of the American College of Sports Medicine are recommended (ACSM 1998a, 1998b). These guidelines advocate appropriate endurance and resistance exercise for developing and maintaining cardiorespiratory fitness, body composition and muscular strength and endurance (ACSM 1998a, 1998b). In addition to these guidelines, there are a number of special considerations specific to individuals with type 2 diabetes, particularly as many people with diabetes have significant coexisting diseases or conditions. Exercise prescription guidelines for ageing people with type 2 diabetes are discussed below. The guidelines include instructions and considerations for both cardiorespiratory (aerobic) training and strength training.

Recommendations for cardiorespiratory exercise

Cardiorespiratory or aerobic exercise training has been shown to produce considerable benefits for individuals with diabetes. Training increases insulin sensitivity and lowers blood glucose levels. Many individuals with type 2 diabetes also exhibit coexisting cardiovascular risk factors, including obesity, hypertension, hypercholesterolaemia (high cholesterol) and dyslipidaemia. In addition to lowering blood glucose, aerobic exercise training targets these co-morbidities. Specifically, aerobic exercise training contributes to weight loss, lowers elevated blood pressure, lowers total cholesterol and improves plasma lipid profile (Albright et al 2000). Therefore individuals with type 2 diabetes benefit more widely from aerobic exercise training than simply improved blood glucose control.

Mode of exercise

Training involving large muscle groups in rhythmic sustained exercise is most recommended for individuals with type 2 diabetes. Walking/running, swimming and cycling are common forms of aerobic exercise that are generally appropriate. However, under some circumstances care should be taken when recommending these modes of exercise to those with type 2 diabetes. The presence of diabetic complications or coexisting disease such as peripheral neuropathy, diabetic retinopathy and osteoarthritis may require alternative modes of exercise to be utilized. For example, cycling requires considerable balance and visual acuity, whilst walking or running may be particularly inappropriate for individuals with peripheral neuropathy or osteoarthritis. Under these circumstances, exercise bikes, rowing machines and aquatic activities may provide viable and effective exercise alternatives. As always, personal interest and individual goals should be taken into account when considering the exercise mode to be utilized, as these are very important in maintaining interest and motivation towards ongoing participation in physical activity.

Frequency

All individuals with type 2 diabetes should endeavour to perform aerobic exercise at least 3 non-consecutive days per week, and ideally 5 or more days per week. Improvements in aerobic fitness increase with increased frequency of training (ACSM 1998b), but the added improvement that comes with training more than 5 days per week is minimal (ACSM 1998b). Frequent exercise should favourably affect cholesterol and lipid profile, lower blood pressure and aid weight (fat) loss. The acute effect of a single exercise session to increase insulin sensitivity and lower plasma glucose lasts for less than 72 hours (Schneider et al 1984), and therefore to obtain the optimal glucose lowering benefits of aerobic exercise, individuals with type 2 diabetes should always exercise within the last 72 hours of the previous exercise bout, and preferably within 48 hours.

Intensity

The American College of Sports Medicine recommends that the minimum training intensity required to improve aerobic fitness is approximately 40–50% of maximum oxygen uptake reserve (VO_2R) or heart rate reserve (HRR) (ACSM 1998b). These guidelines specifically recognize that any person with an initially low level of fitness, as is often the case in those with type 2 diabetes, may achieve fitness improvements with relatively low intensity aerobic exercise training. VO_2R is the difference between maximum oxygen consumption (VO_{2max}) and resting oxygen consumption. Heart rate reserve (HRR) is the difference between maximal heart rate and resting heart rate. For example, in an older person with a resting heart rate of 60 beats per minute, and a maximum heart rate of 160 beats per minute, 50% HRR is equal to 110 beats per minute (i.e. 50% of the difference between 60 and 160). Aerobic exercise programmes of such intensity have been shown to improve aerobic fitness (ACSM 1998b), and improve plasma glucose levels in type 2 diabetes (Albright et al 2000). Being able to commence exercise training in individuals with type 2 diabetes at such low-to-moderate intensity minimizes the risks of exercise, whilst ensuring health benefits are obtained. Furthermore, there is likely to be increased adherence to an exercise programme that is not overly uncomfortable at the outset. Once an exercise programme has been commenced, it is important to progress the exercise intensity as the individual's fitness improves. Individuals should progress towards exercising at 60–70% of VO_2R or HRR.

Whilst these guidelines have been demonstrated to induce improved fitness and other health benefits in individuals with and without diabetes, the practicalities of monitoring exercise intensity in those with type 2 diabetes may be more difficult. The use of heart rate monitoring is appropriate in most individuals, but the development of autonomic neuropathy in some with type 2 diabetes, and the associated effect on heart rate, may mean that heart rate is a poor indicator of exercise intensity in these people. Under these circumstances perceived exertion is a more appropriate means of monitoring exercise intensity. The ACSM suggests that a rating of perceived exertion (RPE) of approximately 11–12 on the original Borg scale (Borg 1982) equates to exercise of low-to-moderate intensity (ACSM 1998b).

Duration

Older people with type 2 diabetes commencing an exercise programme should initially aim to complete at least 10 minutes of continuous exercise. Exercise time should be progressively increased to at least 30 minutes, to optimize improvements in blood glucose control and weight loss, and to provide other health benefits. Exercise duration of up to 60 minutes is most appropriate for individuals with type 2 diabetes. Exercise duration longer than 60 minutes may mean exercise is performed at too low an intensity to significantly improve glucose levels. Longer duration exercise may also provide significant musculoskeletal stresses, and increase the chance of injury.

Progression

There is wide variation in the rate at which exercise programmes can be progressed. However, the following guidelines are useful. Initial changes in training should focus on increasing frequency and duration rather than intensity. As already stated, individuals should initially exercise at least 3 days per week. Progression to exercising 5 days per week can be achieved within the first few weeks of starting a programme. Similarly, an important aim is to progress exercise bouts from 10 minutes up to 30 minutes of continuous exercise. Most people with type 2 diabetes should be able to perform continuous aerobic exercise for 30 minutes within 2–4 weeks of commencing a training programme. Throughout the phase of concurrently increasing frequency and duration, those with type 2 diabetes should participate at a comfortable level, indicating they are exercising at a low-to-moderate exercise intensity. When frequency and duration reach desired levels, it may be appropriate to increase intensity. In older people with type 2 diabetes any increases in intensity should be small and monitored to avoid undue fatigue, injury or deterrence.

Recommendations for strength training

Strength training improves muscular strength and increases muscle mass in all people, including those who are ageing and with diabetes. In particular, the increase in muscle mass may be of benefit to people with type 2 diabetes, as there is greater muscle available for glucose disposal, and therefore clearance of blood glucose is enhanced. As reviewed in Chapter 7 of this book, strength training is viable, safe and effective in older people. Programmes that follow the guidelines outlined below have been shown to increase muscle strength and mass. Although some modification may be necessary for individuals with more severe diabetic disease, the majority of those with diabetes should be able to adhere to these guidelines with the promise of strength gains, and the likelihood of improved diabetic control.

Mode of exercise

In many older individuals, muscle strength can be very low prior to commencing strength training. Under these circumstances relatively light, and readily available free weights, and the use of body weight to provide resistance, may be an appropriate way to start strength training. However, as strength improves and the resistance required to overload muscles increases, machine weights are the safest and most beneficial equipment to use. Machine weights are usually designed to minimize stresses placed on the back, allow resistance to be applied throughout the range of motion, and do not require the participant to balance or control the weight (Feigenbaum and Pollock 1999). Machine weights also often avoid handgripping. Handgripping can unduly elevate blood pressure during resistance exercise. Any programme should include exercises that use large muscle groups, often in combined movement exercises such as leg press or bench press. A total of 8–10 exercises is generally recommended (Feigenbaum and Pollock 1999); 3–4 exercises for the upper body, 3–4 exercises for the legs and 2 exercises for the trunk (back and abdominal muscles) would be ideal.

Frequency

As with aerobic exercise training, strength training on 3 non-consecutive days is generally recommended. This allows at least 48 hours rest or recovery between any two consecutive strength training sessions. There is no clear evidence that strength training more frequently than 3 days per week produces any greater improvements in strength. On the other hand, individuals who train only twice per week will typically achieve 80–90% of the strength benefits of more frequent training (Feigenbaum and Pollock 1999). Therefore, the frequency of strength training should be at least two, but preferably three, times per week.

Intensity

Intensity is probably the most important factor determining strength gains in response to resistance training. To be effective, a strength training programme should include at least one set of each exercise to fatigue or near-fatigue. Frequently, the amount of weight used is based on the one repetition maximum (1 RM). The 1 RM is the amount of weight that can be lifted once, whilst maintaining good lifting form. Many studies in older individuals have prescribed exercise at an intensity of 70–80% 1 RM. This intensity of exercise should allow people to complete 8–12 repetitions to fatigue, and is consistent with the ACSM guidelines (ACSM 1998b). Resistance that allows 8–12 repetitions is described as 'moderate' strength training. Whilst moderate strength training of this type will be appropriate for most people, less intense programmes may be more appropriate for those with more severe diabetes or overt co-morbidities. In these cases, lighter resistance that allows 12–15 repetitions per set is advised.

Sets

There is conjecture as to the number of sets that need to be performed to maximize the benefits of strength training. Historically three sets of 8–12 repetitions constituted a typical weight training programme. However, it now appears that only one set of each exercise is required to achieve most of the strength gains (Feigenbaum and Pollock 1999). Having said that, there is some suggestion that strength gains and muscle mass gains are achieved through different strength training parameters. The total volume of training (i.e. sets × repetitions × resistance) appears to be important for increasing muscle mass (Feigenbaum and Pollock 1999), and increased muscle mass is particularly beneficial to those with type 2 diabetes. Clinicians are clearly faced with making a decision between using one or more sets, depending upon the individual needs of their clients. One set of each exercise achieves most of the strength gains of more sets and may minimize the chance of injury. Performing only one set of each exercise also increases the likelihood of programme adherence, as programmes lasting more than 1 hour are associated with higher drop-out rates (Feigenbaum and Pollock 1999). On the other hand, the increased training volume associated with more than one set of each exercise may be associated with greater increases in muscle mass, and ultimately be more beneficial for diabetic control. The decision between one or more sets needs to be made based on the motivation of the individual, the perceived risks and benefits to an individual, and any time constraints imposed upon the programme.

Progression

Given the importance of exercise intensity in determining the strength gains achieved from a resistance training programme, the amount of resistance used is the main component that is progressed. At the outset of a programme, strength gains are often abrupt and dramatic. Such strength gains are generally attributed to neural adaptations and not muscle hypertrophy. Therefore at the beginning of a programme it may be necessary to frequently increase the resistance being used. A practical way to increase resistance is to use a weight until it can be lifted 12 or more times in one set. Once this goal is achieved, increasing the weight will lead to a reduced number of repetitions before fatigue. The resistance should be increased by a relatively small amount that still allows the weight to be lifted 7–8 times. Over ensuing training sessions, the participant will be able to lift the weight more and more, until they can again lift the weight for at least 12 repetitions. At this point the resistance should again be increased.

Risks and complications of exercise

Hypoglycaemia

In individuals without diabetes, blood glucose levels remain relatively stable during exercise, especially for exercise up to 60 minutes duration. In those with diabetes, blood glucose levels generally decrease during exercise, but these reductions lower blood glucose concentrations from initially high levels to normal levels, and not to hypoglycaemic levels.

Hypoglycaemia during exercise is rare in people with type 2 diabetes. When present, it is usually in people being treated with oral sulfonylurea medications and/or insulin, and those participating in unusually strenuous or prolonged exercise (Albright et al 2000). To decrease the likelihood of hypoglycaemia in individuals using oral diabetic medications or insulin, exercise should generally not be performed within 1 hour following medication. When required, insulin should be injected into a non-exercising site (e.g. the abdomen), and the dose may need to be reduced. Blood glucose monitoring is advisable for those individuals using diabetic medication, particularly at the onset of an exercise programme, or when participating in unusually vigorous or prolonged exercise. There is generally no need to increase carbohydrate consumption before or during exercise to prevent hypoglycaemia in these individuals (Albright et al 2000). Just as for people without diabetes, fluid intake during exercise is important, but plain water is appropriate for exercise of up to 60 minutes. For exercise lasting longer than 1 hour, water and carbohydrate are preferable to help maintain hydration, and minimize the chances of hypoglycaemia. Carbohydrate solutions of 6–8%, as available in most commercial sports drinks, provide adequate glucose intake during exercise without causing gastrointestinal discomfort or compromising gastric water absorption. Despite taking these actions, hypoglycaemia remains a possible complication of exercise in type 2 diabetes. People using medication to control their diabetes should be educated on the recognition and appropriate treatment of hypoglycaemia.

Cardiovascular complications

Macrovascular disease is common in people, particularly older people, with type 2 diabetes. However, the presence of cardiovascular disease, such as coronary artery disease or hypertension, does not absolutely contraindicate exercise. Given the high incidence of co-morbidities and disease complications in people with type 2 diabetes, it is currently recommended that all individuals with diabetes have a thorough medical assessment prior to commencing an exercise programme. The examination should assess the presence and extent of any macrovascular and microvascular disease, glucose control, physical limitations, and medications.

An exercise stress test is recommended for all people with diabetes over 35 years of age to determine the extent of any coronary disease. In addition, the stress test will help identify appropriate training intensities and target heart rates. In those patients with stable angina, the target heart rate during exercise should be at least 10 beats below the ischaemic/angina threshold (Albright et al 2000). The stress test may also detect those individuals who have exercise-induced hypertension. If present, exercise-induced hypertension does not exclude participation in an exercise programme, but does necessitate the need to modify exercise selection.

Autonomic neuropathy impairs normal heart rate regulation: resting heart rate is elevated and maximum heart rate is reduced. Patients with autonomic neuropathy have relatively low fitness levels (Albright et al

2000) and are at increased risk of exercise-induced hypotension (Zola et al 1986). In addition, the early warning signs of myocardial ischaemia may be absent or diminished in those with autonomic neuropathy (Albright et al 2000). Therefore, exercise programmes for individuals with autonomic neuropathy should be of low-to-moderate intensity, and conducted with the approval of their physician.

Peripheral vascular disease (PVD) may be associated with intermittent claudication during exercise. Individuals who experience claudication should exercise to pain tolerance, and rest intermittently during exercise as required. Activities that avoid the weight-bearing of walking/running, and exclusive lower-limb exercise of cycling, may be of benefit in these people. Swimming and water aerobics are ideal exercise alternatives.

Peripheral neuropathy

Peripheral neuropathy is a recognized complication of diabetes. The reduction or loss of distal sensation, especially in the legs and feet, can predispose to injury and infection. As many people with peripheral neuropathy also have peripheral vascular disease, which may impair wound healing, the prevention of lower leg trauma is particularly important in this subgroup of people with diabetes. In general, non-weight-bearing exercises are encouraged in people with known peripheral neuropathy, and the use of well-fitting appropriate footwear for all activities of daily living is recommended. The feet should be inspected daily by the individual, frequently by health professionals, and any skin lesions attended to immediately.

Nephropathy and retinopathy

There is no known association between exercise and progression of nephropathy and retinopathy. However, there is some uncertainty whether the increases in blood pressure experienced during exercise exacerbate these conditions (Albright et al 2000). Therefore as a general recommendation, those with nephropathy and/or retinopathy should avoid exercises that unduly increase blood pressure. These precautions include avoiding high resistance strength exercise (especially upper limb exercise), avoiding intense aerobic exercise, and not performing the Valsalva manoeuvre during exercise (Albright et al 2000).

Factors affecting the adoption and maintenance of exercise

It is now recognized that regular physical activity can play an important role in the prevention and treatment of type 2 diabetes, and its associated co-morbidities. Despite this, exercise training remains an under-utilized therapy in the management of type 2 diabetes. It is clear that performance of regular exercise by those with type 2 diabetes needs to be optimized.

The factors influencing the likelihood of people with type 2 diabetes adopting and maintaining exercise programmes have been discussed in the American College of Sports Medicine position stand on 'Exercise and type 2 Diabetes' (Albright et al 2000). The ACSM describes factors that influence the contemplation, action and maintenance stages of an exercise programme. The factors influencing these three stages are discussed below.

The contemplation stage

It is considered that an individual's likelihood of adopting a particular behaviour is dependent upon their perceived benefits of that behaviour (Albright et al 2000). Therefore it is important that clinicians discuss the health benefits of regular physical exercise with those advised to increase exercise participation. These health benefits include the improvements in diabetic control, fitness, blood pressure, body fat and plasma lipids. The benefits also include the psychological benefits of reduced stress, anxiety and depression, and the social benefits of participation and interaction with family, friends and community-based organizations (Albright et al 2000). Equally, any concerns about the adverse effects of exercise need to be discussed, to enable the individual to recognize that the health benefits exceed any potential short-term discomforts or potential complications. Finally, the clinician should help plan a programme that meets the goals of the individual, whilst taking into account any limitations that may impede an optimal programme. These restrictions may include the availability of support or facilities, financial and time constraints, or other social issues.

The action stage

It is important to provide specific exercise guidelines in order to increase adherence to exercise training (Albright et al 2000). The general recommendation that a person with type 2 diabetes should 'do some exercise' provides no appropriate guidelines for the selection, duration or sustainability of exercise. The goals and physical activity interests of the individual, together with the advice of the clinician, should be considered when devising an appropriate exercise strategy. Further, the appropriateness of any programme in terms of access to facilities, equipment, supervision and sporting partners needs to be considered.

The maintenance stage

The American College of Sports Medicine Position Stand lists seven factors that can help people with type 2 diabetes adopt and maintain an exercise programme (Albright et al 2000). These include:

1. Using appropriate exercise and equipment to avoid injury.
2. Setting realistic exercise goals.
3. Setting an exercise schedule in advance and sticking to it.
4. Using an exercise partner.
5. Encouraging the use of self-rewards.
6. Identifying alternative exercise activities to reduce boredom.
7. Understanding the difference between failure and 'backsliding'.

Table 15.2 Exercise guidelines

Cardiorespiratory exercise		Resistance exercise	
Intensity	Moderate	Intensity	Moderate
VO$_2$R or HRR	40–60%	Sets	1 or more
RPE	12–13	Repetitions	8–12 RM
Duration	30–60 min	No. of exercises	8–10
Frequency	3–5 days/wk	Frequency	2–3 days/wk

VO$_2$R, oxygen uptake reserve; HRR, heart rate reserve; RPE, rating of perceived exertion using Borg 6–20 scale; RM, repetition maximum.

Summary of exercise guidelines

People with type 2 diabetes should endeavour to exercise on most or all days of the week. Exercise should consist of both cardiorespiratory exercise and resistance training. Table 15.2 summarizes the guidelines to exercise.

Conclusions

Exercise provides well-recognized acute and chronic benefits for individuals with type 2 diabetes. Acute exercise reduces blood glucose levels, and increases insulin sensitivity for a period of up to 72 hours. Exercise training improves blood glucose regulation, increases skeletal muscle mass, helps control and lose body fat, lowers blood pressure, and improves plasma lipid profile. Endurance-type exercise has generally been recommended for people with type 2 diabetes. It is now recognized that strength training also improves diabetic control. Therefore, it is currently recommended that people with type 2 diabetes perform a combination of endurance exercise and strength exercise. Older people with type 2 diabetes are generally able to follow the guidelines of the American College of Sports Medicine for 'exercise for developing and maintaining cardiorespiratory and muscular fitness in healthy adults'. Some people with diabetes, particularly older individuals, or those with severe diabetic disease or other co-morbidities, may need to modify their exercise choices to make their exercise programme viable and safe.

References

ACSM 1998a American College of Sports Medicine Position Stand. Exercise and physical activity for older adults. Medicine and Science in Sports and Exercise 30(6):992–1008

ACSM 1998b American College of Sports Medicine Position Stand. The recommended quantity and quality of exercise for developing and maintaining cardiorespiratory and muscular fitness, and flexibility in healthy adults. Medicine and Science in Sports and Exercise 30(6):975–991

Alberti K G, Zimmet P Z 1998 Definition, diagnosis and classification of diabetes mellitus and its complications. Part 1: diagnosis and classification of diabetes mellitus – provisional report of a WHO consultation. Diabetic Medicine 15(7):539–553

Albright A, Franz M, Hornsby G, et al 2000 American College of Sports Medicine position stand. Exercise and type 2 diabetes. Medicine and Science in Sports and Exercise 32(7):1345–1360

Amos A F, McCarty D J, Zimmet P 1997 The rising global burden of diabetes and its complications: estimates and projections to the year 2010. Diabetic Medicine 14 (Suppl 5):S1–85

Andersson A, Sjodin A, Olsson R, Vessby B 1998 Effects of physical exercise on phospholipid fatty acid composition in skeletal muscle. American Journal of Physiology 274(3 Pt 1):E432–438

Baron A D, Brechtel G, Wallace P, Edelman S V 1988 Rates and tissue sites of non-insulin- and insulin-mediated glucose uptake in humans. American Journal of Physiology 255(6 Pt 1):E769–774

Baron A D, Laakso M, Brechtel G, et al 1990 Reduced postprandial skeletal muscle blood flow contributes to glucose intolerance in human obesity. Journal of Clinical Endocrinology and Metabolism 70(6):1525–1533

Blotner H 1945 Effect of prolonged physical inactivity on tolerance of sugar. Archives of Internal Medicine 75:39–44

Boden G, Jadali F, White J, et al 1991 Effects of fat on insulin-stimulated carbohydrate metabolism in normal men. Journal of Clinical Investigation 88(3):960–966

Boden G, Chen X, DeSantis R A, Kendrick Z 1993 Effects of age and body fat on insulin resistance in healthy men. Diabetes Care 16(5):728–733

Bonen A, Clune P A, Tan M H 1986 Chronic exercise increases insulin binding in muscles but not liver. American Journal of Physiology 251(2 Pt 1): E196–203

Borg G A 1982 Psychophysical bases of perceived exertion. Medicine and Science in Sports and Exercise 14(5):377–381

Borkman M, Storlien L H, Pan D A, et al 1993 The relation between insulin sensitivity and the fatty-acid composition of skeletal-muscle phospholipids. New England Journal of Medicine 328(4):238–244

Campbell P J, Mandarino L J, Gerich J E 1988 Quantification of the relative impairment in actions of insulin on hepatic glucose production and peripheral glucose uptake in non-insulin-dependent diabetes mellitus. Metabolism 37(1):15–21

Caro J F, Sinha M K, Raju S M, et al 1987 Insulin receptor kinase in human skeletal muscle from obese subjects with and without noninsulin dependent diabetes. Journal of Clinical Investigation 79(5):1330–1337

Cartee G D, Young D A, Sleeper M D, et al 1989 Prolonged increase in insulin-stimulated glucose transport in muscle after exercise. American Journal of Physiology 256(4 Pt 1):E494–499

Coggan A R, Spina R J, Kohrt W M, Holloszy J O 1993 Effect of prolonged exercise on muscle citrate concentration before and after endurance training in men. American Journal of Physiology 264(2 Pt 1):E215–220

Cononie C C, Goldberg A P, Rogus E, Hagberg J M 1994 Seven consecutive days of exercise lowers plasma insulin responses to an oral glucose challenge in sedentary elderly. Journal of the American Geriatrics Society 42(4):394–398

Craig B W, Hammons G T, Garthwaite S M, Jarett L, Holloszy J O 1981 Adaptation of fat cells to exercise: response of glucose uptake and oxidation to insulin. Journal of Applied Physiology 51(6):1500–1506

Davidson P C, Shane S R, Albrink J M 1966 Decreased glucose tolerance following a physical conditioning program. Circulation 33:3–11

DeFronzo R A, Jacot E, Jequier E, et al 1981 The effect of insulin on the disposal of intravenous glucose. Results from indirect calorimetry and hepatic and femoral venous catheterization. Diabetes 30(12):1000–1007

Deitrick J E, Whedon G D, Shorr E 1948 Effects of immobilization upon various metabolic and physiologic functions of normal men. American Journal of Medicine 4:3–36

Dela F, Mikines K J, von Linstow M, Secher N H, Galbo H 1992 Effect of training on insulin-mediated glucose uptake in human muscle. American Journal of Physiology 263(6 Pt 1):E1134–1143

Dela F, Handberg A, Mikines K J, Vinten J, Galbo H 1993 GLUT 4 and insulin receptor binding and kinase activity in trained human muscle. Journal of Physiology (London) 469:615–624

Dela F, Ploug T, Handberg A, et al 1994 Physical training increases muscle GLUT4 protein and mRNA in patients with NIDDM. Diabetes 43(7):862–865

Dela F, Larsen J J, Mikines K J, et al 1995 Insulin-stimulated muscle glucose clearance in patients with NIDDM. Effects of one-legged physical training. Diabetes 44(9):1010–1020

Despres J P, Tremblay A, Nadeau A, Bouchard C 1988 Physical training and changes in regional adipose tissue distribution. Acta Medica Scandinavica Supplement 723:205–212

Dohm G L, Sinha M K, Caro J F 1987 Insulin receptor binding and protein kinase activity in muscles of trained rats. American Journal of Physiology 252(2 Pt 1): E170–175

Dolkas C B, Greenleaf J E 1977 Insulin and glucose responses during bed rest with isotonic and isometric exercise. Journal of Applied Physiology 43(6):1033–1038

Ebeling P, Bourey R, Koranyi L, et al 1993 Mechanism of enhanced insulin sensitivity in athletes. Increased blood flow, muscle glucose transport protein (GLUT-4) concentration, and glycogen synthase activity. Journal of Clinical Investigation 92(4):1623–1631

Edelman S V, Laakso M, Wallace P, et al 1990 Kinetics of insulin-mediated and non-insulin-mediated glucose uptake in humans. Diabetes 39(8):955–964

Eriksson K F, Lindgarde F 1991 Prevention of type 2 (non-insulin-dependent) diabetes mellitus by diet and physical exercise. The 6-year Malmo feasibility study. Diabetologia 34(12):891–898

Feigenbaum M S, Pollock M L 1999 Prescription of resistance training for health and disease. Medicine and Science in Sports and Exercise 31(1):38–45

Fink R I, Kolterman O G, Griffin J, Olefsky J M 1983 Mechanisms of insulin resistance in aging. Journal of Clinical Investigation 71(6):1523–1535

Fluckey J D, Hickey M S, Brambrink J K, et al 1994 Effects of resistance exercise on glucose tolerance in normal and glucose-intolerant subjects. Journal of Applied Physiology 77(3):1087–1092

Garetto L P, Richter E A, Goodman M N, Ruderman N B 1984 Enhanced muscle glucose metabolism after exercise in the rat: the two phases. American Journal of Physiology 246(6 Pt 1):E471–475

Golay A, Swislocki A L, Chen Y D, Reaven G M 1987 Relationships between plasma-free fatty acid concentration, endogenous glucose production, and fasting hyperglycemia in normal and non-insulin-dependent diabetic individuals. Metabolism 36(7):692–696

Hardin D S, Azzarelli B, Edwards J, et al 1995 Mechanisms of enhanced insulin sensitivity in endurance-trained athletes: effects on blood flow and differential expression of GLUT 4 in skeletal muscles. Journal of Clinical Endocrinology and Metabolism 80(8):2437–2446

Hartley L H, Mason J W, Hogan R P, et al 1972 Multiple hormonal responses to prolonged exercise in relation to physical training. Journal of Applied Physiology 33(5):607–610

Heath G W, Hagberg J M, Ehsani A A, Holloszy J O 1981 A physiological comparison of young and older endurance athletes. Journal of Applied Physiology 51(3):634–640

Heath G W, Gavin J, Hinderliter J M 1983 Effects of exercise and lack of exercise on glucose tolerance and insulin sensitivity. Journal of Applied Physiology 55(2):512–517

Helmrich S P, Ragland D R, Leung R W, Paffenbarger R S Jr 1991 Physical activity and reduced occurrence of non-insulin-dependent diabetes mellitus. New England Journal of Medicine 325(3):147–152

Henriksen E J, Bourey R E, Rodnick K J, et al 1990 Glucose transporter protein content and glucose transport capacity in rat skeletal muscles. American Journal of Physiology 259(4 Pt 1):E593–598

Holloszy J O 1975 Adaptation of skeletal muscle to endurance exercise. Medicine and Science in Sports 7(3):155–164

Holloszy J O, Narahara H T 1965 Studies of tissue permeability. X. Changes in permeability to 3-methylglucose associated with contraction of isolated frog muscle. Journal of Biological Chemistry 240(9):3493–3500

Holloszy J O, Schultz J, Kusnierkiewicz J, Hagberg J M, Ehsani A A 1986 Effects of exercise on glucose tolerance and insulin resistance. Brief review and some preliminary results. Acta Medica Scandinavica Supplement 711:55–65

Holm G, Krotkiewski M 1988 Potential importance of the muscles for the development of insulin resistance in obesity. Acta Medica Scandinavica Supplement 723:95–101

Houmard J A, Shinebarger M H, Dolan P L, et al 1993 Exercise training increases GLUT-4 protein concentration in previously sedentary middle-aged men. American Journal of Physiology 264(6 Pt 1):E896–901

Houmard J A, Shaw C D, Hickey M S, Tanner C J 1999 Effect of short-term exercise training on insulin-stimulated PI 3-kinase activity in human skeletal muscle. American Journal of Physiology 277(6 Pt 1):E1055–1060

Hughes V A, Fiatarone M A, Fielding R A, et al 1993 Exercise increases muscle GLUT-4 levels and insulin action in subjects with impaired glucose tolerance. American Journal of Physiology 264(6 Pt 1):E855–862

Ivy J L 1997 Role of exercise training in the prevention and treatment of insulin resistance and non-insulin-dependent diabetes mellitus. Sports Medicine 24(5):321–336

Ivy J L, Holloszy J O 1981 Persistent increase in glucose uptake by rat skeletal muscle following exercise. American Journal of Physiology 241(5):C200–203

Ivy J L, Zderic T W, Fogt D L 1999 Prevention and treatment of non-insulin-dependent diabetes mellitus. Exercise and Sport Science Review 27:1–35

James D E, Kraegen E W, Chisholm D J 1985 Effects of exercise training on in vivo insulin action in individual tissues of the rat. Journal of Clinical Investigation 76(2):657–666

Katsuki A, Sumida Y, Murashima S, et al 1998 Serum levels of tumor necrosis factor-alpha are increased in obese patients with non-insulin-dependent diabetes mellitus. Journal of Clinical Endocrinology and Metabolism 83(3):859–862

Katz L D, Glickman M G, Rapoport S, Ferrannini E, DeFronzo R A 1983 Splanchnic and peripheral disposal of oral glucose in man. Diabetes 32(7):675–679

Kelley D E, Mokan M, Mandarino L J 1992 Intracellular defects in glucose metabolism in obese patients with NIDDM. Diabetes 41(6): 698–706

Kelley D E, Mintun M A, Watkins S C, et al 1996 The effect of non-insulin-dependent diabetes mellitus and obesity on glucose transport and phosphorylation in skeletal muscle. Journal of Clinical Investigation 97(12):2705–2713

Kern M, Wells J A, Stephens J M, et al 1990 Insulin responsiveness in skeletal muscle is determined by glucose transporter (Glut4) protein level. Biochemical Journal 270(2):397–400

King D S, Dalsky G P, Clutter W E, et al 1988 Effects of exercise and lack of exercise on insulin sensitivity and responsiveness. Journal of Applied Physiology 64(5):1942–1946

Kohrt W M, Kirwan J P, Staten M A, et al 1993 Insulin resistance in aging is related to abdominal obesity. Diabetes 42(2):273–281

Kriska A M, LaPorte R E, Pettitt D J, et al 1993 The association of physical activity with obesity, fat distribution and glucose intolerance in Pima Indians. Diabetologia 36(9):863–869

Krotkiewski M, Bjorntorp P 1986 Muscle tissue in obesity with different distribution of adipose tissue. Effects of physical training. International Journal of Obesity 10(4):331–341

Krotkiewski M, Bylund-Fallenius A C, Holm J, et al 1983 Relationship between muscle morphology and metabolism in obese women: the effects of long-term physical training. European Journal of Clinical Investigation 13(1):5–12

LeBlanc J, Nadeau A, Richard D, Tremblay A 1981 Studies on the sparing effect of exercise on insulin requirements in human subjects. Metabolism 30(11):1119–1124

Lillioja S, Mott D M, Zawadzki J K, et al 1986 Glucose storage is a major determinant of in vivo 'insulin resistance' in subjects with normal glucose tolerance. Journal of Clinical Endocrinology and Metabolism 62(5):922–927

Lillioja S, Young A A, Culter C L, et al 1987 Skeletal muscle capillary density and fiber type are possible determinants of in vivo insulin resistance in man. Journal of Clinical Investigation 80(2):415–424

Lipman R L, Schnure J J, Bradley E M, Lecocq F R 1970 Impairment of peripheral glucose utilization in normal subjects by prolonged bed rest. Journal of Laboratory and Clinical Medicine 76(2):221–230

Lipman R L, Raskin P, Love T, et al 1972 Glucose intolerance during decreased physical activity in man. Diabetes 21(2):101–107

Lohmann D, Liebold F, Heilmann W, Senger H, Pohl A 1978 Diminished insulin response in highly trained athletes. Metabolism 27(5):521–524

Lutwak L, Whedon G D 1959 The effect of physical conditioning on glucose tolerance. Clinical Research 7:143–144

Lynch J, Helmrich SP, Lakka T A, et al 1996 Moderately intense physical activities and high levels of cardiorespiratory fitness reduce the risk of non-insulin-dependent diabetes mellitus in middle-aged men. Archives of Internal Medicine 156(12):1307–1314

Lynch N A, Metter E J, Lindle R S, et al 1999 Muscle quality. I. Age-associated differences between arm and leg muscle groups. Journal of Applied Physiology 86(1):188–194

Mandroukas K, Krotkiewski M, Hedberg M, et al 1984 Physical training in obese women. Effects of muscle morphology, biochemistry and function. European Journal of Applied Physiology 52(4):355–361

Manson J E, Rimm E B, Stampfer M J, et al 1991 Physical activity and incidence of non-insulin-dependent diabetes mellitus in women. Lancet 338:774–778

Manson J E, Nathan D M, Krolewski A S, et al 1992 A prospective study of exercise and incidence of diabetes among US male physicians. JAMA 268(1):63–67

Marin P, Andersson B, Krotkiewski M, Bjorntorp P 1994 Muscle fiber composition and capillary density in women and men with NIDDM. Diabetes Care 17(5):382–386

Mikines K J, Sonne B, Tronier B, Galbo H 1989 Effects of training and detraining on dose–response relationship between glucose and insulin secretion. American Journal of Physiology 256(5 Pt 1):E588–596

Miles P D, Romeo O M, Higo K, et al 1997 TNF-alpha-induced insulin resistance in vivo and its prevention by troglitazone. Diabetes 46(11):1678–1683

Miller J P, Pratley R E, Goldberg A P, et al 1994 Strength training increases insulin action in healthy 50- to 65-yr-old men. Journal of Applied Physiology 77(3):1122–1127

Miller W J, Sherman W M, Ivy J L 1984 Effect of strength training on glucose tolerance and post-glucose insulin response. Medicine and Science in Sports and Exercise 16(6):539–543

Misbin R I, Moffa A M, Kappy M S 1983 Insulin binding to monocytes in obese patients treated with carbohydrate restriction and changes in physical activity. Journal of Clinical Endocrinology and Metabolism 56(2):273–278

Myllynen P, Koivisto V A, Nikkila E A 1987 Glucose intolerance and insulin resistance accompany immobilization. Acta Medica Scandinavica 222(1):75–81

O'Dea K 1984 Marked improvement in carbohydrate and lipid metabolism in diabetic Australian aborigines after temporary reversion to traditional lifestyle. Diabetes 33(6):596–603

Pan D A, Lillioja S, Milner M R, et al 1995 Skeletal muscle membrane lipid composition is related to adiposity and insulin action. Journal of Clinical Investigation 96(6):2802–2808

Panzram G 1987 Mortality and survival in type 2 (non-insulin-dependent) diabetes mellitus [published erratum appears in Diabetologia 1987, 30(5):364]. Diabetologia 30(3):123–131

Phillips S M, Han X X, Green H J, Bonen A 1996 Increments in skeletal muscle GLUT-1 and GLUT-4 after endurance training in humans. American Journal of Physiology 270(3 Pt 1):E456–462

Pratley R E, Hagberg J M, Rogus E M, Goldberg A P 1995 Enhanced insulin sensitivity and lower waist-to-hip ratio in master athletes. American Journal of Physiology 268(3 Pt 1):E484–490

Reitman J S, Vasquez B, Klimes I, Nagulesparan M 1984 Improvement of glucose homeostasis after exercise training in non-insulin-dependent diabetes. Diabetes Care 7(5):434–441

Richter E A, Garetto L P, Goodman M N, Ruderman N B 1982 Muscle glucose metabolism following exercise in the rat: increased sensitivity to insulin. Journal of Clinical Investigation 69(4):785–793

Rodnick K J, Haskell W L, Swislocki A L, Foley J E, Reaven G M 1987 Improved insulin action in muscle, liver, and adipose tissue in physically trained human subjects. American Journal of Physiology 253(5 Pt 1):E489–495

Ruderman N B, Ganda O P, Johansen K 1979 The effect of physical training on glucose tolerance and plasma lipids in maturity-onset diabetes. Diabetes 28 (Suppl 1):89–92

Saltin B, Henriksson J, Nygaard E, Andersen P, Jansson E 1977 Fiber types and metabolic potentials of skeletal muscles in sedentary man and endurance runners. Annals of the New York Academy of Sciences 301:3–29

Saltin B, Lindgarde F, Houston M, et al 1979 Physical training and glucose tolerance in middle-aged men with chemical diabetes. Diabetes 28 (Suppl 1):30–32

Schalin-Jantti C, Harkonen M, Groop L C 1992 Impaired activation of glycogen synthase in people at increased risk for developing NIDDM. Diabetes 41(5):598–604

Schneider S H, Amorosa L F, Khachadurian A K, Ruderman N B 1984 Studies on the mechanism of improved glucose control during regular exercise in type 2 (non-insulin-dependent) diabetes. Diabetologia 26(5):355–360

Seals D R, Hagberg J M, Allen W K, et al 1984 Glucose tolerance in young and older athletes and sedentary men. Journal of Applied Physiology 56(6):1521–1525

Segal K R, Edano A, Abalos A, et al 1991 Effect of exercise training on insulin sensitivity and glucose metabolism in lean, obese, and diabetic men. Journal of Applied Physiology 71(6):2402–2411

Shimokata H, Muller D C, Fleg J L, et al 1991 Age as independent determinant of glucose tolerance. Diabetes 40(1):44–51

Storlien L H, Jenkins A B, Chisholm D J, et al 1991 Influence of dietary fat composition on development of insulin resistance in rats. Relationship to muscle triglyceride and omega-3 fatty acids in muscle phospholipid. Diabetes 40(2):280–289

Stuart C A, Shangraw R E, Prince M J, Peters E J, Wolfe R R 1988 Bed-rest-induced insulin resistance occurs primarily in muscle. Metabolism 37(8):802–806

Vaag A, Alford F, Henriksen F L, Christopher M, Beck-Nielsen H 1995 Multiple defects of both hepatic and peripheral intracellular glucose processing contribute to the hyperglycaemia of NIDDM. Diabetologia 38(3):326–336

Van Pelt R E, Jones P P, Davy K P, et al 1997 Regular exercise and the age-related decline in resting metabolic rate in women. Journal of Clinical Endocrinology and Metabolism 82(10):3208–3212

Vessby B, Tengblad S, Lithell H 1994 Insulin sensitivity is related to the fatty acid composition of serum lipids and skeletal muscle phospholipids in 70-year-old men. Diabetologia 37(10):1044–1050

Wallberg-Henriksson H, Holloszy J O 1984 Contractile activity increases glucose uptake by muscle in severely diabetic rats. Journal of Applied Physiology 57(4):1045–1049

Wei M, Gibbons L W, Mitchell T L, et al 1999 The association between cardio-respiratory fitness and impaired fasting glucose and type 2 diabetes mellitus in men. Annals of Internal Medicine 130(2):89–96

WHO 1994 Prevention of diabetes mellitus. Report of WHO study group. Technical report series 844. WHO, Geneva

Williamson J R, Browning E T, Scholz R 1969 Control mechanisms of gluconeo-genesis and ketogenesis. I. Effects of oleate on gluconeogenesis in perfused rat liver. Journal of Biological Chemistry 244(17):4607–4616

Yamanouchi K, Nakajima H, Shinozaki T, et al 1992 Effects of daily physical activity on insulin action in the elderly Journal of Applied Physiology 73(6):2241–2245

Zola B, Kahn J K, Juni J E, Vinik A I 1986 Abnormal cardiac function in diabetic patients with autonomic neuropathy in the absence of ischemic heart disease. Journal of Clinical Endocrinology and Metabolism 63(1):208–214

Appendix: WHO classifications for overweight and obesity

WHO classification of overweight and obesity	
Description	**BMI* range**
Normal	18.5–24.9
Overweight	25.0–29.9
Obesity class I (moderate)	30.0–34.9
Obesity class II (severe)	35.0–39.9
Obesity class III (very severe)	⩾40.0

*Body Mass Index (BMI) is calculated as weight in kilograms divided by the square height in metres.
Reproduced with kind permission of World Health Organization 2000.

Reference

World Health Organization 2000 WHO Obesity Classification. Obesity: preventing and managing the global epidemic. Report of a WHO Consultation. WHO Technical Report Series 894, Geneva

Index

Please note that all entries in the index refer to older people and physical activity unless otherwise stated. Page numbers in *italics* refer to tables and figures.

OA: osteoarthritis; TFOA: tibiofemoral osteoarthritis; NSAIDs: non-steroidal anti-inflammatory drugs; PA: physical activity.

A

AA (Active Australia) 15
Achilles tendon injury, precautions for exercise 293
ACL transection *see* anterior cruciate ligament (ACL) transection
Active Australia (AA) 15
  women, levels of PA 31
activities of daily living (ADL) 13, 19
  footwear 319
  grip strength and 162
  moderate strength benefits 91
  post-surgery improvements 89, 90
Activity Counseling Trial (ACT) Research Group 55
ACT Research Group 55
adherence, to exercise
  barriers 52, xi
    see also barriers, to PA
  clinical and community 51–53
  coping mechanisms for 52
  fall prevention programmes 259–260
  incentives for 133
  long-term study, women 33, 34
  maintenance phase techniques 53
  OA therapy outcome 221

  optimization xi
  type of activity impact 52
  workforce 67
adipocytes, diabetes type 2 aetiology 305–306, 310
aerobic capacity, strength training 137
aerobic training
  bone density studies 105–106
  cardiorespiratory fitness 6
  diabetes type 2 *see* diabetes mellitus (type 2)
  effect on depression 14–15
  functional outcome improvement 14
  impaired glucose tolerance 308
  injury rate, strength training *vs* 134
  osteoarthritis 218
    resistance exercise *vs* 220
  post-fracture 205
AIMS (Arthritis Impact Measurement Scale) 217
air pollution, PA precautions 298, *298*
Ajzen and Fishbein's model 42–43
akinesia 279
alcohol, effect on bones 116
Alzheimer's disease
  dual task interference 275
  movement 278, 280
  women 30

American College for Sports Medicine
  aerobic capacity required, cardiorespiratory fitness 137
  bone mass augmentation, principles of training 103
  cardiovascular conditions guidelines 290
  healthy adults, guidelines for 175, 189, *189*
  intensity of training guidelines 314–315
  strength training guidelines 175
American College of Rheumatology, guidelines for management of OA 214
American Gerontological Society, motto 13
angina pectoris
  exercise precautions/ limitations 289, 292
  medication-related precautions 296
anterior cruciate ligament (ACL) transection 83–84
  afferent nerve role in animal models 87
  quadriceps inhibition 86
anti-anginals, precautions 296
antifungal treatments 234
antioxidant vitamins, osteoporosis prevention 116

anxiety 29
   dual task interference 271
aquatic exercises *see* hydrotherapy
arthritis
   prevention 11–12
   see also osteoarthritis (OA);
      tibiofemoral osteoarthritis
      (TFOA)
Arthritis Impact Measurement
   Scale (AIMS) 217
avoidance gait 87
azoles 234

B

back pain
   PA precautions/
      contraindications 294
   prevention 11
      secondary programmes 11
   work-related 65, 68
balance
   complex function 258
   maintenance 272–274
   secondary task interference on
      see dual task interference
   training *see* fall prevention
barriers, to PA 42
   access/structural 42, 52
   demographic variables
      41
   health professionals
      overcoming *see* health
      professionals
   individual factors 51
   initiation factors 51–52
      classification 51
   maintenance factors 52
      see also adherence, to exercise
   negative messages/advice 52
   older women 32–33
   older workers 68
   perceived costs 40–41, *41*
   perceived risks 33, 42, 68
   self-control/self-efficacy beliefs
      44–45
   social factors 51–52
      appropriateness 43
basal ganglia disease, dual task
      interference 278–279
behaviour
   changes *see* behaviour change
      (below)

planned, theory *see* theory of
   planned behaviour
   policies to influence ix–x
behavioural contracting 45
behavioural intention 17–18, *18,* 43
   barriers to *see* barriers, to PA
   preceding action (theory) 42–43
behavioural interventions 54–56,
   257
behavioural shaping 44
behaviour change
   based on theory of planned
      behaviour 43
   effective interventions 34
   GPs' role 53
   health professionals instigating
      see health professionals
   interventions for older adults
      53–54
      see also programmes/
      interventions
   management method 44
   models 40–49
      assumptions *48*
      strategies required *48*
      summary *48*
      see also specific models
   in self-management 49, 50, 51
   transtheoretical model *see*
      stages of change model
   in workplace 69
beta-blockers, precautions 296
blood pressure, reductive effect of
   PA 6
body awareness exercises 81
body mass index (BMI)
   in osteoarthritis 217
   overweight/obesity
      classification *328*
bone(s)
   adaptive response
      mechanical strain 79, 102
      optimal characteristics 102–103
   alcohol effect 116
   caffeine effect 116
   formation 79
      people with greatest potential
      80
      resistance training effect 81
   integrity 79
   loss *see* osteoporosis
   modelling and remodelling
      during growth and ageing
      100–101, *101*

   influence of load 79
   rate of loss 78
   resorption 79
   soft drinks effect 116
   see also musculoskeletal system
bone mineral density (BMD)/
   bone mass
   age-related reduction 12, 28, 79
   augmentation in osteoporosis
      see osteoporosis
   children and adolescents 12,
      104–105
   clinically important increases
      103
   factors affecting 100
   fall prevention programmes
      and 255
   femoral neck and fracture risk
      103
   impact activities effect 104
   inactivity and 12
   levels and exercise prescription
      111
   low
      association factors 100
      osteoporotic fracture risk 100
      see also osteoporosis
   maintenance targeting
      programme 255
   measurement 80
   negative effect, factors 107
   peak mass
      calcium intake and variance
      112
      growth effect 101, *101*
   postmenopausal women
      28, 79
      exercise effect 80, *81*
   strength and variance 174
   strength training effect *see*
      strength training
Borg Rating of Perceived Exertion
   Scales 291, 295, 315
breast cancer 11
   moderate physical activity
      effect 28

C

caffeine, effect on bones 116
calcium
   absorption 113
      vitamin D role 113, 114

exercise enhancement 110
osteoporosis prevention
112–113
supplements 113, 255
callus *see* hyperkeratosis
cancer
breast *see* breast cancer
colon 10
prevention 10–11
carbohydrate solutions,
hypoglycaemia 318
carbonated soft drinks 116
cardiorespiratory fitness 6
aerobic training 6
outcome in Activity Counseling
Trial 55–56
physical activity level
relationship *8*
cardiorespiratory system,
physiological effect of PA 6
cardiorespiratory training *see*
aerobic training
cardiovascular disease/conditions
activity increments 9
angina and breathlessness,
limitation on intensity
292
benefits of PA 7–9
mechanisms 9
incidence 289
ischaemic heart disease
289–290, *290*
multiple chronic 291–292
neurological disorders 291
PA outcome among older adults
7–9, *8*
perceived exertion 291
peripheral vascular disease *see*
peripheral vascular disease
(PVD)
precautions and
contraindications (for PA)
289–292, *290*
diabetes type 2 318–319
medication 296
monitoring activity
290–291
prevention 7–9
protocol for high risk signs 290,
290
cardiovascular fitness
programmes, falls
prevention 252–253
Cardiovascular Health Study 8

case-control studies 3, *4*
centre of pressure (COP) *see* dual
task interference
CHAMPS project 34
individual tailoring 55
Charcot arthropathy 87
CHD *see* coronary heart disease
cholecalciferol 114
chondroitin 223
chronic disease
cardiovascular 291–292
inactivity as risk factor 27
incidence (WHO) ix
prevention, health benefits of
PA 9–11
claudication 319
cognitive function 14
impairment *see* Alzheimer's
disease
cohort studies 2, *4*
colon cancer 10
Community Healthy Activity
Model Program for Seniors
see CHAMPS project
compliance, with exercise *see*
adherence, to exercise
computerization, repetitive office
work 65
concentric contraction 171, 176
condylar lift, knee joint 83,
85–86
confidence levels 14
consciousness-raising, stages of
change model 45, 46
cool-down periods 295
coordination of movement 92
coping mechanisms, adherence to
PA 52
corns *see* hyperkeratosis
coronary heart disease (CHD)
benefit potential of PA 9, 19
diabetes type 2 304–305
OA risk 217
risk factors 7
sedentary lifestyle risk 7–8
see also cardiovascular disease/
conditions
corporate fitness programmes
67–68
cortisone, plantar heel pain
237
costs
falls 247–248
healthcare ix

hip fractures 248
osteoarthritis (OA) 213–214
perceived, barriers to PA
40–41, *41*
workplace injuries 65, 66
counter-conditioning
maintenance phase 53
stages of change model 45,
46
cue to action 42
cytokines, sarcopenia 166

D

dairy foods 113
dementia
Lewy body, dual task
interference 275
see also Alzheimer's disease
demographic factors ix
health belief model factors
and 41
depression
aerobic training 14–15
gender differences 29
OA association 214
PA effect on 14–15, 19
resistance training 15, 107
strength training 139, *140*
DEXA scan sites 80
diabetes mellitus (type 2)
abdominal fat risk factor
309–310
activity improvement with
Internet intervention 56
adipocytes, aetiological role
305–306, 310
adoption and maintenance of
exercise 319–320
aerobic training
recommendations 313–315,
321
body fat control 310
duration 315
frequency 314
intensity 314–315
mode of exercise 313–314
progression 315
studies on benefit 309
aetiology 305–306, 310
aging effect 307–308
bedrest studies 307
complications 304–305

diabetes mellitus (type 2) (*contd*)
coronary heart disease 304–305
diagnosis 304, *304*
epidemiology 306–307
exercise guidelines *321*
fluid intake 318
free fatty acids, aetiological role 305, 306, 310
genetic predisposition 305
handgripping 316
health belief model application *41*, 41–42
heels
dry skin on 235
podiatric intervention 240
shock attenuation 237
hypoglycaemia 317–318
incidence 303
Internet-based intervention 56
maximum risk reduction 10
mechanism of improved glucose tolerance with PA 309–313
body fat control 309–310
capillary density 312
glucose transportation efficiency 311
hepatic glucose output control 309
insulin signalling 311
muscle blood flow control 312–313
muscle fibre type 312
muscle mass control 6, 310
skeletal muscle and biochemical changes 310–312
nephropathy 319
PA precautions/ contraindications 317–319
cardiovascular complications 318–319
see also cardiovascular disease/conditions
peripheral vascular disease *see* peripheral vascular disease (PVD)
personal coach 56
physical inactivity causing possible mechanisms 305–306
studies supporting 307–308

prevention 10, 306–307
recommended exercise for 313–317
retinopathy 319
risk factors for cardiovascular conditions 313
strength training recommendations 315–317
frequency 316
intensity 316
machine weights 316
mode of exercise 316
progression 317
sets 317
training cessation studies 307
women 28
Diabetes Network Internet-based Physical Activity Intervention programme 56
Diabetes Prevention Program (DPP) 10
dietary factors
carbohydrate solutions for hypoglycaemia 318
loss of appetite 165
low protein diets 165
malnutrition 117
nutrients 117–118
nutritional supplementation drinks 118
resistance training 170
osteoporosis prevention *see* osteoporosis, dietary prevention
recommendations 20
reduction in food 117
vitamin D deficiency status 114
reasons 113
disablement process, musculoskeletal system 158–159, *159*
diseases(s)
chronic *see* chronic disease
incidence ix
perceived seriousness/ susceptibility, behaviour change *see* health belief model
prevention programmes, primary, secondary and tertiary 11
dogs, walking and 32–33

drugs, PA precautions 296
dual task interference 267–287
akinesia 279
attention aspects 268–269
aging effect on 269, 272
capacity limitation 268
demand increase with sensory cues 270
gait requirement 275
tests 282
backward digit recall 270, 279
balance impairment 275–278
balance maintenance 272–274
centre of pressure
balance-impaired elders *vs* healthy elders 276, 277
measurement 270, *273*
sway-referenced surface *273*, 274
clinical assessment 281–282
clinical interventions for 282–284
balance re-education 282
guidelines 283
rehabilitation 282
cognitive task 270
definition 267
dual task methodology 268
frontal lobe function 275
healthy older people 272–275
balance maintenance 272–274
centre of pressure 276, 277
human locomotion 275
reactive balance 274
healthy younger adults, task complexity 269–270
incidence 267, 284
individual factors influencing 271–272
physiological arousal 271
prioritization 272, 274, 284
locomotion 269, 271, 275
gait tasks 275
ground clearance 279
stride control 280
virtual obstacle task 275
movement disorders 278–280
akinesia 279
primary task complexity 279
multiple tasks test 281, 283
optokinetic stimulation 274
physiological arousal 271

postural stability
  old people *vs* young adults
    272
  spatial and non-spatial tasks
    on 270
postural task 270
  articulation during 271
rate-limiting factors 268
rhythmic movements 269
sensory cues 268, 270
  alteration for assessment 274
  gait hypokinesia 280
spatial memory task 270
speech 269
structural limitation 268,
    269, 270
task factors influencing 269–271
  reaction time 270, 271
  rehabilitation 283–284
  stimulus introduction timing
    270, 274
  type of secondary task 270,
    279, 281
tests/assessment 281–282
theories on 268, 269
timed up and go (TUG) test 281
timing of secondary task 271
  studies on impact 274
walking while talking test
    275–276, 282
dual task methodology 268
dual task timed up and go test
    (DTTUG) 281
dynamic standing balance,
    strength training
    149–151, *150*
dystonia 271

E

eccentric contraction 176
elastic tubing/bands
  resistance training 177
  strength training 132
elderly, groupings 1
electronic databases, study
    searches 126
emotional well-being, women 29
empowerment of patients 50
endurance, strength training
    137–138

endurance training, insulin
    sensitivity 308, 309, 311
energy balance, obesity control 7
environmental factors,
    precautions 297, 297–298,
    298
environmental re-evaluation,
    stages of change model 45
epidemiology (methods)
  approaches to analysis 3
  case-control studies 3, *4*
  cohort studies 2, *4*
  definition 1
  descriptive 15–19
    methods 15–16
  evidence
    appraisal principles 2
    criteria 3
    quality 2, *4*
    source 2–3
  experimental designs 2
  health benefits (evidence-based)
    1–25
    biomedical outcomes 5
    classification system 5
    conceptual model 4–5, *5*
    methods to ascertain 1–4
    social outcome domain 5
  measurements of exposure 3
  measures of association 3, *3*
  observational studies 2
  participation in PA by elderly
    15–19, *16*
  randomized controlled trials
    2, *4*
  research design(s) 2–3
    examples *4*
  selection bias 3
  study factors 2
    definition 2
    identification/selection *see*
      strength training, studies
  surveillance difficulties 19
  surveys
    elderly-specific 18
    of PA levels 15–16
    relevance of population
      monitoring 18–19
  women *see* women
error strain distribution theory,
    mechanical strain on
    musculoskeletal system 79
executive functioning 14

exercise(s)
  biomechanical considerations
    76–98
  definition 2
  effect on peak bone strength
    103–105
  guidelines for rehabilitation
    after fractures *see* fractures
  high acetabular pressures,
    cartilage damage 218
  hormone replacement therapy
    effect 109–110
  osteoporosis risk reduction *see*
    osteoporosis
  precautions and
    contraindications
    cardiovascular conditions *see*
      cardiovascular disease/
      conditions
    cold and heat 297, *297*
    diabetes type 2 *see* diabetes
      mellitus (type 2)
    environmental factors
      297–298
    hydrotherapy 298–299, *299*
    medication 296
    musculoskeletal conditions
      292–295
    pollution 298, *298*
  programmes *see* programmes/
    interventions
  progression regimes, osteogenic
    effect 81–82
  role across lifespan, improved
    bone health 112
  types 2
  workplace programmes 67–68
  see also physical activity (PA);
    specific types

F

fall(s)
  bunions risk 231
  community dwelling elderly
    174
  costs 247–248
  epidemiology 247–248
  exercise programme types 12
  fears over 51
  incidence 187

fall(s) (*contd*)
  prevention *see* fall prevention
  reduced BMD effect 28
  risk factors 100, 174
    dual task interference *see* dual
      task interference
    extrinsic and intrinsic *249,*
      249–250
    reduced BMD 28
  risk reduction 6, 28
faller(s)
  foot problems associated 231
  hospital stay 248
  instigating PA, theory of
    planned behaviour
    application 43, *43*
  lower extremity muscle
    strength, *vs* non-fallers 174
  mental health 28, 248
  prospective prediction studies
    275–276, 282
fall prevention 12–13
  balance training 12, 34–35
    activities for 174, 258
    evidence for 251–252
    musculoskeletal factors
      250–251
    programme incorporation
      256, 258
  BMD maintenance programmes
    255
  cardiovascular fitness
    programmes 252–253
  combination programmes
    253–255
  criteria for developing
    programmes 256–257
  decision factors on types 257
  important considerations
    256–257
  evidence for 251–255
  exercise regimes 81
  general movement coordination
    92
  group/supervised programmes
    254–255
  home programmes 253–254
  important/successful
    components 255–256
  lifestyle modification 259
  lower limb exercises 176
  minimum PA dosage required
    256

  muscle activation 91–92
  options 251
  participation factors 259–260
  settings (environment) for
    programmes 251, 260–261
  strength training 90–91
    balance effect 149–151, *150*
    combined programmes
      253, 254
    evidence for 252
    key muscles to target 259
    potential gain 174–175
    programme incorporation
      258–259
    steadiness 173
  sustainability factors 260
  tai chi 34–35
    evidence for 254–255
    types 254
  walking activity 34–35, 253
Falls Efficacy Scales 248
fears, about PA
  in OA 89
  in women 33
fears, of falling 51
FFAs, diabetes type 2 aetiology
  305, 306, 310
FHSQ 240
fibres of muscle *see* muscle(s),
  fibres
FICSIT projects, balance and fall
  reduction 34–35
flatfoot deformity 238
flexibility, strength training 138
foot
  ageing effect 231–233
  disorders *see* foot problems
  emollient preparations 235
  epidermis 231–232
  flexibility 232
  hygiene 233, 234
  ligamentous changes 232
  medial arch 232, 238
  muscles 232–233
  orthoses 235, 237
  pads 235
  role in weight-bearing 229
  surgery, considerations 235
Foot Function Index 240
Foot Health Status Questionnaire
  (FHSQ) 240
foot problems 229–246
  blood supply reduced 232

  common types 230
    management 233–234
  corns and calluses *see*
    hyperkeratosis
  diabetes type 2 235, 319
  digital neuritis 238
  dry skin 235
  exercise for 239–240
  falls risk 231
  fissuring 231–232, 235
  flatfoot deformity 238
  forefoot 238
  fractures 238
  functional types 237–238
  gender differences 230
  heel
    dry skin on 235
    plantar pain 230, 237, 240
    shock attenuation 237, 240
  midfoot 238
  mobility effect 231, 240
  nail disorders *see* nail(s)
  pain 231
  podiatric treatment *see* podiatric
    treatment
  prevalence 230
  prevention 239–240
  quality of life 240
  reporting of 229–230
    discrepancies 230
  skin disorders 234–235
  structural types 236–237
  toes 238
  treatment on quality of life 240
  walking difficulties 231
  see also specific examples
footwear
  appropriate
    overuse injury prevention
      295
    peripheral neuropathy 319
  fashion/ill-fitting
    changing behaviour difficulty
      235, 239
    corns and calluses 234–235
    nail problems 233
    prevalence 235, 239
    structural foot problems 236
    women 230
fractures
  ankle 190
  bed exercises 201
  cast immobilization 199

cause 194–195
client safety 191
common sites 294
co-morbidities 205
disability 188
distal radius 188, 189
  extension range 192
exercise prescription guidelines
    189–192, *190*
  adaptive soft tissue changes
    196–199
  decision algorithm for
    192–194, *193*
  exercise aim 191–192, 205
  pain/inhibition 191, 195–196
exercise types
  aerobic training 205
  isometric exercise 204
  low-intensity resistance
    training 190
  pendular exercises 196, *196*
  weight-bearing exercises 190
exercising muscles after
    199–205
  decision algorithm 199–200,
    200
  impairment or activity
    limitation identification
    200–201, *201*
  muscle activation skill
    201–202
  muscle strengthening *see*
    strength training
  specificity of training 200–201
falls risk 250
  see also fall(s)
fixation 190
fixed exercise equipment 191
foot bone 238
gender differences 28, 77, 101
health consequences in older
    people 187–188
hip *see* hip fractures
incidence 187
irritability of joints 195–196
low bone mineral density and
    100, 103
mortality 188
movement loss 192–195
  causes 194–195
oscillatory exercises 195
passive joint mobilization
    principle 195

physiotherapy 189
preventing future problems 205
quadriceps control exercises
    201–202, *202*
rehabilitation 188–189
restrictions on exercise
    190–191
stage of healing 189–191, *190*
strength training 202–205
  double quarter-squat 203, *203*
  endurance improvement
    204–205
  isometric exercises 204
  key principles 202–203
  loads 204
stretching exercises 196–199
  hold–relax focus 199
stride standing 202
subsequent fractures 188
susceptibility 187
un-unified, appropriate training
    protocol 201–202
vertebral
  co-morbidity 100
  subsequent fracture risk
    100, 188
weight-bearing exercises 190
Frailty and Injuries – Cooperative
    Studies Intervention
    Techniques, balance and
    falls reduction 34–35
Framingham study, OA risk 222
  criticisms 215
free fatty acids (FFAs), diabetes
    type 2 aetiology 305,
    306, 310
functional status
  moderate intensity effect 35
  physical activity relationship
    13–14
  see also activities of daily living
    (ADL)

G

gait
  avoidance patterns 87
  coordination of movement 92
  hip extension strength 91
  hypokinesia 280
  pattern retraining 88

requirements, attention aspects
    275
symmetry and muscle
    imbalance 90
see also walking activity
GALM (Groningen Active Living
    Model) 55
gastrointestinal problems, OA
    association 214
gender differences
  activity patterns 16, *16*
  depression 29
  foot problems 230
  fractures 28, 77, 101
  life expectancy 26
  osteoarthritis 214
  osteopenia 188
  osteoporosis 188
  see also women
general medical practitioners (GPs)
  as gatekeepers 53
  key position to help older
    adults 53
  requirements for health
    promotion 39
  see also health professionals
glucosamine 223
glucose tolerance, impaired (IGT)
  correction 308
  diagnosis 304, *304*, 305
  exercise training benefit 308
  improvement with PA *see under*
    diabetes mellitus (type 2)
  prevention 306–307
glucose tolerance test, oral
    (OGTT) 309, 310
GLUT4
  exercise training on 311
  fibre type difference 312
golf, contraindications 293, 294
Good Life Club 50
GPs, *see* general medical
    practitioners (GPs); health
    professionals
grip strength
  accelerated decline with age
    160
  larger-than-normal, OA
    susceptibility 85
  loss due to fracture 188
  muscle mass correlation 161
  as muscle strength measure 14
  performance measures 162

Groningen Active Living Model
(GALM) 55
growth hormone (GH), decline
165–166
gymnasiums, workforce
membership 67

H

haemostatic factors, physiological
effect of PA 6
hamstrings
inhibition 86
osteoarthritis 86
hand grip strength *see* grip
strength
head arms and trunk (HAT) 91
health behaviour, changes *see*
behaviour change
health belief model 40–42
application model *41*, 41–42
assumptions 40–41, *48*
criticism of 42
intervention guidelines 57
health benefits of PA 1–25
cardiovascular 7–9
chronic disease prevention 9–11
epidemiology *see* epidemiology
(methods)
falls prevention 12–13
mental health 14–15
musculoskeletal disorder
prevention 11–13
psychosocial *see* mental
health/psychosocial factors
quality of life 13–14
stroke prevention 9–10
in workforce 64
*see also individual diseases and
benefits*
healthcare costs ix
see also costs
healthcare policies, to influence
behaviour ix–x
health insurance, premiums 66
health locus of control/self-
efficacy 44–45
application 44–45
assumptions 44, *48*
intervention guidelines 58
health perception 17

health policy makers, Australian
initiatives 50
health professionals
adherence in clients *see*
adherence, to exercise
barriers acknowledgement 52
see also barriers, to PA
behavioural change instigation
39, 40, 52
guidelines for interventions
57–58
increasing motivation for 49
models 40–49
patient empowerment 50
self-management model *see*
self-management
stage of change
determination 46–47, 257
strategies required *48*
challenging negative attitudes
43
client self-management 39–40
communication methods 39
designing programmes for
older adults 56–57
see also programmes/
interventions; *specific
examples*
information provision 39
gatekeeper role 53
health belief model 42
individualizing 53–54
promotion of PA 38–62
clinical and community
setting 51–53
see also promotional strategies
role 38, 51
opportunity for modifying
risk factors 53
training 39
see also general medical
practitioners (GPs)
health promotion programmes ix
health professionals' role *see*
health professionals
workplace 64–65, 66, 67, 71
see also workplace
see also promotional strategies
(of PA)
heel problems *see* foot problems
helping relationships
maintenance phase 53
stages of change model 45

hexokinase, increased activity
with exercise 311
hip
arthroplasty 89, 89–90
extension strength 91
hip fractures
antidepressant medication 107
complications 100
exercise prescription *see*
fractures
falls and incidence 174
see also fall(s)
healthcare costs 248
inactivity as risk factor 12–13
incidence 77, 99–100
institutionalization 188
mortality 188
optimal model for prevention
77
prevention 12–13
calcium and vitamin D 114
see also fall prevention
risk factors 100
falls 250
therapeutic programmes 77
walking activity effect 29
women at risk 28, 29
see also fractures; osteoporosis
hold–relax technique 199
home-based programmes 52
hormone replacement therapy
(HRT) 109–110
adverse consequences
165–166
Huntington's disease, dual task
interference 278, 279
hydrotherapy
OA 82, 88, 222
precautions and
contraindications 298,
298–299, 299
hyperkeratosis (calluses and
corns)
callus and corn differentiation
234
causes 234–235
medicated pads avoidance 235
onychophosis accompaniment
233
surgical intervention
consideration 235
temporary relief 235
types 234

hypoglycaemia, diabetes (type 2)
317–318
hypokinesia 271
gait 280

I

impact exercise
bone density studies 107
jumping 102, 104
resistance training
incorporation 108
impaired glucose tolerance (IGT)
see glucose tolerance,
impaired (IGT)
inactivity see sedentariness/
sedentary lifestyle
inflammation, sarcopenia 166
information technology
electronic databases 126
programmes/interventions 56
repetitive office work, injury
association 65
insulin
resistance
definition 304
muscle mass affecting 6
obesity 309–310
see also diabetes mellitus
(type 2)
sensitivity
endurance training 308, 309,
311
healthy individuals 308
muscle fibres 312
signalling, diabetes
improvement 311
insulin-like growth factor one
(IGF-1)
decline in level 165
strength training effect 145
interdigital neuritis 238
intermittent claudication 319
internet, physical activity
interventions 56
ischaemic heart disease,
PA precautions/
contraindications 289–290,
290
isokinetic muscle-strength
training, OA 218

isometric exercise
fractures 204
light-resistance 190

J

Jebsen Test of Hand Function 193
jogging, loading cycles 79
joint
degeneration 293–294
loading
knee 84
model benefit/damage 78
osteoarthritis 84–86
see also musculoskeletal
system, loading
see also specific joints
jumping see impact exercise

K

knee joint
condylar lift 83, 85–86
increased varus moments
84–85
injury 88
proprioception 87, 88
muscle stabilizers see
quadriceps
OA see osteoarthritis (OA);
tibiofemoral osteoarthritis

L

Lamisil 234
leg atherosclerosis, reduction by
PA 10
Lewy body dementia, dual task
interference 275
life expectancy 26, 76
lifestyle
modification, fall prevention 259
sedentary see sedentariness/
sedentary lifestyle
lipid levels, physiological effect of
PA 6, 9
loading see musculoskeletal
system

Lorig's chronic disease self-
management model 50
lower limb strength see strength
training

M

machine weights, diabetes type 2
316
magnesium, osteoporosis
prevention 116
maintenance, of PA see adherence,
to exercise
maximal voluntary contraction
(MVC) 204
mechanical strain see
musculoskeletal system
mechanostat theory, mechanical
strain on musculoskeletal
system 79
medication, PA precautions
296
meniscectomy 84
menopause/postmenopause
bone loss 12, 79, 101
per year 101
see also osteoporosis
bone mineral density see bone
mineral density (BMD)/
bone mass
bone modelling 80
calcium/vitamin D
supplementation 113, 255
strength training 80
weighted vest resistance
exercise 177
mental health/psychosocial
factors
anxiety 29
depression see depression
dual task interference 271
effect of PA 14–15, 19
mechanism 29
falls effect 28, 248
fungal nail effect 234
strength training effect 139,
140
women 29, 30
MES theory see minimum
effective strain (MES)
theory

meta-analysis
  definition 2
  example 4
metatarsalgia 238
metatarsal osteotomy, corns and
      calluses, careful
      consideration for 235
Mini Mental State Examination
      (MMSE) 282
minimum effective strain (MES)
      theory
  mechanical strain on
      musculoskeletal system
      79, 102
  sensitivity and oestrogen levels
      109
MMSE 282
mobility
  foot problems effect 231
  limited, strength-training for
      177–178
  physiological effect of PA 6
  reduced independence 11
  see also walking activity
moods, PA effect on 14–15
Morton's neuroma 238
motivation, for physical activity xi
  increasing, by practitioners 49
  older women 32
  workforce/workplace 66, 69
motor neuron disease,
      cardiopulmonary function
      compromised 291
movement
  coordination 92
  loss, fractures 192–195
  see also mobility; walking
      activity
movement disorders
  akinesia 279
  dual task interference see dual
      task interference
  PA precaution/
      contraindication 291
  see also Parkinson's disease
multiple sclerosis, dual task
      interference 275
muscle(s)
  age-related changes
    dual task interference 272
    endurance 161–162
    factors responsible for
      163–166

mass 159–160, 160, 308
  power 161
  strength 6, 160–161
  ultrastructure findings 160
blood flow, glucose tolerance
      312–313
capillary density, oral glucose
      tolerance 312
co-activation, fall prevention
      91–92
diet
  insufficiency effect 165
  supplementation and training
      170
endurance
  age-related changes 161–162
  increasing in post-fracture
      204–205
exercise, functional restoration
      effect/role 166–174
  guidelines see resistance
      training, guidelines
  prescription 175–179
  see also specific types of exercise
fibres
  age-related changes 159–160,
      160
  insulin sensitivity 312
  potential conversion 312
  rapid force production loss
      161
  reduced PA, effect 164
  strength training 141–142, 142
  type I 159
  type II 159–160
function 160–162
functional decline 158–186
  see also muscle(s), mass;
      muscle(s), strength
glucose transportation 311
glucose transporter protein see
      GLUT4
hormonal decline effect
      165–166
inflammation effect 166
insulin-resistance
  biochemical defects 310–311
  diabetes type 2 aetiology 306
mass
  age-related changes 159–160,
      160, 308
  decrease affecting insulin
      resistance 6

glucose tolerance with
      increase 310
  stages in disablement process
      158–159, 159
  strength training effect see
      strength training
motor unit loss and
      remodelling 163–164
neuropathic change 163–164
performance, preservation with
      higher PA 164–165
power
  age-related changes 161
  functional performance factor
      162
  high-velocity movements 176
  resistance training 172
reduced PA effect 164–165
sarcomere changes post-
      fracture 198
strength
  age-related changes 6,
      160–161
  fall protection 90–91
  grip see grip strength
  increasing see strength
      training
  physical performance
      benefits 172–173
  physiological effect of PA 6–7
  proxy measures 14
  resistance training effect see
      resistance training
weakness
  cast immobilization 199
  diminished daily task
      performance 162–163, 163
  exercise in prevention see
      resistance training;
      strength training
  fall risk 174
  OA 86–87, 219
  post-fracture 199
  Z band disruption 160
  see also musculoskeletal system
musculoskeletal conditions
  back pain see back pain
  fractures see fractures
  joint degeneration 293–294
  PA precautions/
      contraindications 292–295
  tendon injury 293
  see also osteoarthritis (OA)

musculoskeletal system
  activity benefit/damage
      balance 77, *78*
  disablement process 158–159,
      159
  effective mechanical loading,
      characteristics 102–103
  injury 76, 77
      common types 293–294
      prevention during exercise
          295
  injury management 294–295
      acute 294
      overuse 295
      RICE 294
      subacute 295
  joint and tissue loading
      model *78*
  loading
      bone modelling and
          remodelling 79
      cartilage changes 84
      effective, characteristics
          102–103
      excessive 77
      optimal adaptive bone
          response 102–103
      osteogenic effect 79
      sports injury 86
  mechanical strain 78–80
      exercise effect 80
      minimum effective 79
      rate frequency and gradient
          79–80
  mobility *see* mobility
  repetitive strain 79
  risks of exercise 292–293
  strength training effect *see*
      strength training
  see also bone(s); muscle(s)
MVC (maximal voluntary
      contraction) 204
myofibrillar disruption 160

N

nail(s)
  cutting 233
  disorders and treatment
      233–234
  fungal infection 234
  ingrown 233–234
  thickening 233
nephropathy, PA precautions/
      contraindications 319
neurological disorders
  cardiopulmonary function
      compromised 291
  dual task interference
      balance impairment 272–278
      movement disorders 278–280
  PA precautions/
      contraindications 291
neurological factors
  dual task processing 268–269
      see also dual task interference
  locomotion 269
  speech 269
neuromuscular factors
  ageing effect 91
  facilitation techniques 199
  osteoarthritis 86–87
      knee injury and
          proprioception 87, 88
  resistance training effect
      170–171
  strength training effect 91,
      92, 173
non-insulin-dependent diabetes *see*
      diabetes mellitus (type 2)
non-steroid anti-inflammatory
      drugs (NSAIDs), OA 219,
      221
Nurses' Health Study 28
nutrition *see* dietary factors

O

OA *see* osteoarthritis
obesity
  insulin resistance 309–310
      see also diabetes mellitus
          (type 2)
  prevention, physiological effect
      of PA 7
  tibiofemoral osteoarthritis
      and 84
  WHO classification *328*
  women, TFOA *see* tibiofemoral
      osteoarthritis
observational studies,
      epidemiological methods 2
occupational therapists,
      requirements for health
      promotion 39
odds ratios (OR) 3
oestrogen
  reduced levels effect 79, 109
  replacement 109–110, 166
  see also menopause/
      postmenopause
onychauxis 233
onychocryptosis 233–234
onychogryphosis 233
onychomycosis 234
onychophosis, hyperkeratosis
      accompaniment 233
optokinetic stimulation, dual task
      interference 274
oral glucose tolerance test (OGTT)
      309, 310
osteoarthritis (OA) 82–86, 213–228
  activity avoidance 89
  adherence, effect on outcome
      221
  aerobic training 218
      resistance exercise *vs* 220
  aetiology 82, 214–216
  alternative modes of exercise
      314
  anterior cruciate ligament
      transection *see* anterior
      cruciate ligament (ACL)
      transection
  aquatic exercises 82
  arthroplasty, fitness after 218
  articular cartilage 83, 214
  avoidance gait 87
  balance training 88
  biomechanical considerations
      82–86
  clinical recommendations
      (for exercise) 222–223
  co-morbidities 214
  condylar lift 83, 85–86
  coronary heart disease 217
  costs 213–214
  definition 82
  epidemiology 214
  gait retraining 88
  gastrointestinal problems 214
  genetic predisposition 215
  hamstrings 86
  heavy PA, risk 12, 82, 215–216
      programme cautions 218

osteoarthritis (OA) *(contd)*
  hydrotherapy 88, 222
  impact 214
  incidence 82, 213–214
  joint changes 83, 215
  joint loading and 84–86
  knee joint 83–84
    see also tibiofemoral
      osteoarthritis (TFOA)
  locomotion force linked
    susceptibility 85
  mean body mass index 217
  medication influence and effect
    on pain 221
  muscle weakness 86–87
  neuromuscular factors 86–87
  NSAIDs with exercise 219, 221
  nutriceutical recommendations
    223
  occupational therapy 222
  PA effects 11, 217–220
  PA precautions/
    contraindications 293–294
  patient education and self
    management 222
  pharmacological intervention
    recommendations 222–223
  physiotherapy 222
  pre- and post-surgery recovery
    89, 89–90
  prevention and rehabilitation
    implications 87–88
  proprioception 87, 88
  protection from falls 90–91
  quadriceps 86–87
    target training 88
  radiographic changes 216–217
  resistance training 87–88
    aerobic *vs* 220
  risk with vigorous activity 12
  strength training
    isokinetic 218
    pain and disability reduction
      219–220
  study of risk, criticisms 215
  symptoms *216*, 216–217
  therapeutic exercise for
    management 217–221
    clinical recommendations 222
    combination programmes 220
    physiological effects 217–218
    roles for 218–220
    setting 217
  traumatic impacts 86
  weight bearing 88
  weight loss recommendations
    222
  weight support devices 219
  see also tibiofemoral
    osteoarthritis (TFOA)
osteoblasts 100
osteocalcin, strength training
  effect 145
osteoclasts 100
osteopenia 80
  back pain reduction 108
  definition 188
  exercise regimes, effects 81
  gender differences 188
  incidence 188
  individualized exercise
    prescription 108–109
  prescribing exercise 80–81
    recommendations 110
osteophytes 83, 215
osteoporosis
  absolute risk in populations 78
  biomechanical considerations
    77–82
  bone mass augmentation
    children and adolescents
      104–105
    exercise regimes and effects
      81–82
    recommendations 103,
      107–108
    resistance training for *see*
      resistance training
    studies on effect, different
      exercises 105–108
  definition 77, 188
  dietary prevention 112–118
    antioxidant vitamins 116
    calcium *see* calcium
    magnesium and sodium 116
    phosphorus 115–116
    protein 116–117
    recommendations 118
    vitamin D *see* vitamin D
    vitamin K 115
    zinc 116
  epidemiology 99, 188
  exercise in prevention 101–112
    stage of life factor 101–102
  foot fractures 238
  fracture of hip *see* hip fractures
  frail individuals 109
  gender prevalence differences
    188, 248
  hormone replacement, exercise
    enhancement 109–110
  incidence 99, 188
  individualized exercise
    prescription 108–109
  pathogenesis and early life
    origin 101
  postmenopausal 28
  prescription for exercise
    recommendations
      110–111
    algorithm guide *111*
    risk level and recommendations
      111
  vertebral fracture association
    100
osteoporotic fractures *see* hip
  fractures
overuse injury
  management 295
  prevention, appropriate
    footwear 295

P

paced auditory serial addition test
  (PASAT) 282
PACE programme 54
pain
  back *see* back pain
  exercise prescription guideline
    for fractures 191, 195–196
  foot, walking speed 231
  osteoarthritis and strength
    training 219–220
  plantar 230, 237, 240
  tibiofemoral osteoarthritis
    (TFOA) 86
  work-related 65
parathyroid hormone, strength
  training effect 145
Parkinson's disease
  cardiopulmonary function
    compromised 291
  dual task interference
    akinesia 279
    balance impairment 275,
      277–278

movement disorders 278, 279–280
physiotherapy 291
patient empowerment 50
PEDro scale 127
pendular exercises, fractures 196, *196*
peripheral neuropathy, PA precautions/ contraindications 319
peripheral vascular disease (PVD), PA precautions/ contraindications 291
claudication 319
mode of exercise 313–314
personal coaches 56
phosphorus, osteoporosis prevention 115–116
physical activity (PA) 218
activity patterns *16*, 16–17
adherence *see* adherence, to exercise
aerobic training *see* aerobic training
barriers *see* barriers, to PA
benefit/damage balance 77, *78*
see also health benefits of PA
definition *2*, 214
domains *2*, 19
increasing needs ix–xi
knowledge of current recommendations 17, *18*
participation 15–19, *16*
results 16–18
surveys 15–16
see also epidemiology (methods)
physiological effect 5–7, 19
programmes *see* programmes/ interventions
trends in prevalence rates 17, *18*
types *2*, x
vigorous programmes *see* vigorous programmes
women *see* women
work issues *see* workplace
see also exercise; *specific types*
Physical Activity Readiness Questionnaire 289
Physical Activity Scale for the Elderly (PASE) 18

physical inactivity *see* sedentariness/sedentary lifestyle
Physician-based Assessment and Counseling for Exercise (PACE) programme 54
physiotherapists, requirements for health promotion 39
physiotherapy
fractures 189
osteoarthritis 222
Parkinson's disease 291
phytochemicals 116
plantar pain 230, 237, 240
podiatric treatment
corns and calluses 235, 239
nail disorders treatment 233
podiatrist, requirements for health promotion 39
pollution of air, PA precautions 298, *298*
population studies *see* epidemiology (methods)
postmenopause *see* menopause/ postmenopause
postural control, dual task interference effects *see* dual task interference
Prochaska and Di Clemente, model *see* stages of change model
progesterone, replacement 109–110
programmes/interventions
adherence *see* adherence, to exercise
behavioural change incorporation 54–56, 257
clear purpose for 69
effectiveness for women 33–35
enjoyment factors 55, 69
evaluation building 57
future provision 56
home-based 34, 52, 177–179, 253–254
individualized advice 53–54
Internet provision 56
intervention guidelines 57–58
methodological problems 33
older adults 53–56
designing for 56–57
screening and evaluation prior to *see* screening
specificity principle 175

targeting and tailoring 54–55
telephone strategies 34, 52
vigorous *see* vigorous programmes
workplace 68–71
worker involvement 69
see also workplace
see also specific examples
progressive resistance training 175
promotional strategies (of PA)
addressing perceived risks 33
see also barriers, to PA
health professionals *see* health professionals
women 27
at work *see* workplace, health promotion programmes
see also health promotion programmes
proprioception 87
improvement activities 88
knee injury 87, 88
proprioceptive neuromuscular facilitation (PNF) technique 199
protein
low in diet, muscle mass loss 165
osteoporosis prevention 116–117
proximal femur fracture *see* hip fractures
psychological factors *see* mental health/psychosocial factors

Q

quadriceps
'avoidance gait' patterns 87
inhibition 87
anterior cruciate ligament transection 86
muscle mass reduction 160
OA role *see* osteoarthritis
people with long-term training, ultrasound imaging results 164
post-fracture control 201–202, *202*
strength and steadiness 173
target exercises 176

quality of life (QOL) 5, 13–14
  dose–response relationship 13
  foot problems 240
  fungal nail infection 234
  measures *see* SF-36 QOL
  muscle function, compromise
    with decline 162, *163*

R

randomized controlled trials
  (RCTs) 2, *4*
rehabilitation, after fractures *see*
  fractures
reinforcement management
  maintenance phase 53
  stages of change model 45, 46
relative risks (RR) 3
repetitions, strength training 317
repetitive office work, injury
  association 65
repetitive strain, musculoskeletal
  79
research designs *see* epidemiology
  (methods)
resistance training
  bone density studies 106–107
  bone modelling stimulus 80
  definition 2
  depression, effect on 15, 107
  detraining and retraining *171,*
    171–172
  duration 177
  elastic bands for 177
  exercises for osteogenic effect
    81, 82
  exercise targeting 176
  frequency 177, *178*
  functional mobility
    improvements 170, 178, *178*
  guidelines for prescription
    176–179
    diabetes type 2 *321*
  high-intensity 82, 176
  high velocity *vs* conventional
    172
  home-based 177–179
    equipment to provide
      resistance 174, 177, 179
  impact exercise incorporation
    108
  intensity 176–177

high-intensity 82, 176
low-intensity 81, 176
  fractures 190
mobility limited individuals
  177–178
muscle power 172
muscle strength and
  hypertrophy 167–172, *168*
  frail and healthy participants
    169, 169–170
  lower-intensity training 176
neuromuscular effects 170–171
osteoarthritis 87–88
  aerobic walking *vs* 220
  free unweighted exercise *vs*
    219
osteoporosis prevention
  107–108
physical performance benefits
  172–173
prescription 175
  goal for 175
progressive 175
purpose/benefits 6
sarcopenia, countermeasures
  159
sequence 176
stair climbing 177–178
steadiness 173
types 2
walking 173
weighted vests 177
see also strength training
rest, ice, compression and
  elevation (RICE), acute
  injury management 294
resting metabolic rate (RMR) 7
retinopathy, PA precautions/
  contraindications 319
reward strategies 58
rheumatoid arthritis, muscle
  strengthening 11
RICE, musculoskeletal injury
  management 294
rotator cuff tears 293
rowing 82

S

sarcopenia 158
screening 134, 175–176
  stress testing 175, 318

sedentariness/sedentary lifestyle
  BMD association 12
  bone formation potential 80
    children and adolescents 104
  chronic disease risk 27
  compensatory effect after
    vigorous exercise 7
  coronary heart disease risk 7–8
  deaths per year 38
  diabetes type 2 aetiology
    305–306
    see also diabetes mellitus
      (type 2)
  group identification 15
  health benefits and intensity of
    PA 288
  hip fractures risk 12–13
  initiators for women 32–33
  initiators of *see* barriers, to PA
  muscle alterations 164
  negative effects x–xi
  as obstacle to health x
  pre-participation assessment
    289
  rate increase with age 17, *17*, x
  reasons for x
  sedentary leisure activities x
  work economics 64–65
self-care *see* functional status
self-efficacy
  measures 17–18, *18*
  model *see* health locus of
    control/self-efficacy
self-esteem 14
self-liberation, stages of change
  model 45–46
self-management
  behaviour change incorporation
    49, 50, 51
  coaches, and learning 50
  concept 39–40, 49, 58
  definitions 49
  interventions
    educational 49–50
    integration 58
  model 49–51
  programmes 49
self-re-evaluation, stages of
  change model 45, 46
SF-36 QOL 13
  foot health status 240
  women PA participants
    29–30, *30*
  see also quality of life

shoes *see* footwear
sit-to-stand maneuver, strength training 147–148, *148*
social barriers 51–52
social liberation, stages of change model 45, 46
social support
  for activity in women 35
  lack of *see* barriers, to PA
  providing and receiving, motivating PA 32, 69, 257
  workplace 70
sodium, osteoporosis prevention 116
soft drinks 116
somatosensation 87
soy products 116
spatial memory task 270
spinach 115
spinal cord injured persons, dual task interference 277
spinal disc degeneration 294
stages of change model 45–49
  action 47, 320
  application 46–47, 47, 54
  assumptions 45, 48
  contemplation 45, 46, 47, 320
  decisional balance 46
  first tenet 45
  guidelines 57
  intervention targeting and tailoring 54, 55
    guidelines 57
  maintenance 45, 47, 320
    techniques for 53
  pre-contemplation 45, 46, 47
  preparation 45, 47
  processes required for change 45–46
  progress direction 46
  second tenet 45–46
  sequence of changes 45
  third tenet 46
stair-climbing
  resistance training, weighted vests 177–178
  strength training, changes in activity 148–149, *149*
static balance, strength training 149–151, *150*
stimulus control
  maintenance phase 53
  stages of change model 46

strain frequency 79
strain gradient 79
strain history, concept 80
strain magnitude, mechanical strain on musculoskeletal system 79
strain rate 79
strength training 125–157
  activity changes 146–151
  adverse incidents 133–134
  aerobic capacity 137
  body fat changes *144*, 144–145
  body function changes 134–138
  body structure changes 139–142
  bone mineral density effect 142–144, *143*
    measuring 80
  data analysis 127
  depression, effect on 139, *140*
  diabetes type 2 *see* diabetes mellitus (type 2)
  endurance 137–138
  environmental factors 132–133
  falls protection *see* fall prevention
  flexibility 138
  foot problems 239
  fractures *see* fractures
  graduated elastic tubing 132
  guidelines, providers of 175
  haematology *145*, 145–146
  injury rate, aerobic training *vs* 134
  isokinetic 218
  lower limb strength 134–137, *136, 137*
    exercises for 176
    OA rehabilitation 87–88
    quadriceps *see* quadriceps
  muscle mass 140, *141*
    sets of repetitions 317
  neuromuscular effects 91, 92, 173
  OA, pain and disability reduction 219–220
  participation changes 151
  personal factors 133
  psychological function effect 139, *140*
  screening and evaluation prior to 134, 175

sit-to-stand 147–148, *148*
skeletal muscle 139–140
  cross-sectional area 141, *142*
  fibres 141–142, *142*
stair-climbing, changes in activity 148–149, *149*
static and dynamic balance 149–151, *150*
studies
  electronic databases 126
  evaluation of effects 126
  identification and selection 126–128
  inclusion criteria 126
  programme content 128–132, *129–131*
  quality 128
  theory of planned behaviour application 43, *43*
  upper body strength 134, *135*
    exercises for 176
  walking 91, 146–147
  weight-lifting stress test 175
  weight types *129–131*
  see also resistance training
stress testing *see* screening
stress, workplace 65, 68
stretching exercises
  fractures *see* fractures
  heel pain 237
  osteoarthritis 218
stroke
  cardiopulmonary function compromised 291
  dual task interference 277
  prevention 9–10
    mechanism 10
  types 9–10
sunlight exposure 113–114
surgery
  corns and calluses, careful considerations for 235
  postoperative recovery, OA *89*, 89–90

T

tai chi, falls reduction *see* fall prevention
tarsal tunnel syndrome 238
team inclusiveness, in workplace 69

telephone reminder, strategies 34
telephone support 52
tendon injury, precautions for exercise 293
terbinafine 234
testosterone, replacement 165–166
TFOA see tibiofemoral osteoarthritis
theory of planned behaviour 42–43, 54
  application of model 43, *43*
  assumptions 42–43, *48*
  criticism of 43
  intervention guidelines 57–58
theory of reasoned action see theory of planned behaviour
Theraband™ resistance exercises 81, 177
thrombus, risk reduction by PA 10
Thurstone's Word-Fluency Test 275
tibialis posterior dysfunction 238
tibiofemoral osteoarthritis (TFOA) 83
  aetiology 85–86
  cartilage 83–84
  impact loading 83
  injury 87, 88
  knee varus moments 84–85, 88
  obesity/overweight people 84, 85, 88
    risk of development 215
    weight loss recommendations 222
  pain 86
  stance phase 83
  see also osteoarthritis (OA)
timed up and go test (TUG) 281
toe(s)
  gait pattern retraining 88
  nail problems see nail(s)
  see also foot; foot problems
tolnaftate 234
total hip arthroplasty (THA), exercise programme after *89*, 89–90
tumour necrosis factor-α (TNF-α) 310

U

undecenoic acid 234
US Surgeon General's Report on Physical Activity and Health, importance of PA 27, 64

V

vertebral fractures see fractures
vigorous programmes
  compensatory sedentariness 7
  osteoarthritis risk 12, 82, 215–216
    programme cautions 218
vitamin D 113–115
  cutaneous synthesis 113–114, *114*
  deficiency status in elderly 114
    reasons 113, 115
  recommended dietary intake 114–115
vitamin K, osteoporosis prevention 115

W

walking activity
  biomechanics 91
  dogs and 32–33
  falls reduction 34–35, 253
  foot problems effect 231
  hip fracture reduction 29, 188
  individual programmes for women 34
  large heel strike, OA susceptibility 85, 87
  loading cycles 79
  lower injury rate *vs* sports 12
  neurological control 269
  OA see aerobic training
  resistance training effect 173
  secondary task interference on see dual task interference
  strength training effect 91, 146–147
  toe-out 88
  vigorous 292
  see also gait
walking speed
  foot pain 231
  measure for muscle strength 14, 162
walking while talking test, dual task interference 275–276, 282
warm-up periods 295
water activities 81
  osteoarthritis 82
  see also hydrotherapy
weight
  loss recommendations, OA 222
  overweight classification *328*
weight-bearing
  exercises, after fractures 190
  foot role 229
  osteoarthritis 88
weighted vests 177
weight-lifting stress test 175
weights, types *129–131*
weight support devices 219
white collar workers 65
women 26–37
  Alzheimer's disease 30
  attitudes to activity 32
  barriers to PA see barriers, to PA
  common participation activities 32
  disease prevalence 27
  effectiveness of interventions 33–35
  health behaviour effect on longevity 30
  individual tailoring of activities 34, 35
  levels of PA *31*, 31–32
  life expectancy 26
  menopause see menopause/postmenopause
  mental health 29
  osteoporosis see osteoporosis
  premature death reduction 27–28
  promotional (of PA) strategies 27
  reasons for PA 32
  reasons for PA promotion 27–30
  stereotypes 32
  study bias 27

workforce
  age and performance 63–64, 66
  age statistics 63
  health benefits of activity 64
  manual tasks 68
  physical inactivity 64–65
workplace
  claims 66
  culture 70
  employers' responsibilities 66
  environment 64
  exercise/fitness programmes 67–68
  expenses/costs 65, 66
  gyms 67
  health insurance 66
  health promotion programmes 64–65, 66
    financial return 66–67
    health outcome 66
    international examples 71
    motivating factors 66
    types of activity 67

injuries 65
  costs 65
  prevention 68
PA programmes 68–71
  barriers 68
  clear purpose 69
  leadership and commitment 69
  measure outcomes 70–71
  opportunities for PA 70
  social support 70
  team inclusiveness 69
  worker involvement 69
physically demanding jobs, changes with technology 64
repetitive work 65
strenuous PA, joint damage 216
stress 65
World Health Organization (WHO)
  chronic disease incidence ix

incidence of chronic conditions 303
International Classification of Functioning (ICF), target therapy 191
obesity and overweight classification 328
PA role 19

Y

Yale measure 18

Z

Z band disruption 160
zinc, osteoporosis prevention 116